Acknowledgments

I wish to express my appreciation to the staff of Elsevier, Inc., especially Kellie White and Laura Bayless, for assisting me with this text. I wish to express also my continued admiration and gratitude to Kevin Patton for another outstanding edition of *The Human Body in Health & Disease*. Your time and dedication to science education will hopefully inspire potential caregivers and improve the quality of health care for the future.

To Bill, who is always there, my thanks for the whispers of inspiration and encouragement.

Finally, to the designer of the human body, this book is dedicated. What a miraculous creation!

Linda Swisher, RN, EdD

Preface

TO THE INSTRUCTOR

This Study Guide is designed to help your students master basic anatomy and physiology. It works in two ways. First, the section of the preface titled "To the Student" contains detailed instructions on:

- How to achieve good grades in anatomy and physiology
- How to read the textbook
- How to use the exercises in this Study Guide
- How to use visual memory as a learning tool
- How to use mnemonic devices as learning aids
- How to prepare for an examination
- How to take an examination
- How to find out why questions were missed on an examination

Second, the Study Guide itself contains features that facilitate learning:

1. SUBJECT DIVISIONS, designed to break down the process of learning into small units. The questions in this Study Guide have been developed to help the student master the learning objectives identified at the beginning of each chapter in the text. The Guide is also sequenced to correspond to key areas of each chapter. A variety of questions has been prepared to cover the material effectively and expose the student to multiple learning approaches.
2. CROSSWORD PUZZLES and KNOW YOUR MEDICAL TERMS, to encourage the use of new vocabulary words and emphasize the proper spelling of these terms.
3. OPTIONAL APPLICATION QUESTIONS, particularly targeted for the health occupations student but appropriate for any student of anatomy and physiology because questions are based upon information contained within the chapter.
4. DIAGRAMS with key features indicated by numbers for identification. Students can easily check their work by comparing the diagram in the workbook with the equivalent figure in the text and with the answer key in the back of the Study Guide.
5. PAGE NUMBER REFERENCES in the answer section. Each answer is cross-referenced to the appropriate text page. In addition, questions are grouped into specific topics that correspond to the text. Each major topic of the Study Guide provides references to specific areas of the text, so that students having difficulty with a particular group of questions have a specific reference area to assist them with remedial work. This is of great assistance to both instructor and student, because remedial work is made easier and more effective when the area of weakness is identified accurately.

These features should make mastery of the material a rewarding experience for both instructor and student.

TO THE STUDENT

How to Achieve Good Grades in Anatomy and Physiology

This Study Guide is designed to help you be successful in learning anatomy and physiology. Before you begin using the Study Guide, read the following suggestions. Successful students understand effective study techniques and have good study habits.

How to Read the Textbook

Keep up with the reading assignments. Read the textbook assignment before the instructor covers the material in a lecture. If you have failed to read the assignment beforehand, you may not grasp what the instructor is talking about in the lecture. When you read, consider using some of the following helpful hints.

1. As you finish reading an area, ask yourself if you understand the material. If you do not, put a question mark in the margin by that sentence. If the instructor does not clarify the material in lecture, ask him or her to explain it to you further.
2. Complete the learning objectives in the text. A learning objective is a specific task that you are expected to be able to complete after you have read a chapter. It sets specific goals for the student and breaks down learning into small units. It emphasizes the key points that the author is making in the chapter.
3. Underline and make notes in the margin to highlight key ideas, mark something you need to reinforce at a later time, or indicate areas that you do not understand.

iv

4. If you come to a word you do not understand, look it up in a dictionary. Write the word on one side of an index card and its definition on the other side. Carry these cards with you, and when you have a spare minute, use them like flash cards. If you do not know how to spell or pronounce a word, you will have a difficult time remembering it.
5. Carefully study each diagram and illustration as you read. Many students ignore these aids. The author included them to help students understand the material.
6. Summarize what you read. After finishing a paragraph, try to restate the main ideas. Repeat this again when you finish the chapter. Identify and mentally restate the main concepts of the chapter. Check to see if you are correct. In short, be an active reader. Do not just stare at a page or read it superficially.
7. Finally, attack each unit of learning with a positive mental attitude. Motivation and perseverance are prime factors in achieving good grades. The combination of your instructor, the text, the Study Guide, and your dedicated work will lead to success in anatomy and physiology.

How to Use the Exercises in This Study Guide

After you have read a chapter and learned all of the new words, begin working with the Study Guide. Read the overview of the chapter, which summarizes the main points.

Familiarize yourself with the "Topics for Review" section, which emphasizes the learning objectives outlined in the text. Complete the questions and diagrams in the Study Guide. After completing the exercises in a chapter, you can check your answers in the back of the book. Each answer is referenced to the appropriate text page. Additionally, questions are grouped into specific topics that correspond to the text. Each major topic of the Study Guide provides references to specific areas of the text, so if you are having difficulty with a particular grouping of questions, you have a specific reference area to assist you with remedial work. This feature allows you to identify your area of weakness accurately. A variety of questions is offered throughout the Study Guide to help you cover the material effectively. The following examples are among the exercises that have been included to assist you.

Multiple Choice Questions

Multiple choice questions will have only one correct answer for you to select from the several possibilities presented. There are two types of multiple choice questions that you need to be acquainted with:

1. "None of the above is correct" questions. These questions test your ability to recall rather than recognize the correct answer. You would select the "none of the above" choice only if all the other choices in that particular question were incorrect.
2. Sequence questions. These questions test your ability to arrange a list of structures in the correct order. In this type of question, you are asked to determine the sequence of the structures given in the various choices, and then you are to select the structure listed that would be third in that sequence, as in this example:

   Which one of the following structures is the third through which food passes?
   A. Stomach
   B. Mouth
   C. Large intestine
   D. Esophagus
   E. Anus

   The correct answer is *A.*

Matching Questions

Matching questions ask the student to select the correct answer from a list of terms and to write that answer in the space provided.

True or False Questions

True or false questions ask you to write "T" in the answer space if you agree with that statement. If you disagree with the statement, you will circle the incorrect word(s) and write the correct word(s) in the answer space.

Identify the Term That Does Not Belong

In questions that ask you to identify the incorrect term, three words are given that relate to each other in structure or function, and one more word is included that has no relationship or has an opposing relationship to the other three terms. You are asked to circle the term that does not relate to the others. An example might be: iris, cornea, stapes, retina. You would circle the word *stapes* because all of the other terms refer to the eye.

Fill-in-the-Blank Questions

Fill-in-the-blank questions ask you to recall one or more missing words and to insert them into the answer blanks. These questions may involve sentences or paragraphs.

Applying What You Know Questions

Application questions ask you to make judgments about a situation based on the information in the chapter. These questions may ask how you would respond to a situation or ask you to suggest a possible diagnosis for a set of symptoms.

Charts

Several charts have been included that correspond to figures in the text. Areas have been omitted so that you can fill them in and test your recall of these important concepts.

Word Find Puzzles

The Study Guide includes word find puzzles that allow you to identify key terms in the chapter in an interesting and challenging way.

Crossword Puzzles and Know Your Medical Terms

Vocabulary words from the Language of Science and Language of Medicine sections at the beginning and end of each chapter of the text have been developed into crossword puzzles and know your medical terms. This encourages recall and proper spelling. Each chapter additionally contains an exercise with scrambled words. This also emphasizes recall and proper spelling in a challenging and interesting way.

Labeling Exercises

Labeling exercises present diagrams with areas that are not identified. For each of these diagrams, you are to print the name of each numbered part on the appropriately numbered line. You may choose to further distinguish the structures by coloring them with a variety of colors. After you have written down the names of the structures to be identified, check your answers. When it comes time to review for an examination, you can place a sheet of paper over your answers to test yourself.

After completing the exercises in the Study Guide, check your answers. If they are not correct, refer to the answers page and review it for further clarification. If you still do not understand a question or an answer, ask your instructor for further explanation or assistance.

If you have difficulty with several questions from one section, refer to the pages listed at the end of the section. After reviewing the section, try to answer the questions again. If you are still having difficulty, talk to your instructor.

Check Your Knowledge

This section selects questions from throughout the chapter to provide you with a final review. This mini-test gives you an overview of your knowledge of the entire chapter after completing all of the other sections. It emphasizes the main concepts of the unit but should not be attempted until the specific topics of the chapter have been mastered.

How to Use Visual Memory

Visual memory is another important tool in learning. If I asked you to picture an elephant in your mind, with all its external parts labeled, you could do that easily. Visual memory is a powerful key to learning. Whenever possible, try to build a memory picture. Remember: A picture is worth a thousand words.

Visual memory works especially well with the sequencing of items, such as circulatory pathways and the passage of air or food. Students who try to learn sequencing by memorizing a list of words do poorly on examinations. If they forget one word in the sequence, they then may forget the remaining words as well. With a memory picture you can pick out the important features.

How to Use Mnemonic Devices

Mnemonic devices are little jingles that you memorize to help you remember things. If you make up your own, they will stick with you longer. Here are three examples of such devices:

"On Old Olympus' towering tops a Finn and German viewed some hops." This one is used to remember the cranial nerves. Each word begins with the same letter as does the name of one of the nerves: olfactory, optic, oculomotor, trochlear, trigeminal, abducens, facial, auditory, glossopharyngeal, vagus, sensory (accessory), hypoglossal.

"C. Hopkins CaFe where they serve Mg NaCl." This mnemonic device reminds you of the chemical symbols for the biologically important electrolytes: carbon, hydrogen, oxygen, phosphorus, potassium, iodine, nitrogen, sulfur, calcium, iron, magnesium, sodium, chlorine.

"Roy G. Biv." This mnemonic device helps you remember the colors of the visible light spectrum: red, orange, yellow, green, blue, indigo, violet.

How to Prepare for an Examination

Prepare far in advance for an examination. Actually, your preparation for an examination should begin on the first day of class. Keeping up with your assignments daily makes the final preparation for an examination much easier. You should begin your final preparation at least three nights before the test. Last-minute studying usually means poor results and limited retention.

1. Make sure that you understand and can answer all of the learning objectives for the chapter on which you are being tested.
2. Review the appropriate questions in this Study Guide. Review is something that you should do after every class and at the end of every study session. It is important to keep going over the material until you have a thorough understanding of the chapter and rapid recall of its contents. If review becomes a daily habit, studying for the actual examination will not be difficult. Go through each question and write down an answer. Do the same with the labeling of each structure on the appropriate diagrams. If you have already done this as part of your daily review, cover the answers with a piece of paper and quiz yourself again.
3. Check the answers that you have written down against the correct answers in the back of the Study Guide. Go back and study the areas in the text that refer to questions that you missed and then try to answer those questions again. If you still cannot answer a question or label a structure correctly, ask your instructor for help.
4. As you read a chapter, ask yourself what questions you would ask if you were writing a test on that unit. You will most likely ask yourself many of the questions that will show up on your examinations.
5. Get a good night's sleep before the test. Staying up late and upsetting your biorhythms will only make you less efficient during the test.

How to Take an Examination
The Day of the Test
1. Get up early enough to avoid rushing. Eat appropriately. Your body needs fuel, but a heavy meal just before a test is not a good idea.
2. Keep calm. Briefly look over your notes. If you have prepared for the test properly, there will be no need for last-minute cramming.
3. Make certain that you have everything you need for the test: pens, pencils, test sheets, and so forth.
4. Allow enough time to get to the examination site. Missing your bus, getting stuck in traffic, or being unable to find a parking space will not put you in a good frame of mind to do well on the examination.

During the Examination
1. Pay careful attention to the instructions for the test.
2. Note any corrections.
3. Budget your time so that you will be able to finish the test.
4. Ask the instructor for clarification if you do not understand a question or an instruction.
5. Concentrate on your own test paper and do not allow yourself to be distracted by others in the room.

Hints for Taking a Multiple Choice Test
1. Read each question carefully. Pay attention to each word.
2. Cross out obviously wrong choices and think about those that are left.
3. Go through the test once, quickly answering the questions you are sure of; then go back over the test and answer the rest of the questions.
4. Fill in the answer spaces completely and make your marks heavy. Erase answers completely if you make a mistake.
5. If you must guess, stick with your first hunch. Most often, students will change right answers to wrong ones.
6. If you will not be penalized for guessing, do not leave any blanks.

Hints for Taking an Essay Test
1. Budget time for each question.
2. Write legibly and try to spell words correctly.
3. Be concise, complete, and specific. Do not be repetitious or long-winded.
4. Organize your answer in an outline—this helps not only you but also the person who grades the test.
5. Answer each question as thoroughly as you can, but leave some room for possible additions.

Hints for Taking a Laboratory Practical Examination
Students often have a hard time with this kind of test. Visual memory is very important here. To put it simply, you must be able to identify every structure you have studied. If you are unable to identify a structure, then you will be unable to answer any questions about that structure.

Questions that could appear on an examination of this type might include:

1. Identification of a structure, organ, or feature
2. Identification of the function of a structure, organ, or feature

3. Sequence questions for air flow, passage of food or urine, and so forth
4. Disease questions (for example, if an organ fails, what disease will result?)

How to Find Out Why Questions Were Missed on an Examination

After the examination, go over your test after it has been scored to see what you missed and why you missed it. You can pick up important clues that will help you on future examinations. Ask yourself these questions:

1. Did I miss questions because I did not read them carefully?
2. Did I miss questions because I had gaps in my knowledge?
3. Did I miss questions because I did not understand scientific words?
4. Did I miss questions because I did not have good visual memory of things?

Be sure to go back and learn the things you did not know. Chances are these topics will come up on the final examination.

Your grades in other classes will improve as well when you apply these study methods. Learning should be fun. With these helpful hints and this Study Guide, you should be able to achieve the grades you desire. Good luck!

Contents

1 Introduction to the Body

A command of terminology is necessary for a student to be successful in any area of science. This chapter defines the terminology and concepts that are basic to the field of anatomy and physiology. Building a firm foundation in these language skills will assist you with all future chapters.

The study of anatomy and physiology involves the structure and function of an organism and the relationship of its parts. It begins with a basic organization of the body into different structural levels. Beginning with the smallest level (the cell) and progressing to the largest, most complex level (the system), this chapter familiarizes you with the terminology and the levels of organization needed to facilitate the study of the body as a part or as a whole.

It is also important to be able to identify and describe specific body areas or regions as we progress in our study of this field. The anatomical position is used as a reference position when dissecting the body into planes, regions, or cavities. The terminology defined in this chapter allows you to describe the areas efficiently and accurately.

Finally, the process of homeostasis is reviewed. This state of relative constancy in the chemical composition of body fluids is necessary for good health. In fact, the very survival of the body depends on the successful maintenance of homeostasis.

TOPICS FOR REVIEW

Before progressing to Chapter 2, you should have an understanding of the structural levels of organization; the planes, regions, and cavities of the body; the terminology used to describe these areas; and the concept of homeostasis as it relates to the survival of the species.

SCIENTIFIC METHOD

Fill in the blanks.

1. A systematic approach to discovery is known as the _____.

2. A tentative explanation in research is known as a _____.

3. The testing of a hypothesis is _____.

4. In clinical trials, a group getting a drug is the _____.

5. In clinical trials, a group getting a substitute is the _____.

LEVELS OF ORGANIZATION

Match each term on the left with its corresponding description on the right.

_____ 6. Organism   A. Many similar cells that act together to perform a common function

_____ 7. Cells   B. The most complex units that make up the body

_____ 8. Tissue   C. A group of several different kinds of tissues arranged to perform a special function

_____ 9. Organ   D. Denotes a living thing

_____ 10. Systems   E. The smallest "living" units of structure and function in the body

If you had difficulty with this section, review pages 4-6.

1

ANATOMICAL POSITION

Match each term on the left with its corresponding description on the right.

_____ 11. Body   A. At the sides

_____ 12. Arms   B. Face upward

_____ 13. Feet   C. Erect

_____ 14. Prone   D. Face downward

_____ 15. Supine   E. Forward

If you had difficulty with this section, review page 7.

ANATOMICAL DIRECTIONS

Planes or Body Sections
Fill in the crossword puzzle.

ACROSS
17. Lower or below
18. Horizontal plane
21. Toward the midline of the body

DOWN
16. Upper or above
19. Toward the belly
20. Toward the side of the body
22. Farthest from the point of origin of a body point

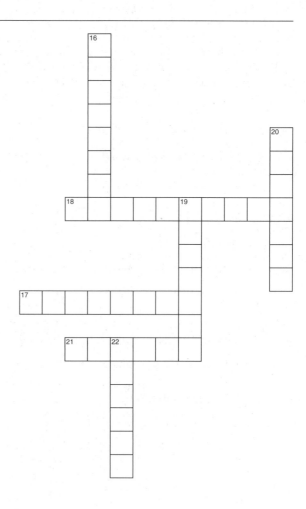

Circle the correct answer.
23. The stomach is (*superior* or *inferior*) to the diaphragm.
24. The nose is located on the (*anterior* or *posterior*) surface of the body.
25. The lungs lie (*medial* or *lateral*) to the heart.
26. The elbow lies (*proximal* or *distal*) to the forearm.
27. The skin is (*superficial* or *deep*) to the muscles below it.
28. A midsagittal plane divides the body into (*equal* or *unequal*) parts.
29. A frontal plane divides the body into (*anterior and posterior* or *superior and inferior*) sections.
30. A transverse plane divides the body into (*right and left* or *upper and lower*) sections.
31. A plane that is not parallel to other places and is a diagonal cut is a/an (*oblique* or *coronal*) plane.

If you had difficulty with this section, review pages 7-9.

BODY CAVITIES

Match each term with its body cavity location and write "A" or "B" in the answer blank.

A. Ventral cavity   B. Dorsal cavity

_____ 32. Thoracic

_____ 33. Cranial

_____ 34. Abdominal

_____ 35. Pelvic

_____ 36. Mediastinum

_____ 37. Spinal

_____ 38. Pleural

If you had difficulty with this section, review page 9.

BODY REGIONS

Circle the word in each word group that does not belong.

39.	Axial	Head	Trunk	Extremities
40.	Axillary	Cephalic	Brachial	Antecubital
41.	Frontal	Orbital	Plantar	Nasal
42.	Carpal	Crural	Plantar	Pedal
43.	Cranial	Occipital	Tarsal	Temporal

If you had difficulty with this section, review pages 11-14.

TRUE OR FALSE

For each of the following statements, write "T" in the answer blank if the statement is true. If the statement is false, circle the incorrect word(s) and write the correct word(s) in the answer blank.

_____ 44. The term *autopsy* comes from the Greek words *auto* (self) and *opsis* (view).

_____ 45. Autopsies are usually performed in four stages.

_____ 46. In the first stage of an autopsy, the exterior of the body is examined for abnormalities such as wounds or scars.

_____ 47. The face, arms, and legs are usually dissected during the second stage of an autopsy.

_____ 48. Microscopic examination of tissues occurs during all stages of an autopsy.

_____ 49. Tests to analyze the chemical content of body fluids or to determine the presence of infectious organisms also may be performed during an autopsy.

If you had difficulty with this section, review page 12.

BALANCE OF BODY FUNCTIONS

Fill in the blanks.

50. _____ depends on the body's ability to maintain or restore homeostasis.

51. *Homeostasis* is the term used to describe the relative constancy of the body's _____.

52. During exercise, homeostasis is disrupted and may cause the body's temperature to _____.

53. Changes and functions that occur during the early years are called _____.

54. Changes and functions that occur after young adulthood are called _____

    _____.

55. Homeostatic control mechanisms are categorized as either _____ or

    _____ feedback loops.

56. Negative feedback loops are _____ mechanisms.

57. Positive feedback control loops are _____.

If you had difficulty with this section, review pages 14-15.

UNSCRAMBLE THE WORDS

58. **L X A A I**

    ⬡ ☐ ☐ ☐ ☐

59. **Y Y G P H I O O S L**

    ☐ ☐ ☐ ⬡ ☐ ⬡ ☐ ☐ ☐

60. **N O R L A T F**

    ☐ ☐ ⬡ ☐ ☐ ☐

61. **A S R O D L**

    ☐ ⬡ ☐ ☐ ☐ ☐

Take the circled letters, unscramble them, and fill in the solution.

What was Becky's favorite music?

62. ☐ ☐ ☐ ☐ ☐

APPLYING WHAT YOU KNOW

63. Mrs. Hunt has had an appendectomy. The nurse is preparing to change the dressing. She knows that the appendix is located in the right iliac inguinal region, the distal portion extending at an angle into the hypogastric region. Place an X on the diagram where the nurse will place the dressing.

64. Mrs. Wiedeke noticed a lump in her breast. Dr. Reeder noted on her chart that a small mass was located in the left breast medial to the nipple. Place an X where Mrs. Wiedeke's lump would be located.

65. Heather was injured in a bicycle accident. X-ray films revealed that she had a fracture of the right patella. A cast was applied beginning at the distal femoral region and extending to the pedal region. Place one X where Heather's cast begins and another where it ends.

66. **Word Find**

Find and circle 18 terms presented in this chapter. Words may be spelled top to bottom, bottom to top, right to left, left to right, or diagonally.

Anatomy	Posterior
Atrophy	Proximal
Homeostasis	Sagittal
Medial	Superficial
Mediastinum	Superior
Organ	System
Organization	Thoracic
Physiology	Tissue
Pleural	Ventral

```
N H L T E B W N G N M M Y X A
O O H A V U U C L W E P N G L
I M U N I T S A I D E M W A L
T E R T V C T S I C J S R T K
A O N O P T I A I W A T Y R H
Z S Q S I R L F A T N R G O W
I T W G P R O I R E T S O P F
N A A Z J E E X V E E H L H Z
A S N L M C T P I C P D O Y T
G I C A Y U O X U M N U I V P
R S M R T N U K B S A Y S V M
O R C U R O I R B S Q L Y U G
L H X E M P M E T S Y S H V S
U W L L Q D U Y Y N E E P J B
Q N Z P K D B O D C G I N J A
```

DID YOU KNOW?

■ Many animals produce tears, but only humans weep as a result of emotional stress.
■ The brain is the body's computer. In terms of memory storage, your brain holds approximately 1,000 terabytes. That's the equivalent of 3 million hours of video—you'd have to watch it continuously for 300 years to see it all!

KNOW YOUR MEDICAL TERMS

Using the prefixes, root words, and suffixes below, develop new medical terms from this chapter. Words may be used more than once.

Prefixes	Roots	Suffixes
hypo	ped	ic
super	stasis	(i)or
dia	ventr	al
homeo	thesis	phragm
epi	later	
ante	gastric	
	brachial	

67. under or below; placing or proposition   _____

68. upon; stomach; relating to   _____

69. front; arm   _____

70. same or equal; standing still   _____

71. side; relating to   _____

72. foot; relating to   _____

73. over or about; quality   _____

74. across; enclose   _____

75. belly; relating to   _____

If you had difficulty with this section, review pages 3, 17 and 18.

CHECK YOUR KNOWLEDGE

Multiple Choice
Circle the correct answer.

1. The body's ability to respond continuously to changes in the environment and to maintain consistency in the internal environment is called:
   A. homeostasis
   B. superficial
   C. structural levels
   D. none of the above

2. The regions frequently used by health professionals to locate pain or tumors divide the abdomen into four basic areas called:
   A. planes
   B. cavities
   C. pleural
   D. quadrants

3. Which of the following organs or structures does *not* lie within the mediastinum?
   A. Thymus
   B. Liver
   C. Esophagus
   D. Trachea

4. A lengthwise plane running from front to back that divides the body into right and left sides is called:
   A. transverse
   B. coronal
   C. frontal
   D. sagittal

5. A study of the functions of living organisms and their parts is called:
   A. physiology
   B. chemistry
   C. biology
   D. none of the above

6. The thoracic portion of the ventral body cavity is separated from the abdominopelvic portion by a muscle called the:
   A. latissimus dorsi
   B. rectus femoris
   C. diaphragm
   D. pectoralis

7. An organization of varying numbers and kinds of organs arranged together to perform a complex function is called a:
   A. cell
   B. tissue
   C. system
   D. region

8. The plane that divides superior from inferior is known as the _____ plane.
   A. transverse
   B. sagittal
   C. frontal
   D. none of the above

9. Which of the following structures does *not* lie within the abdominal cavity?
   A. Spleen
   B. Most of the small intestine
   C. Urinary bladder
   D. Stomach

10. Which of the following is an example of an upper abdominal region?
    A. Right iliac region
    B. Left hypochondriac region
    C. Left lumbar region
    D. Hypogastric region

11. The dorsal body cavity contains components of the:
    A. reproductive system
    B. digestive system
    C. respiratory system
    D. nervous system

12. Which of the following organs is *not* found in the pelvic cavity?
    A. Bladder
    B. Stomach
    C. Rectum
    D. Colon

13. Similar cells acting together to perform a common function exist at a level of organization called a/an:
    A. organ
    B. chemical
    C. tissue
    D. system

14. Which of the following planes would be considered coronal?
    A. A plane that divides the body into anterior and posterior portions
    B. A plane that divides the body into upper and lower portions
    C. A plane that divides the body into right and left sides
    D. A plane that divides the body into superficial and deep portions

15. If your reference point is "nearest to the trunk of the body" versus "farthest from the trunk of the body," where does the elbow lie in relation to the wrist?
    A. Anterior
    B. Posterior
    C. Distal
    D. Proximal

16. In the anatomical position:
    A. the dorsal body cavity is anterior to the ventral
    B. palms face toward the back of the body
    C. the body is erect
    D. all of the above

17. The buttocks are often used as intramuscular injection sites. This region can be called:
    A. sacral
    B. buccal
    C. cutaneous
    D. gluteal

18. In the human body, the chest region:
    A. can be referred to as the thoracic cavity
    B. is a component of the ventral body cavity
    C. contains the mediastinum
    D. all of the above

19. Which of the following is *not* a component of the axial subdivision of the body?
    A. Upper extremity
    B. Neck
    C. Trunk
    D. Head

20. The scientific study of disease is:
    A. dissection
    B. volar
    C. pathology
    D. pathogens

Matching

Match each term in column A with the most appropriate term in column B. Write the corresponding letter in the answer blank. (Only one answer is correct for each.)

Column A

_____ 21. Ventral

_____ 22. Skin

_____ 23. Transverse

_____ 24. Anatomy

_____ 25. Superficial

_____ 26. Pleural

_____ 27. Appendicular

_____ 28. Posterior

_____ 29. Midsagittal

_____ 30. System

Column B

A. Equal

B. Cutaneous

C. Lung

D. Extremities

E. Respiratory

F. Anterior

G. Structure

H. Surface

I. Back

J. Horizontal

DORSAL AND VENTRAL BODY CAVITIES

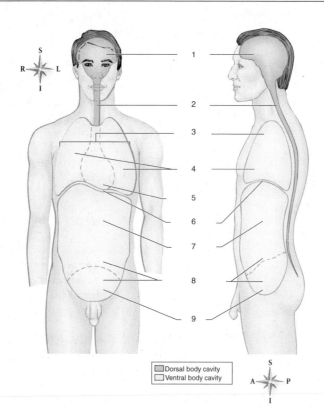

1. _____

2. _____

3. _____

4. _____

5. _____

6. _____

7. _____

8. _____

9. _____

DIRECTIONS AND PLANES OF THE BODY

1. _____
2. _____
3. _____
4. _____
5. _____
6. _____

7. _____
8. _____
9. _____
10. _____
11. _____
12. _____

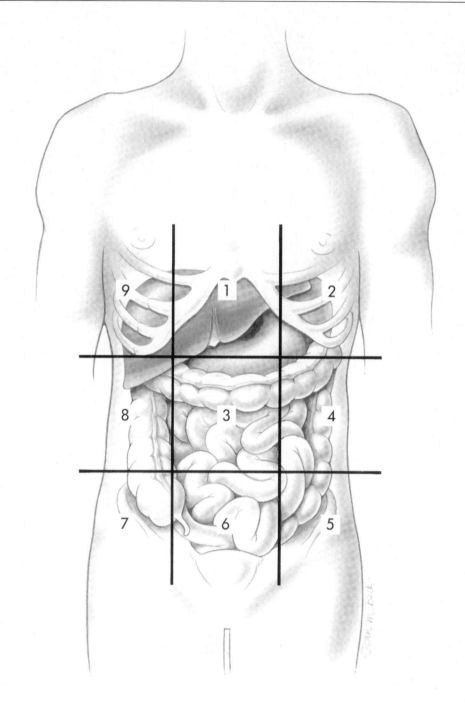

1. _____   6. _____

2. _____   7. _____

3. _____   8. _____

4. _____   9. _____

5. _____

Chapter **1**   **Introduction to the Body**

2 Chemistry of Life

Although anatomy can be studied without knowledge of the principles of chemistry, it is hard to imagine having an understanding of physiology without a basic comprehension of chemical reactions in the body. Trillions of cells make up the various levels of organization in the body. Our health and survival depend upon the proper chemical maintenance in the cytoplasm of our cells.

Chemists use the terms *elements* or *compounds* to describe all of the substances (matter) in and around us. What distinguishes these two terms is their basic structure. An element cannot be broken down. A compound, on the other hand, is made up of two or more elements and can be broken down into the elements that form it.

Organic and inorganic compounds are equally important to our survival. Without organic compounds, such as carbohydrates, proteins, and fats, and without inorganic compounds, such as water, we could not sustain life.

Because we cannot see many of the chemical reactions that take place daily in our bodies, it is sometimes difficult to comprehend the principles involved in initiating them. Chemicals are responsible for directing virtually all of our bodily functions. Therefore, it is important to master the fundamental concepts of chemistry in order to understand physiology.

TOPICS FOR REVIEW

Before progressing to Chapter 3, you should have an understanding of the basic chemical reactions in the body and of the fundamental concepts of biochemistry.

LEVELS OF CHEMICAL ORGANIZATION

Multiple Choice
Circle the correct answer.

1. Which of the following is *not* a subatomic particle?
   A. Proton
   B. Electron
   C. Isotope
   D. Neutron

2. Electrons move about within certain limits called:
   A. energy levels
   B. orbitals
   C. chemical bonding
   D. shells

3. The number of protons in the nucleus is an atom's:
   A. atomic mass
   B. atomic energy level
   C. atomic number
   D. none of the above

4. The number of protons and neutrons combined is the atom's:
   A. atomic mass
   B. atomic energy level
   C. orbit
   D. chemical bonding

5. Which of the following is *not* one of the major elements present in the human body?
   A. Oxygen
   B. Carbon
   C. Nitrogen
   D. Iron

6. Atoms usually unite with each other to form larger chemical units called:
   A. energy levels
   B. mass
   C. molecules
   D. shells

7. Substances whose molecules have more than one element in them are called:
   A. compounds
   B. orbitals
   C. elements
   D. neutrons

11

True or False

For each of the following statements, write "T" in the answer blank if it is true. If the statement is false, circle the incorrect word(s) and write the correct word(s) in the answer blank.

_____ 8. *Matter* is anything that occupies space and has mass.

_____ 9. In the body, most chemicals are in the form of electrons.

_____ 10. At the core of each atom is a nucleus composed of positively charged protons and negatively charged neutrons.

_____ 11. Orbitals are arranged into *energy levels* depending on their distance from the nucleus.

_____ 12. The *formula* for a compound contains symbols that represent each element in the molecule.

If you had difficulty with this section, review pages 25-27.

CHEMICAL BONDING

Multiple Choice

Circle the correct answer.

13. Ionic bonds are chemical bonds formed by the:
    A. sharing of electrons between atoms
    B. donation of protons from one atom to another
    C. donation of electrons from one atom to another
    D. acceptance of protons from one atom to another

14. Molecules that form ions when dissolved in water are called:
    A. covalent bonds
    B. electrolytes
    C. isotopes
    D. ionic bonds

15. When atoms share electrons, a/an _____ forms.
    A. covalent bond
    B. electrolyte
    C. ionic bond
    D. isotope

16. Covalent bonds:
    A. break apart easily in water
    B. are not easily broken
    C. donate electrons
    D. none of the above

17. An example of an ionic bond is:
    A. NaCl
    B. Ca
    C. O
    D. P

18. If a molecule "dissociates" in water, it:
    A. has taken on additional ions
    B. has eliminated ions
    C. separates to form free ions
    D. forms a covalent bond

If you had difficulty with this section, review pages 27-28.

INORGANIC CHEMISTRY

Match each term with its corresponding description or definition.

_____ 19. A type of compound

_____ 20. Compound essential to life

_____ 21. Dissolves solutes

_____ 22. Water plus common salt

_____ 23. Reactants combine only after (H) and (O) atoms are removed

_____ 24. Combine to form a larger product

_____ 25. The reverse of dehydration synthesis

_____ 26. Yields energy for muscle contraction

_____ 27. Alkaline compound

_____ 28. A measure of the H^+ concentration

_____ 29. Easily dissociates to form H^+ ions

_____ 30. Dissociates very little

A. Aqueous solution

B. Water

C. ATP

D. Base

E. Solvent

F. pH

G. Dehydration synthesis

H. Inorganic

I. Weak acid

J. Hydrolysis

K. Strong acid

L. Reactants

If you had difficulty with this section, review pages 29-31.

ORGANIC CHEMISTRY

Match each numbered term with its category. Write the corresponding letter in the blank.

A. Carbohydrate   B. Lipid   C. Protein   D. Nucleic acid

_____ 31. Monosaccharide

_____ 32. Triglyceride

_____ 33. DNA

_____ 34. Cholesterol

_____ 35. Amino acid

_____ 36. Glycogen

_____ 37. Sucrose

_____ 38. Phospholipid

_____ 39. Contains C, O, H, and N

_____ 40. RNA

If you had difficulty with this section, review pages 31-35.

41. **N T E I P O R**

□□□◯□□□

42. **S E B A**

□◯□□

43. **K L A L A N I E**

□□□◯□□□□

44. **D L P I I**

◯□□□□

Take the circled letters, unscramble
them, and fill in the solution.

**What was missing from the Thanksgiving
dinner?**

45. □□□□□

Fill in the crossword puzzle.

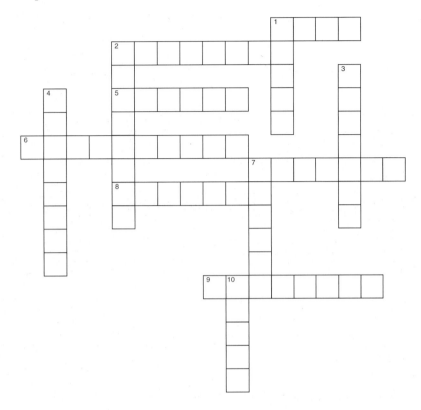

ACROSS

1. Below 7.0 on pH scale
2. Bond formed by sharing electrons
5. Occupies space and has mass
6. Reverse of dehydration synthesis
7. Substances composed of one type of atom
8. Uncharged subatomic particle
9. Subatomic particle

DOWN

1. Combine to form molecules
2. Substances whose molecules have more than one element
3. Amino acid
4. Polysaccharide
7. Chemical catalyst
10. Fat

KNOW YOUR MEDICAL TERMS

Select the correct term for the given literal definitions below.

46. _____ apart; unite; action   a. buffer

47. _____ cushion; actor   b. hydrogen

48. _____ many; sugar; chemical   c. cholesterol

49. _____ bile; solid; oil   d. dissociate

50. _____ band   e. polysaccharide

51. _____ not; natural; to assemble   f. inorganic compound

52. _____ water; produce   g. bond

If you had difficulty with this section, review pages 36-37.

15

53. Annmarie just finished preparing a meal of pan-fried hamburgers for her family. While the frying pan was still hot, she poured the liquid grease into a metal container to cool. Later, she noticed that the liquid oil had solidified as it cooled. Explain the chemistry of why the then room-temperature fat was solid.

54. Carol was gaining weight, yet she was eating very little. Her physician suspected hypothyroidism and suggested a test that measures radiation emitted by the thyroid when radioactive iodine is introduced into the gland. Describe what the radiologist will do to evaluate Carol's thyroid function.

55. India was concerned. She had just returned from the doctor's office after her yearly physical and was reviewing her blood results before filing them away. She noted that her blood results were 7.36. She is aware that cytoplasm has a pH of 7.0. Shouldn't blood have the same pH as cytoplasm, or is this still within the normal range?

56. Word Find

Find and circle 12 terms presented in this chapter. Words may be spelled top to bottom, bottom to top, right to left, left to right, or diagonally.

Alkaline	Electrolyte
Atomic mass	Molecule
Base	Nucleic acid
Carbohydrate	Proton
Dehydration	Reactant
Dissociation	Solvent

```
E  T  A  R  D  Y  H  O  B  R  A  C  E
T  B  H  S  I  H  L  I  N  A  T  O  D
B  N  E  H  S  G  O  U  L  P  O  T  E
R  Z  A  M  S  F  R  K  U  S  M  T  H
P  R  O  T  O  N  A  I  E  C  I  X  Y
B  R  N  U  C  L  E  I  C  A  C  I  D
C  A  F  T  I  A  E  W  G  G  M  W  R
L  E  S  N  A  B  E  C  E  E  A  E  A
G  Q  E  E  T  E  A  R  U  S  S  F  T
Q  R  P  V  I  B  Y  K  I  L  S  W  I
E  T  Y  L  O  R  T  C  E  L  E  B  O
S  B  U  O  N  E  S  P  N  B  R  B  N
O  P  J  S  T  D  J  M  O  L  U  H  D
```

DID YOU KNOW?

■ After a vigorous workout, your triglycerides fall 10% to 20%, and your HDL increases by the same percentage for 2 to 3 hours.

■ Being right-handed can prolong your life. Right-handed people live 5 to 9 years longer than left-handed people.

CHECK YOUR KNOWLEDGE

Fill in the blanks.

1. In order to describe which atoms are present in a compound, a chemical _____ is used.

2. Atoms are composed of protons, electrons, and _____.

3. The farther an orbital extends from the nucleus, the _____ its energy level.

4. Substances can be classified as _____ or _____.

5. Chemical bonds form to make atoms more _____.

6. A(n) _____ is an electrically charged atom.

7. Few _____ compounds have carbon atoms in them, and none have C—C or C—H bonds.

8. _____ _____ is a reaction in which water is lost from the reactants.

9. Chemists often use a _____ _____ to represent a chemical reaction.

10. High levels of _____ in the blood make the blood more acidic.

11. _____ are compounds that produce an excess of H^+ ions.

12. _____ maintain pH balance by preventing sudden changes in the H^+ ion concentration.

13. _____ literally means "carbon" and "water."

14. _____ is a steroid lipid.

15. Collagen and keratin are examples of _____ proteins.

16. Two atoms that have the same atomic number but different atomic masses are _____ the same element.

17. _____ are chemical catalysts.

18. In the DNA molecule, nucleotides are arranged in a twisted strand called a _____ _____.

19. RNA uses the same set of bases as DNA except for the substitution of _____ for thymine.

20. Glycogen and starch are examples of _____.

Chapter **2** **Chemistry of Life**

3 | Cells

Cells are the smallest structural units of living things. Therefore, because we are living, we are made up of a mass of cells. Human cells, which vary in shape and size, can be seen only under a microscope. The three main parts of a cell are the cytoplasmic membrane, the cytoplasm, and the nucleus. As you review this chapter, you will be amazed at the correlation between a cell and the body as a whole. You will identify miniature circulatory systems, reproductive systems, digestive systems, power plants (much like muscular systems), and many other structures that will aid in your understanding of these body systems in future chapters.

Cells—just like humans—require water, food, gases, the elimination of wastes, and numerous other substances and processes in order to survive. The movement of these substances into and out of cells is accomplished by two primary methods: passive transport processes and active transport processes. In passive transport processes, no cellular energy is required to effect movement through the cell membrane. However, in active transport processes, cellular energy is required to provide movement through the cell membrane.

The study of cell reproduction completes this chapter's overview of cells. A basic explanation of DNA, "the hereditary molecule," illuminates the due respect for the amazing capability of the cell to transmit physical and mental traits from generation to generation. Reproduction of the cell—mitosis—is a complex process made up of several stages. These stages are outlined and diagrammed in the text to facilitate learning.

This chapter concludes with a discussion of changes that may occur during cell growth and reproduction. Knowledge of the structure, characteristics, and function of cells is necessary to continue your understanding of the levels of organization in the body.

TOPICS FOR REVIEW

Before progressing to Chapter 4, you should have an understanding of the structure and function of the smallest living unit in the body—the cell. Your review should also include the methods by which substances move through the cell membrane and the stages that occur during cell reproduction. As you finish this chapter, you should have an understanding of tonicity and how the concentration of body fluids impacts cellular health.

OVERVIEW OF CELLS

PARTS OF CELLS

Match each term on the left with its corresponding description on the right.

Group A

1. Cytoplasm   A. Component of plasma membrane

2. Plasma membrane   B. Controls genetic code of the cell

3. Cholesterol   C. "Living matter"

4. Nucleus   D. Organizes and moves structures within the cell

5. Centrosome   E. Surrounds cells

Group B

6. Ribosomes   A. "Power plants"

7. Endoplasmic reticulum   B. "Digestive bags"

8. Mitochondria   C. "Chemical processing and packaging center"

9. Lysosomes   D. "Protein factories"

10. Golgi apparatus   E. "Smooth and rough"

18

Fill in the blanks.

11. The fat molecule _____ helps stabilize the phospholipid molecules to prevent breakage of the plasma membrane.

12. A procedure performed before transplanting an organ from one individual to another is

    _____.

13. Fine, hairlike extensions found on the exposed or free surfaces of some cells are called

    _____.

14. Which organelle is distinguished by the fact that it has two types; it can be either smooth or rough.

    _____

15. _____ are usually attached to the rough endoplasmic reticulum and produce enzymes and other protein compounds.

16. The _____ provide energy-releasing chemical reactions that go on continuously.

17. The organelles that can digest and destroy microbes that invade the cell are called

    _____.

18. Mucus is an example of a product manufactured by the _____.

19. Rod-shaped structures, known as _____, play an important role during cell division.

20. _____ are threadlike structures made up of proteins and DNA.

21. Movement of the _____ of a sperm cell is an example of a specialized organelle having a specialized function.

22. _____ increase the absorption rate of nutrients in the blood.

If you had difficulty with this section, review pages 44-50.

MOVEMENT OF SUBSTANCES THROUGH CELL MEMBRANES

Circle the correct answer.

23. The energy required for active transport processes is obtained from:
    A. ATP
    B. DNA
    C. diffusion
    D. osmosis

24. An example of a passive transport process is:
    A. permease system
    B. phagocytosis
    C. pinocytosis
    D. diffusion

25. Movement of substances from a region of high concentration to a region of low concentration is known as:
    A. active transport
    B. passive transport
    C. cellular energy
    D. concentration gradient

26. Osmosis is similar to diffusion and is a special case of:
    A. filtration
    B. equilibrium
    C. active transport
    D. passive transport

27. _____ involves the movement of solutes across a selectively permeable membrane by the process of diffusion.
   A. Osmosis
   B. Filtration
   C. Dialysis
   D. Phagocytosis

28. One of the processes responsible for urine formation in the kidney is:
   A. osmosis
   B. permease system
   C. filtration
   D. diffusion

29. Which movement always occurs down a hydrostatic pressure gradient?
   A. Osmosis
   B. Filtration
   C. Dialysis
   D. Facilitated diffusion

30. The uphill movement of a substance through a living cell membrane is:
   A. osmosis
   B. diffusion
   C. active transport process
   D. passive transport process

31. The ion pump is an example of what type of movement?
   A. Gravity
   B. Hydrostatic pressure
   C. Active transport process
   D. Passive transport process

32. An example of a cell capable of phagocytosis is the:
   A. white blood cell
   B. red blood cell
   C. muscle cell
   D. bone cell

33. A salt solution that contains a higher concentration of salt than living red blood cells would be:
   A. hypotonic
   B. hypertonic
   C. isotonic
   D. homeostatic

34. A red blood cell becomes engorged with water and will eventually lyse, releasing hemoglobin into the

   solution. This solution is _____ to the red blood cell.
   A. hypotonic
   B. hypertonic
   C. isotonic
   D. homeostatic

If you had difficulty with this section, review pages 50-54.

CELL GROWTH AND REPRODUCTION

Circle the word in each word group that does not belong.

35.	DNA	Adenine	Uracil	Thymine
36.	Complementary base pairing	Guanine	RNA	Cytosine
37.	Anaphase	Specific sequence	Gene	Base pairs
38.	RNA	Ribose	Thymine	Uracil
39.	Translation	Protein synthesis	mRNA	Interphase
40.	Cleavage furrow	Anaphase	Prophase	2 daughter cells
41.	Preparatory stage	Prophase	Interphase	DNA replication
42.	Identical	Two nuclei	Telophase	Metaphase
43.	Metaphase	Prophase	Telophase	Gene

If you had difficulty with this section, review pages 56-62.

UNSCRAMBLE THE WORDS

44. **T H I R A E E N P S**

   ☐ ☐ ◯ ☐ ◯ ☐ ☐ ☐ ☐

45. **E R I L C T E O N**

   ☐ ☐ ◯ ☐ ☐ ☐ ◯ ☐ ☐

46. **U I I F O N S D F**

   ☐ ◯ ☐ ☐ ☐ ☐ ☐ ◯ ☐

47. **O E E P A T S H L**

   ☐ ◯ ☐ ☐ ☐ ◯ ☐ ☐

48. **R A N L G L E E O**

   ◯ ☐ ☐ ◯ ☐ ☐ ☐ ☐ ☐

Take the circled letters, unscramble them, and fill in the solution.

Why Susie asked Carlos to read a letter from her friend Juan.

49. ☐ ☐ ☐ ☐ ☐ ☐ ☐ ☐ ☐ ☐ ☐ ☐ ☐

APPLYING WHAT YOU KNOW

50. Mr. Fee's boat capsized, and consequently he was stranded on a deserted shoreline for 2 days without food or water. When found, he had swallowed a great deal of seawater. He was taken to the emergency room in a state of dehydration. In the space below, draw the appearance of Mr. Fee's red blood cells as they would appear to the laboratory technician.

51. The nurse was instructed to dissolve a pill in a small amount of liquid medication. Just as she dropped the capsule into the liquid, she was interrupted by the telephone. On her return to the medication cart, she found the medication completely dissolved and apparently scattered evenly throughout the liquid. This phenomenon did not surprise her because she was aware from her knowledge of cell transport that _____ had created this distribution.

52. Ms. Bence has emphysema and has been admitted to the hospital unit with oxygen administered per nasal cannula. Emphysema destroys the tiny air sacs in the lungs. These tiny air sacs, alveoli, provide what function for Ms. Bence?

53. Word Find

Find and circle 16 terms presented in this chapter. Words may be spelled top to bottom, bottom to top, right to left, left to right, or diagonally.

```
A  P  D  I  E  V  E  W  N  P  F  E  H  Y  X
I  G  I  Z  N  S  R  L  X  S  T  W  F  Z  S
R  J  V  N  N  T  A  I  L  M  R  P  H  M  F
D  W  U  E  O  O  E  H  B  E  A  D  U  G  F
N  W  I  U  I  C  I  R  P  O  N  N  F  B  W
O  P  U  R  S  H  Y  T  P  O  S  A  W  X  K
H  X  F  O  U  R  Y  T  A  H  L  O  G  A  W
C  L  Z  N  F  O  Y  P  O  R  A  E  M  R  M
O  U  I  X  F  M  L  F  O  S  T  S  T  E  O
T  T  B  Y  I  A  B  C  O  T  I  L  E  S  D
I  V  S  O  D  T  T  M  I  T  O  S  I  S  U
M  N  A  A  I  I  L  E  N  L  N  N  N  F  R
E  O  K  K  I  D  C  Q  H  B  I  V  I  T  H
E  K  T  X  B  Z  A  E  A  L  S  A  E  C  K
S  B  Z  R  P  M  V  L  X  W  Z  A  Z  C  V
```

Chromatid	Hypotonic	Pinocytosis
Cilia	Interphase	Ribosome
Cuboidal	Mitochondria	Telophase
DNA	Mitosis	Translation
Diffusion	Neuron	
Filtration	Organelle	

KNOW YOUR MEDICAL TERMS

Match the term on the left with the literal translation on the right.

54. _____ Hyperplasia   A. Scalloped process

55. _____ Flagellum   B. Produce entire collection

56. _____ Atrophy   C. Drink cell condition

57. _____ Pinocytosis   D. Apart loosening

58. _____ Crenation   E. Push condition

59. _____ Osmosis   F. Excessive shape

60. _____ Genome   G. Whip

61. _____ Dialysis   H. Without nourishment state

If you had difficulty with this section, review pages 61-64.

DID YOU KNOW?

■ The largest single cell in the human body is the female sex cell, the ovum. The smallest single cell in the human body is the male sex cell, the sperm.

■ Human bodies produce 70 kg of ATP per day.

■ Every human spent about half an hour as a single cell.

CELLS

Fill in the crossword puzzle.

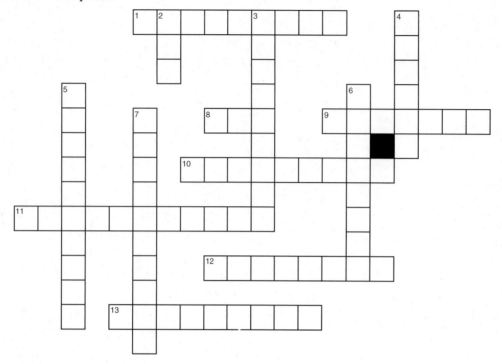

ACROSS

1. Shriveling of cell due to water withdrawal
8. Energy source for active transport
9. Reproduction process of most cells
10. Cell organ
11. Cartilage cell
12. First stage of mitosis
13. Occurs when substances scatter themselves evenly throughout an available space

DOWN

2. Ribonucleic acid (abbreviation)
3. Last stage of mitosis
4. Nerve cell
5. Literally means "center part"
6. Specialized example of diffusion
7. Having an osmotic pressure greater than that of the solution

CHECK YOUR KNOWLEDGE

Multiple Choice

Circle the correct answer.

1. Which of the following cellular structures has the ability to secrete digestive enzymes?
   A. Lysosomes
   B. Mitochondria
   C. Golgi apparatus
   D. Ribosomes

2. Red blood cells do what when placed in a hypertonic salt solution?
   A. Remain unchanged
   B. Undergo crenation
   C. Lyse
   D. None of the above

3. Which of the following statements is true of chromatin granules?
   A. They exist in the cell cytoplasm
   B. They are made up of DNA
   C. They form spindle fibers
   D. All of the above

4. In which stage of mitosis do chromosomes move to opposite ends of the cell along the spindle fibers?
   A. Anaphase
   B. Metaphase
   C. Prophase
   D. Telophase

5. Filtration is a process that involves which of the following?
   A. Active transport
   B. The expenditure of energy
   C. Changes in hydrostatic pressure
   D. All of the above

6. The synthesis of proteins by ribosomes using information coded in the mRNA molecule is called what?
   A. Translation
   B. Transcription
   C. Replication
   D. Crenation

7. The genetic code for a particular protein is passed from DNA to mRNA by a process known as:
   A. transcription
   B. translation
   C. interphase
   D. genome

8. If a strand of DNA has a base sequence of AGGC, the complementary pair for that strand will be:
   A. TCCG
   B. CCTG
   C. TTCG
   D. TUUG

9. Which of the following is not true of RNA?
   A. It is a single strand
   B. It contains uracil rather than thymine
   C. The base pairs are adenine and uracil and guanine and cytosine
   D. It contains deoxyribose sugar

10. All of the DNA in each cell of the body is called the:
    A. tissue typing
    B. genome
    C. gene
    D. genetic code

Matching

Match each term in column A with the most appropriate term in column B. (Only one answer is correct for each.)

Column A	Column B
11. _____ Dialysis	A. Chromatids
12. _____ Plasma membrane	B. Thymine
13. _____ Isotonic	C. Active transport
14. _____ Pinocytosis	D. Energy
15. _____ Prophase	E. Carrier protein
16. _____ Adenine	F. Diffusion
17. _____ Diffusion	G. Phospholipids
18. _____ Hypotonic solution	H. Lyse
19. _____ Mitochondria	I. Passive transport
20. _____ Ion pump	J. Blood cells

Fill in the Blanks

21. The living internal material of cells is _____.

22. DNA and RNA play crucial roles in _____ synthesis.

23. During _____, the DNA of each chromosome replicates itself.

24. "Cell suicide" or cell death is also known as _____.

25. The energy required for active transport processes is obtained from _____.

1. _____

2. _____

3. _____

4. _____

5. _____

6. _____

7. _____

8. _____

9. _____

10. _____

11. _____

12. _____

13. _____

14. _____

15. _____

16. _____

17. _____

18. _____

MITOSIS

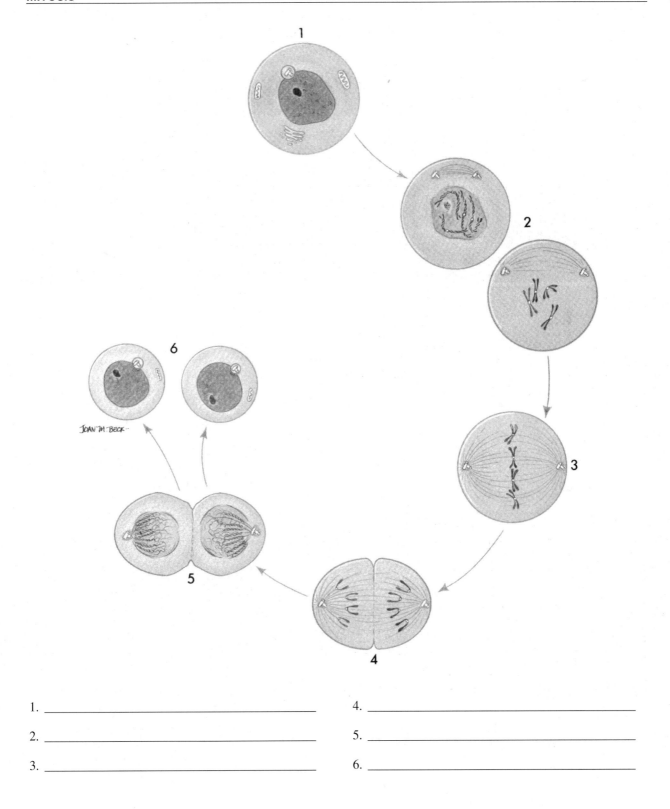

JOAN M BECK

1. _____   4. _____

2. _____   5. _____

3. _____   6. _____

4 Tissues

After successfully completing the study of the cell, you are ready to progress to the next level of anatomical structure: tissues. Four principal types of tissues—epithelial, connective, muscle, and nervous—perform multiple functions to ensure that homeostasis is maintained. Among these functions are protection, absorption, excretion, support, insulation, conduction of impulses, movement of bones, and destruction of bacteria. This variety of functions gives us a real appreciation for the complexity of this level. A macroscopic view confirms this statement as we marvel at the fact that soft, sticky, liquid blood and sturdy compact bone are both considered tissues. As you view the various tissue slides in your text and under a microscope, you will observe the various shapes, arrangement of cells, and general characteristics of each unique type. These numerous distinctions also help explain the varying ability of tissues to regenerate or repair after trauma, disease, or injury.

The chapter concludes with a discussion of changes that may occur during cell growth and reproduction. Knowledge of the characteristics and functions of tissues is necessary to complete your understanding of this structural level of organization and to successfully bridge your knowledge between the cell and the study of body organs.

TOPICS FOR REVIEW

Before progressing to Chapter 5, you should thoroughly review the types of tissues and the unique characteristics of each one. You should also have a basic understanding of how tissue repair is accomplished and the possible effect of that repair on the body.

INTRODUCTION TO TISSUES

Multiple Choice

Circle the correct answer.

1. A tissue is:
   A. a membrane that lines body cavities
   B. a group of similar cells that perform a unique function to help the organ do its job
   C. a thin sheet of cells embedded in a matrix
   D. the most complex organizational unit of the body

2. The four principal types of tissues include all of the following *except*:
   A. nervous
   B. muscle
   C. cartilage
   D. connective

3. Tissues differ from each other in the:
   A. size and shape of their cells
   B. amount and kind of material between the cells
   C. special functions they perform
   D. all of the above

4. The matrix of the blood is the:
   A. red blood cells
   B. white blood cells
   C. platelets
   D. plasma

If you had difficulty with this section, review pages 71-72.

EPITHELIAL TISSUE

Circle the correct answer.

5. Which of the following is *not* a function of epithelium?
   A. Secretion
   B. Protection
   C. Absorption
   D. All of the above are functions of the membranous epithelium.

6. Which of the following is *not* a structural example of epithelium?
   A. Stratified squamous
   B. Simple transitional
   C. Simple columnar
   D. Pseudostratified

7. Epithelial cells can be classified according to shape. Which of the following is not a characteristic shape of epithelium?
   A. Cuboidal
   B. Rectangular
   C. Squamous
   D. Columnar

8. Endocrine glands discharge their products into:
   A. body cavities
   B. blood
   C. organ surfaces
   D. none of the above

9. Which statement regarding pseudostratified epithelium is false?
   A. Basement membrane lies beneath pseudostratified epithelium
   B. Pseudo means "false"
   C. Pseudostratified epithelium is several layers thick
   D. Pseudostratified epithelium lines the trachea

Matching

Match the arrangement of epithelial cells with its corresponding description.

10. _____ Single layer of cube-shaped cells

11. _____ Multiple layers of cells with flat cells at the outer surface

12. _____ Single layer of flat, scalelike cells

13. _____ Single layer of tall, thin cells that compose the surface of mucous membranes

14. _____ Cilia from this tissue move mucus along the lining surface of the trachea

15. _____ Typically found in body areas subjected to stress and must be able to stretch

A. Simple squamous

B. Simple cuboidal

C. Simple columnar

D. Pseudostratified

E. Stratified squamous

F. Stratified transitional

Tissue Labeling

Label the following images and identify the principal tissue type of each. Be as specific as possible. Consult your textbook if you need assistance.

1. Tissue type: _____

1 _____

2 _____

3 _____

2. Tissue type: _____

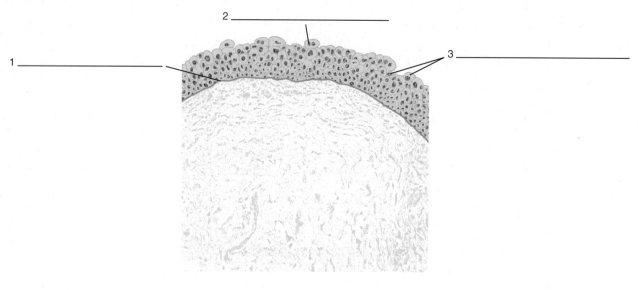

2 _____

1 _____

3 _____

3. Tissue type: _____

If you had difficulty with this section, review pages 72-76.

CONNECTIVE TISSUE

Multiple Choice
Circle the correct answer.

16. Which of the following is *not* an example of connective tissue?
    A. Transitional
    B. Adipose
    C. Blood
    D. Bone

17. Adipose tissue performs which of the following functions?
    A. Insulation
    B. Protection
    C. Support
    D. All of the above

18. The basic structural unit of bone is the microscopic:
    A. osteon
    B. lacunae
    C. lamellae
    D. canaliculi

19. The term *osteon* is synonymous with:
    A. cartilage
    B. chondrocyte
    C. haversian system
    D. osteoblast

20. Dense fibrous connective tissue consists mainly of:
    A. white collagen fibers
    B. liquid matrix
    C. goblet cells
    D. glands

21. Which statement is false regarding connective tissue?
    A. It is the most abundant tissue
    B. It is widely distributed throughout the body
    C. It exists in more varied forms than any of the other tissue types
    D. It is voluntary

Tissue Labeling

Label the following images and identify the principal tissue type of each.

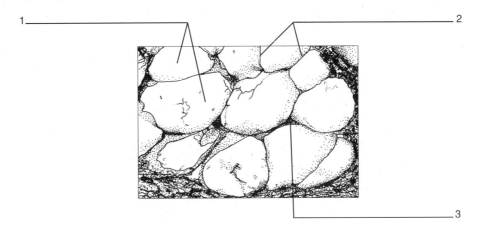

1 _____   2 _____

                                 3 _____

4. Tissue type: _____

1 _____   2 _____

5. Tissue type: _____

6. Tissue type: _____

7. Tissue type: _____

If you had difficulty with this section, review pages 76-81.

MUSCLE TISSUE

Matching

Identify the type of muscle tissue with its corresponding definition.

22. _____ Multiple nuclei, striated, voluntary cells

23. _____ Nonstriated, involuntary, narrow fibers with only one nucleus per fiber

24. _____ Striated, branching, involuntary cells with intercalated disks

25. _____ Responsible for willed body movements

26. _____ Also called *visceral muscle*

27. _____ Found in the walls of hollow internal organs

A. Cardiac muscle

B. Skeletal muscle

C. Smooth muscle

Tissue Labeling

Label the following images and identify the principal tissue type of each.

8. Tissue type: _____

9. Tissue type: _____

If you had difficulty with this section, review pages 81-83.

NERVOUS TISSUE

Matching

Match each term with its corresponding description.

28. _____ Supportive cells   A. Neuron

29. _____ Cell process that transmits nerve impulses away from the cell body   B. Neuroglia

30. _____ The conducting cells of the nervous system   C. Axon

31. _____ Cell process that carries nerve impulses toward the cell body   D. Dendrite

10. Tissue type: _____

If you had difficulty with this section, review pages 83-85.

TISSUES

32. Fill in the missing areas of the chart.

Tissue	Location	Function
Epithelial		
1. Simple squamous	1a. Alveoli of lungs	1a.
	1b. Lining of blood and lymphatic vessels	1b.
2. Stratified squamous	2a.	2a. Protection
	2b.	2b. Protection
3. Simple columnar	3.	3. Protection, secretion, absorption
4.	4. Urinary bladder	4. Protection
5. Pseudostratified	5.	5. Protection
6. Simple cuboidal	6. Glands; kidney tubules	6.
Connective		
1. Areolar	1.	1. Connection
2.	2. Under skin	2. Protection; insulation
3. Dense fibrous	3. Tendons; ligaments; fascia; scar tissue	3.
4. Bone	4.	4. Support, protection
5. Cartilage	5.	5. Firm but flexible support
6. Blood	6. Blood vessels	6.
7.	7. Red bone marrow	7. Blood cell formation

Tissue	Location	Function
Muscle		
1. Skeletal (striated voluntary)	1.	1. Movement of bones
2.	2. Wall of heart	2. Contraction of heart
3. Smooth	3.	3. Movement of substances along ducts; change in diameter of pupils and shape of lens; "gooseflesh"
Nervous		
1.	1.	1. Irritability, conduction

If you had difficulty with this section, review Tables 4-1, 4-2, and 4-3 and pages 72-75, 77-81.

TISSUE REPAIR

Fill in the blanks.

33. _____ is the growth of new tissue (as opposed to scarring).

34. A _____ is an unusually thick scar.

35. Tissues usually repair themselves by allowing _____ cells to remove dead or injured cells.

36. Epithelial and _____ tissues have the greatest capacity to regenerate.

37. Like muscle tissue, _____ tissue has a very limited capacity to regenerate.

38. **E D I N E D T R**

39. **E S T O N O**

40. **U M A S S U O Q**

41. **S I F R D A I E T T**

42. **L A I G**

Take the circled letters, unscramble them, and fill in the solution.

What Madison's friend gave her when she tripped and fell.

43.

APPLYING WHAT YOU KNOW

44. Merrily is 5'4" and weighs 115 lbs. She appears very healthy and fit, yet her doctor advised her that she is "overfat." What might be the explanation for this assessment?

45. Holly is a bodybuilder who is obsessed with her physique. She exercises daily and eats a very low-fat diet. A personal fitness trainer has assessed her body fat at 12%. Determine whether she is too lean or too fat. Explain the relationship between her body-fat percentage and lifestyle.

46. Word Find

Find and circle 16 terms presented in this chapter. Words may be spelled top to bottom, bottom to top, right to left, left to right, or diagonally.

Adipose   Hematopoietic
Axon   Keloid
Cartilage   Matrix
Columnar   Muscle
Connective   Pseudostratified
Cuboidal   Regeneration
Epithelial   Transitional
Fascia

```
C Q E D E M A T R I X L A A N S
D I Y G F S F F C E A U I X O V
S T T X H C O O O N T W C O I C
S E I E O I L P O M P Z S N T C
M J P S I U J I I V T Z A T A A
H U N I M O T J Q D U Z F I R R
R A S N T I P Q W B A F G U E T
I R A C S H L O M I O L U R N I
V R W N L C E H T O B T G L E L
K Q A S P E H L G A O N D T G A
Q R O I V V Q K I D M I P O E G
T L A D I O B U C A O E B H R E
H N N B U Q H O G L L U H P P K
Q F M S C O N N E C T I V E A K
Y H O H I M I K F A J E Q F R V
D E I F I T A R T S O D U E S P
```

DID YOU KNOW?

■ As many as 500,000 Americans die from cancer each year. That's more than all the lives lost in the past 100 years by the U.S. military forces. Half of all cancers are diagnosed in people under the age of 67.

■ Your smell or body odor is unique to you unless you have a twin. Even babies recognize the scent of their mother.

KNOW YOUR MEDICAL TERMS

Fill in the missing medical word or word parts.

47. anti _____ gen _____

48. axle _____

49. cartilage _____ cell _____

50. glue _____ produce _____

51. endo _____ crin _____

52. osteo _____ on _____

53. acorn _____

54. kel _____ oid _____

55. layer _____ made _____

56. scale _____ characterized by _____

If you had difficulty with this section, review pages 71-86.

Fill in the crossword puzzle.

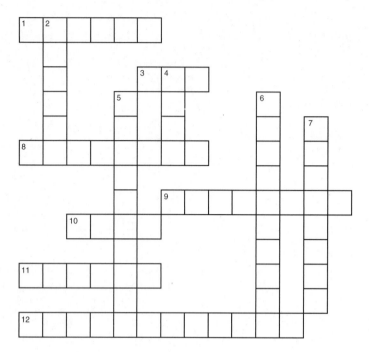

ACROSS

1. Visceral muscle tissue
3. Adipose
8. Glands that release substances through ducts
9. Voluntary
10. Supporting cells of nervous system
11. Unusually thick scar
12. Cartilage cells

DOWN

2. Intracellular substance of a tissue
4. Carries nerve impulses away from the cell body
5. Many layers of epithelial cells
6. Most abundant tissue in body
7. Flat, scalelike epithelial cells

Labeling

Label the following images and identify the principal tissue type of each. Be as specific as possible. Consult your textbook if you need assistance.

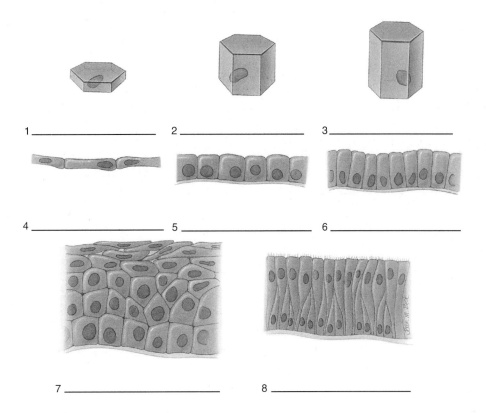

1 _____   2 _____   3 _____

4 _____   5 _____   6 _____

7 _____   8 _____

Multiple Choice

Circle the correct answer.

9. Which of the following is *not* an example of connective tissue?
   A. Striated
   B. Areolar
   C. Reticular
   D. Hematopoietic

10. Which of the following is the most abundant and widely distributed type of body tissue?
    A. Epithelial
    B. Connective
    C. Muscle
    D. Nerve

11. Simple squamous epithelial tissue is made up of which of the following?
    A. A single layer of long, narrow cells
    B. Several layers of long, narrow cells
    C. A single layer of very thin and irregularly shaped cells
    D. Several layers of flat, scalelike cells

12. Which of the following groupings is correct when describing one of the muscle cell types?
    A. Visceral, striated, involuntary
    B. Skeletal, smooth, voluntary
    C. Cardiac, smooth, involuntary
    D. Skeletal, striated, voluntary

13. Which statement is *not* true regarding tissue repair?
    A. Skeletal muscle tissue rarely regenerates itself when injured
    B. Tissues have varying capacity to repair themselves
    C. Nerve tissue has limited capacity to regenerate
    D. Neuroglia produce nerve growth factors that offer promise of treating brain damage

Fill in the Blanks

14. _____ connective tissue is the "glue" that helps keep the organs of the body together.

15. Mucus-producing cells that appear in a simple columnar epithelium are known as

_____ cells.

16. The intracellular substance of a tissue is the _____.

17. The thick, dark bands in cardiac muscle tissue are called _____ _____.

18. A _____ is an unusually thick scar that develops in the lower layer of skin.

19. The growth of new tissue after it has been damaged is accomplished by a process known as

_____.

20. _____ _____ is a screening process used to match donors to recipients when performing organ transplants.

21. _____ is a protein that forms microscopic twisted ropes within the matrix of many tissues and gives the tissues flexible strength.

22. A special kind of adipose tissue called _____ fat actually burns its fuel when the body is cold to produce heat.

23. Spongy bone is also known as _____.

24. Special connecting and supporting cells of the nervous tissue are known as _____.

25. _____ is the strongest and most durable type of cartilage.

5 Organ Systems

A smooth-running automobile is the result of many systems working together harmoniously. The engine, the fuel system, the exhaust system, the brake system, and the cooling system are but a few of the many complex structural units that the automobile as a whole relies on to keep it functioning smoothly. So it is with the human body. We, too, depend on the successful performance of many individual systems working together to create and maintain a healthy human being.

When you have completed your review of the 11 major organ systems and the organs that make up these systems, you will find your understanding of the performance of the body as a whole much more meaningful.

TOPICS FOR REVIEW

Before progressing to Chapter 6, you should have an understanding of the 11 major organ systems and be able to identify the organs that are included in each system. Your review should also include current approaches to organ replacement.

ORGAN SYSTEMS

Match each term on the left with its corresponding term on the right.

Group A

_____ 1. Integumentary	A. Hair
_____ 2. Skeletal	B. Spinal cord
_____ 3. Muscular	C. Hormones
_____ 4. Nervous	D. Tendons
_____ 5. Endocrine	E. Ligaments

Group B

_____ 6. Cardiovascular	A. Esophagus
_____ 7. Lymphatic	B. Ureters
_____ 8. Urinary	C. Larynx
_____ 9. Digestive	D. Genitalia
_____ 10. Respiratory	E. Spleen
_____ 11. Reproductive	F. Capillaries

Circle the word in each word group that does not belong.

12. Pharynx	Trachea	Mouth	Alveoli
13. Uterus	Rectum	Gonads	Prostate
14. Veins	Arteries	Heart	Pancreas
15. Pineal	Bladder	Ureters	Urethra
16. Tendon	Smooth	Joints	Voluntary
17. Pituitary	Brain	Spinal cord	Nerves
18. Cartilage	Joints	Ligaments	Tendons
19. Hormones	Pituitary	Pancreas	Appendix
20. Thymus	Nails	Hair	Oil glands
21. Esophagus	Pharynx	Mouth	Trachea
22. Thymus	Spleen	Tonsils	Liver

23. Fill in the missing areas.

System	Organs	Functions
1. Integumentary	Skin, nails, hair, sense receptors, sweat glands, oil glands	
2. Skeletal		Support, movement, storage of minerals, blood formation
3. Muscular	Muscles	
4.	Brain, spinal cord, nerves	Communication, integration, control, recognition of sensory stimuli
5. Endocrine		Secretion of hormones; communication, integration, control
6. Cardiovascular	Heart, blood vessels	
7. Lymphatic		Transportation, immune system
8.	Kidneys, ureters, bladder, urethra	Elimination of wastes, electrolyte balance, acid-base balance, water balance
9. Digestive		Digestion of food, absorption of nutrients
10.	Nose, pharynx, larynx, trachea, bronchi, lungs	Exchange of gases in the lungs
11. Reproductive		Survival of species; production of sex cells, fertilization, development, birth; nourishment of offspring; production of hormones

If you had difficulty with this section, review pages 93-101 and the chapter summary on page 108-109.

ORGAN REPLACEMENT

Fill in the blanks.

24. An organ not required for life to continue is a _____ _____.

25. Many people suffering from deafness have had their hearing partially restored by "artificial ears" called

_____ _____.

26. One of the earliest devices to augment vital functions was the "artificial kidney" or _____

_____.

27. Electromechanical devices that help keep blood pumping in patients suffering from end-stage heart disease are

known as _____ _____

_____ _____.

28. One approach that offers the hope of a permanent solution to loss of vital organ function is _____

_____.

29. After cancerous breasts are removed, "new" breasts can be formed from skin and muscle tissue using a

method known as _____ _____

_____.

30. The advantage to using a patient's own tissues in organ replacement is that the possibility of

_____ is reduced.

If you had difficulty with this section, review pages 101-105.

UNSCRAMBLE THE WORDS

31. **R T A H E**

32. **I E P L N A**

33. **E E N V R**

34. **S U H E S O P G A**

Take the circled letters, unscramble
them, and fill in the statement.

The more thoroughly you review this chapter, the less

35. [   ] **you will be during your test.**

APPLYING WHAT YOU KNOW

36. Myrna is 15 years old and has not yet started menstruating. Her family physician decides to consult two other physicians, each of whom specializes in a different system. Specialists in the areas of _____ and _____ are consulted.

37. Brian is admitted to the hospital with second- and third-degree burns over 50% of his body. He is placed in isolation. When Jenny visits him, she is required to wear a hospital gown and mask. Why is Brian placed in isolation? Why is Jenny required to wear special attire?

38. Sheila had a mastectomy to remove a cancerous lesion in her breast. Her body rejected the breast implant used to re-construct her breast. Is there another breast reconstruction option that can be offered to Sheila? If so, explain this option.

39. Word Find

Find and circle the names of 11 organ systems. Words may be spelled top to bottom, bottom to top, right to left, left to right, or diagonally.

Circulatory   Nervous
Digestive   Reproductive
Endocrine   Respiratory
Integumentary   Skeletal
Lymphatic   Urinary
Muscular

```
Y R A T N E M U G E T N I R F
H N E R V O U S K I R J M G T
L Y M P H A T I C I S Y Y U I
B N X Y R O T A L U C R I C W
P E L R E O M J M S O M M P S
C C W M A N D L A T E L E K S
R R K E M L I U A A V V U K N
D K X P D J U R C J I R Q E M
C D B V C V I C C T T K W C X
X R Q Q D P H C S O I X P A Z
M F M U S Y D E V U D V Y K E
U E S E C Z G T Q D M N E K O
P Y R A N I R U C T C N E W H
N H T N D E P S I X A Q O I E
```

DID YOU KNOW?

- Muscles comprise 40% of your body weight. Your skeleton, however, only accounts for 18% of your body weight.
- The coccyx (tailbone) has no purpose today. Many scientists believe that it is what is left of the mammal tail that humans used to have in prehistoric years.
- The largest human organ is the skin, with a surface area of about 25 square feet.

KNOW YOUR MEDICAL TERMS

True or False. Indicate in the blank space if the literal translation is true or false for the medical term.

_____ 40. adrenal gland   means   toward/kidney/acorn

_____ 41. digestive   means   stomach/pertaining

_____ 42. capillary   means   hair/relating to

_____ 43. feces   means   waste

_____ 44. hormone   means   excite

_____ 45. integument   means   on/center/result of action

_____ 46. kidney   means   womb

_____ 47. lymphatic   means   flesh/relating

_____ 48. organ   means   relating to system

_____ 49. stem cell   means   tree trunk/storeroom

_____ 50. radiography   means   frequency/drawing

If you had difficulty with this section, review pages 93, and 106-107.

ORGAN SYSTEMS

Fill in the crossword puzzle.

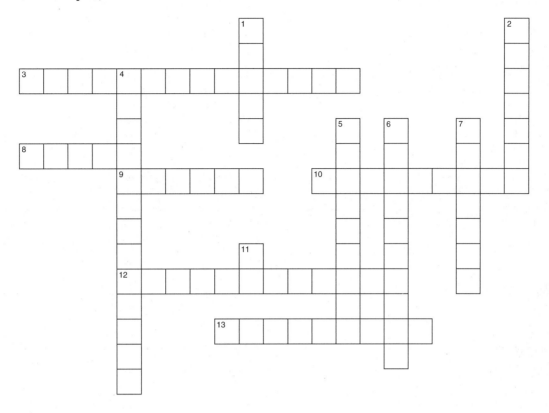

ACROSS

3. Heart and blood vessels
8. Waste product of kidneys
9. Testes and ovaries
10. System of hormones
12. Specialized signal of nervous system (two words)
13. Subdivision of circulatory system

DOWN

1. Undigested residue of digestion
2. Chemical secretion of endocrine system
4. Skin
5. Vulva, penis, and scrotum
6. Device used to replace a body part or improve it
7. Agent that causes change in the activity of a structure
11. Gastrointestinal tract (abbreviation)

CHECK YOUR KNOWLEDGE

Multiple Choice

Circle the correct answer.

1. Which body system serves to clean the blood of waste products?
   A. Digestive
   B. Endocrine
   C. Cardiovascular
   D. Urinary

2. Ovaries and testes are considered components of which system?
   A. Reproductive system
   B. Endocrine system
   C. Both A and B
   D. None of the above

Chapter **5** **Organ Systems**

3. Which of the following organs is classified as an accessory organ of the digestive system?
   A. Mouth
   B. Esophagus
   C. Tongue
   D. Anal canal

4. Factors in the environment such as heat, light, pressure, and temperature that can be recognized by the nervous system are called:
   A. Effectors
   B. Stimuli
   C. Receptors
   D. Nerve impulses

5. Which body system stores the mineral calcium?
   A. Cardiovascular
   B. Digestive
   C. Lymphatic
   D. Skeletal

6. What is undigested material in the gastrointestinal tract called?
   A. Feces
   B. Urine
   C. Lymph
   D. Blood

7. Which body system produces heat and maintains body posture?
   A. Endocrine
   B. Muscular
   C. Cardiovascular
   D. Skeletal

8. Which of the following is *not* a function of the integumentary system?
   A. Integration
   B. Temperature regulation
   C. Ability to serve as a sense organ
   D. Protection

9. Which of the following is *not* a component of the digestive system?
   A. Spleen
   B. Liver
   C. Pancreas
   D. Gallbladder

10. When a group of tissues starts working together to perform a common function, what level of organization is achieved?
    A. Systemic
    B. Tissue
    C. Organ
    D. Cellular

Matching

Match each word in column A with the most appropriate corresponding word in column B. (There is only one correct answer for each.)

Column A

_____ 11. Sweat glands

_____ 12. Heart

_____ 13. Spleen

_____ 14. Vas deferens

_____ 15. Bladder

_____ 16. Gallbladder

_____ 17. Uterine tubes

_____ 18. Trachea

_____ 19. Spinal cord

_____ 20. Adrenals

Column B

A. Endocrine

B. Urinary

C. Integumentary

D. Cardiovascular

E. Respiratory

F. Digestive

G. Male reproductive

H. Lymphatic

I. Female reproductive

J. Nervous

Fill in the Blanks

21. Voluntary muscle may also be called _____.

22. Structures attached to a main part are _____.

23. A _____ is part of a muscle organ that attaches the muscle to a bone.

24. The cranial and spinal nerves and all of their branches make up the _____

_____   _____.

25. The primary function of the cardiovascular system is _____.

6 Mechanisms of Disease

One of our foremost concerns is health. We are fascinated and constantly confronted with information regarding what is necessary to be in good health, what is required for proper maintenance of the body, and what behaviors are responsible for disease.

Organisms play an important role in health. They are microscopic structures that are present everywhere. Many organisms are helpful and may be used for the preparation of foods, in industry and agriculture, to solve problems during the production of shelter and clothing, and in combating disease. However, many other organisms are responsible for producing disease. They attack and disturb the normal homeostasis of the body and adversely affect our health. Many varieties of organisms exist. They are often classified by shape, size, function, or staining properties. To prevent disease, we must prevent pathogenic or disease-producing organisms from entering the body. This is not an easy task because we are surrounded by pathogenic organisms. It is important that we understand the transmission and control of these organisms to fully comprehend the mechanisms of disease.

TOPICS FOR REVIEW

Before progressing to Chapter 7, you should familiarize yourself with disease terminology and patterns of disease. You should continue your review by studying pathophysiology and pathogenic organisms. Finally, an understanding of tumors, cancer, and inflammation is necessary to round out your knowledge of this chapter.

STUDYING DISEASE

PATTERNS OF DISEASE

Match each term on the left with its corresponding description on the right.

Group A

_____ 1. Pathology

_____ 2. Signs

_____ 3. Symptoms

_____ 4. Syndrome

_____ 5. Etiology

A. Subjective abnormalities

B. Study of disease

C. Collection of different signs and symptoms that present a clear picture of a pathological condition

D. Study of factors involved in causing a disease

E. Objective abnormalities

Group B

_____ 6. Latent

_____ 7. Convalescence

_____ 8. Pandemics

_____ 9. Endemic

_____ 10. Pathogenesis

A. Recovery

B. Disease native to a local region

C. "Hidden" stage

D. Epidemics that spread throughout the world

E. Actual pattern of a disease's development

If you had difficulty with this section, review pages 113-114.

PATHOPHYSIOLOGY

Fill in the blanks.

11. _____ is the organized study of the underlying physiological processes associated with disease.

12. Many diseases are best understood as disturbances of _____.

13. Altered or _____ genes can cause abnormal proteins to be made.

14. An organism that lives in or on another organism to obtain its nutrients is called a _____.

15. Abnormal tissue growths may also be referred to as _____.

16. *Autoimmunity* literally means _____.

17. Genetic factors, age, lifestyle, stress, environmental factors, and preexisting conditions are _____ _____ that may be responsible for predisposing a person to disease.

18. Scientists at the _____ _____ _____ _____ _____ _____ continuously track the incidence and spread of disease in this country and worldwide.

19. Conditions caused by psychological factors are sometimes called _____ disorders.

20. A primary condition can put a person at risk for developing a _____ condition.

If you had difficulty with this section, review pages 115-117.

PATHOGENIC ORGANISMS AND PARTICLES

PREVENTION AND CONTROL

Circle the correct answer.

21. The smallest of all pathogens—microscopic nonliving particles—are called:
    A. bacteria
    B. fungi
    C. viruses
    D. protozoa

22. A tiny, primitive cell without a nucleus is called a:
    A. bacterium
    B. fungus
    C. virus
    D. protozoa

23. An example of a viral disease is:
    A. diarrhea
    B. mononucleosis
    C. syphilis
    D. toxic shock syndrome

24. Bacteria that require oxygen for metabolism are classified as:
    A. gram positive
    B. gram negative
    C. aerobic
    D. anaerobic

25. Bacilli are shaped like:
    A. spheres
    B. curves
    C. squares
    D. rods

26. Without chlorophyll, _____ cannot produce their own food, so they must consume or parasitize other organisms.
    A. bacteria
    B. fungi
    C. viruses
    D. protozoa

27. Protozoa include:
    A. amoebas
    B. flagellates
    C. ciliates
    D. all of the above

28. Pathogenic animals include which of the following?
    A. Nematodes
    B. Platyhelminths
    C. Arthropods
    D. All of the above

29. The key to preventing diseases caused by pathogenic organisms is to:
    A. have an annual physical
    B. stop them from entering the body
    C. isolate yourself from all disease-carrying individuals
    D. none of the above

30. The destruction of all living organisms is known as:
    A. disinfection
    B. antisepsis
    C. sterilization
    D. isolation

31. Ways in which pathogens can spread include:
    A. person-to-person contact
    B. environmental contact
    C. opportunistic invasion
    D. transmission by vector
    E. all of the above

32. Compounds produced by certain living organisms that kill or inhibit pathogens are:
    A. antiseptics
    B. antibiotics
    C. disinfectants
    D. sterilizers

If you had difficulty with this section, review pages 118-127.

TUMORS AND CANCER

Circle the correct answer.

33. Benign tumors usually grow (*slowly* or *quickly*).

34. Malignant tumors (*are* or *are not*) encapsulated.

35. An example of a benign tumor that arises from epithelial tissue is a (*papilloma* or *lipoma*).

36. A general term for malignant tumors that arise from connective tissues is (*melanoma* or *sarcoma*).

37. Abnormal, undifferentiated tumor cells are often produced by a process called (*hyperplasia* or *anaplasia*).

38. A cancer specialist is an (*osteologist* or *oncologist*).

39. The Papanicolaou test is a (*biopsy* or *MRI*).

40. (*Staging* or *Grading*) involves classifying a tumor based on its size and the extent of its spread.

41. Cachexia involves a loss of (*appetite* or *hair*).

If you had difficulty with this section, review pages 129-133.

WARNING SIGNS OF CANCER

List the eight warning signs of cancer.

42. _____

43. _____

44. _____

45. _____

46. _____

47. _____

48. _____

49. _____

If you had difficulty with this section, review page 31.

INFLAMMATION

If the statement is true, write "T" in the answer blank. If the statement is false, correct the statement by circling the incorrect term and writing the correct term in the answer blank.

_____ 50. As tissue cells are damaged, they release inflammation mediators such as histamines, prostaglandins, and kinins.

_____ 51. Inflammatory exudate is quickly removed by lymphatic vessels and carried to lymph nodes, which act as filters.

_____ 52. Inflammation mediators can also act as signals that attract red blood cells to the injury site.

_____ 53. The movement of white blood cells in response to chemical attractants is called *chemotaxis*.

_____ 54. Inflammation can be local or systemic.

_____ 55. Fevers usually subside after the irritant has been eliminated.

_____ 56. The fever response in children and in older adults often differs from that in the normal adult.

If you had difficulty with this section, review pages 134-135.

UNSCRAMBLE THE WORDS

57. **N G F U I**

[ ][ ][ ][(○)][(○)]

58. **C E O N O G N E**

[ ][(○)][ ][(○)][ ][ ][ ]

59. **A D E E M**

[ ][(○)][ ][(○)]

60. **R S P O E**

[ ][ ][ ][(○)][ ]

Take the circled letters, unscramble them, and fill in the solution.

Emc^2

$\begin{array}{c} 1 \\ \times 7 \\ \hline 7 \end{array}$ $\begin{array}{c} 1 \\ \times 9 \\ \hline 9 \end{array}$

What Mr. Lynch found to be most difficult as a teacher.

61. [ ][ ][ ][ ][ ][ ][ ][ ]

62. Trent was examined by his doctor and was diagnosed as having a rhinovirus. Does he have need for concern? Why or why not?

63. Julius, a 2-year-old child, was experiencing rectal itching and insomnia. The pediatrician told Julius' mother that he suspected a nematode. What is the common term for the specific nematode that might cause these symptoms?

64. Shirley was cleaning her house and wanted to use the most appropriate and effective aseptic method to prevent the spread of germs. What would you suggest?

65. Mr. and Mrs. Gibbs adopted a child of Chinese descent. Mrs. Gibbs researched the "gene pool" of the child to alert her to any special concerns. What is a "gene pool" and how will this information assist Mr. and Mrs. Gibbs in the rearing of their child?

66. Bill has decided to become a paramedic. When he applied for school, it was suggested that he receive the series of vaccinations for hepatitis B. Why?

67. Word Find

Find and circle 18 terms presented in this chapter. Words may be spelled top to bottom, bottom to top, right to left, left to right, or diagonally.

```
N  P  E  S  D  B  S  L  A  A  C  E  R
W  O  L  S  I  C  I  M  E  D  I  P  E
X  V  I  O  F  S  X  V  R  E  N  A  T
O  D  P  T  U  E  A  D  O  N  C  R  U
H  S  O  V  A  S  T  T  P  O  U  A  C
Y  S  M  P  U  M  O  A  S  M  B  S  A
Y  P  A  R  O  I  M  B  I  A  A  I  I
N  L  I  O  S  R  E  A  F  L  T  T  D
W  V  J  T  C  Z  H  C  L  L  I  E  Y
W  Q  K  O  W  G  C  T  Q  F  O  C  M
V  Q  F  Z  I  F  G  E  R  P  N  F  A
K  E  N  O  Q  E  J  R  B  A  F  I  L
B  B  J  A  F  E  N  I  C  C  A  V  H
W  Z  F  H  R  B  S  U  D  M  Q  D  C
M  X  E  C  K  M  B  M  K  U  O  Z  P
```

Acute	Chlamydia	Metastasis
Adenoma	Ciliate	Parasite
Arthropod	Epidemic	Protozoa
Bacterium	Incubation	Spore
Biopsy	Inflammation	Vaccine
Chemotaxis	Lipoma	Virus

DID YOU KNOW?

- As many as 500,000 Americans die from cancer each year, making it the second-leading cause of death after cardiovascular disease. Half of all cancers are diagnosed in people under the age of 67.
- Scientists have proved that stress can change the bacteria levels in the gut, which can have significant impact on our immunity.
- Bloodsucking hookworms inhabit 700 million people worldwide.
- Israeli scientists have discovered that bacteria can communicate with each other through nanotubes.

KNOW YOUR MEDICAL TERMS

Circle the correct answer.

68. patho   means   (*health* or *disease*)

69. edema   means   (*swelling* or *broad*)

70. amoeba   means   (*change* or *small*)

71. fungus   means   (*mold* or *mushroom*)

72. pus   means   (*rotten* or *stringy*)

73. anthrax   means   (*boil* or *cow*)

74. acute   means   (*quick* or *sharp*)

If you had difficulty with this section, review pages 113 and 136-137.

MECHANISMS OF DISEASE

Fill in the crossword puzzle.

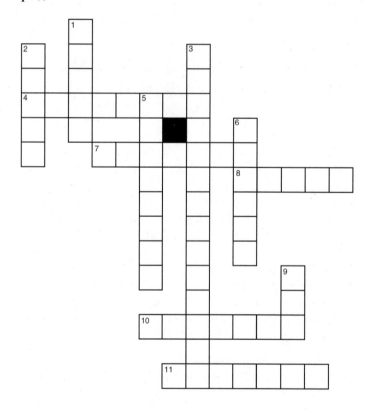

ACROSS	DOWN
4. Roundworm	1. Tissue swelling
7. Microscopic organism	2. Lack chlorophyll
8. Round cells	3. Glandular cancer
10. Possess pseudopodia	5. "Cancer gene"
11. Rod-shaped cells	6. Spreads disease to other organisms
	9. Thick inflammatory exudate

Multiple Choice
Circle the correct answer.

1. Diseases with undetermined causes are:
   A. asymptomatic
   B. idiopathic
   C. psychogenic
   D. predisposing

2. The study of the occurrence, distribution, and transmission of diseases is:
   A. entomology
   B. pathology
   C. oncology
   D. epidemiology

3. Streptomycin is an example of a/an:
   A. antibiotic
   B. vaccine
   C. pathogenic organism
   D. all of the above

4. Reversal of a chronic condition is called:
   A. inflammatory response
   B. predisposing condition
   C. hemostasis
   D. remission

5. If antibodies are found in an immunological test, it is assumed that:
   A. the patient has been exposed to a pathogen
   B. the infection is gone
   C. A and B
   D. none of the above

6. An epidemiologist:
   A. studies the transmission of disease
   B. monitors infection control programs
   C. tracks the spread of disease
   D. all of the above

7. Study of the underlying physiological processes associated with disease leads to:
   A. strategies of prevention
   B. strategies of treatment
   C. A and B
   D. none of the above

8. Severe loss of appetite, weight loss, and general weakness in a cancer patient describe:
   A. secondary infection
   B. cachexia
   C. inflammatory response
   D. chemotaxis

9. Intracellular parasites that are not technically living organisms are characteristics of:
   A. bacteria
   B. fungi
   C. amoebas
   D. viruses

10. Examples of protozoa include all of the following *except*:
    A. bacilli
    B. flagellates
    C. sporozoa
    D. amoebas

Matching
Match each term in column A with the most appropriate definition or description in column B. (Only one answer is correct for each.)

Column A

_____ 11. Syndrome

_____ 12. Metastasis

_____ 13. Anaerobic

_____ 14. Protozoa

_____ 15. Pathogenesis

_____ 16. Fever

_____ 17. Metazoa

_____ 18. Pathology

_____ 19. Neoplasm

_____ 20. Arthropods

Column B

A. Study of disease

B. Require absence of oxygen

C. Collection of signs and symptoms

D. Spread of cancer cells

E. Multicellular organisms that parasitize humans

F. Abnormal cell growth

G. Pattern of disease development

H. Mites

I. Inflammatory response

J. One-celled organisms that parasitize cells

Fill in the Blanks

21. Conditions caused by psychological factors are sometimes called _____.

22. A _____ its RNA to "transcribe backward" to produce the virus's primary genetic code and insert it into the host's DNA genome.

23. The _____ is found almost everywhere and is the second-leading cause of the common cold.

24. _____ large parasites that are also known as _____.

25. _____ technique involves killing or disabling pathogens on surfaces before they can spread to other people.

MAJOR GROUPS OF PATHOGENIC BACTERIA

1. _____

2. _____

3. _____

4. _____

MAJOR GROUPS OF PATHOGENIC PROTOZOA

1.

2.

3.

4.

EXAMPLES OF PATHOGENIC ANIMALS

1.

2.

3.

1.

2.

7 Skin and Membranes

More of our time, attention, and money are spent on the integumentary system than on any other. Every time we look into a mirror we become aware of the integumentary system, as we observe our skin, hair, nails, and the appendages that give luster and comfort to this system. The discussion of the skin begins with the structure and function of the two primary layers called the *epidermis* and *dermis*. It continues with an examination of the appendages of the skin, which include the hair, receptors, nails, sebaceous glands, and sudoriferous glands. The study of skin also includes a review of one of the most serious and frequent threats to the skin—burns. An understanding of the integumentary system provides you with an appreciation of the danger that severe burns can pose to this system.

Membranes are thin, sheetlike structures that cover, protect, anchor, or lubricate body surfaces, cavities, or organs. The two major categories of membranes are epithelial and connective. Each type is located in specific areas of the body, and each is vulnerable to specific disease conditions. Knowledge of the location and function of these membranes prepares you for the study of their relationship to other systems and the body as a whole.

TOPICS FOR REVIEW

Before progressing to Chapter 8, you should have an understanding of the skin, its appendages, major skin disorders, and infections. Your review should include the classification of burns and the method used to estimate the percentage of body surface area affected by burns. A knowledge of the types of body membranes, their location, and their function is necessary to complete your study of this chapter.

BODY MEMBRANES

Match each numbered term or description with its category and write the corresponding letter in the answer blank.

A. Cutaneous   B. Serous   C. Mucous   D. Synovial

_____ 1. Pleura

_____ 2. Lines joint capsules

_____ 3. Respiratory tract

_____ 4. Skin

_____ 5. Peritoneum

_____ 6. Contains no epithelium

_____ 7. Urinary tract

_____ 8. Lines body surfaces that open directly to the exterior

If you had difficulty with this section, review pages 146-147.

FUNCTIONS OF THE SKIN

Match each term on the left with its description or definition on the right.

Group A

_____ 9. Integumentary system	A. Outermost layer of skin
_____ 10. Epidermis	B. Deeper of the two layers of skin
_____ 11. Dermis	C. Hypodermis
_____ 12. Subcutaneous	D. The skin is the primary organ
_____ 13. Cutaneous membrane	E. Composed of dermis and epidermis

Group B

_____ 14. Keratin	A. Protective protein
_____ 15. Melanin	B. Blue-gray color of skin resulting from a decrease in oxygen
_____ 16. Stratum corneum	C. Rows of peglike projections
_____ 17. Dermal papillae	D. Brown pigment
_____ 18. Cyanosis	E. Outer layer of epidermis

Match each numbered term or description with its corresponding skin layer and write "A" or "B" in the answer blank.

A.   Epidermis   B.   Dermis

_____ 19. Tightly packed epithelial cells		_____ 25. Follicle	
_____ 20. Nerves		_____ 26. Sebaceous gland	
_____ 21. Fingerprints		_____ 27. Sweat gland	
_____ 22. Blisters		_____ 28. More cellular than the other layer	
_____ 23. Keratin			
_____ 24. Connective tissue			

If you had difficulty with this section, review pages 148-154.

Fill in the blanks.

29. The most important functions of the skin are _____, _____, _____, _____, and _____.

30. _____ prevents the sun's ultraviolet rays from penetrating the interior of the body.

31. The hair of a newborn infant is called _____.

32. Hair growth begins from a small, cap-shaped cluster of cells called the _____ _____.

33. Hair loss of any kind is called _____.

34. The _____ _____ muscle produces "goose pimples."

35. A birthmark that appears as a bruise at birth and grows rapidly into a bright red nodule is called a _____ _____.

36. The most numerous, important, and widespread sweat glands in the body are the _____ sweat glands.

37. The _____ sweat glands are found primarily in the axilla and in the pigmented skin areas around the genitals.

38. _____ has been described as "nature's skin cream."

If you had difficulty with this section, review pages 149-155.

DISORDERS OF THE SKIN

Circle the correct answer.

39. Any disorder of the skin may be called:
    A. dermatitis
    B. dermatosis
    C. dermatotomy
    D. none of the above

40. Any measurable variation from the normal structure of a tissue is known as a/an:
    A. lesion
    B. burn
    C. blister
    D. erythema

41. An example of a papule is a:
    A. scratch
    B. bedsore
    C. freckle
    D. wart

42. An example of a skin disorder that may produce fissures is:
    A. acne
    B. a bedsore
    C. psoriasis
    D. athlete's foot

43. The skin is the _____ line of defense against microbes that invade the body's internal environment.
    A. first
    B. second
    C. third
    D. fourth

44. Tinea is a fungal infection and may appear as:
    A. ringworm
    B. jock itch
    C. athlete's foot
    D. all of the above

45. Furuncles are local staphylococci infections and are also known as:
    A. scabies
    B. warts
    C. boils
    D. impetigo

46. The most common type of skin cancer is:
    A. squamous cell
    B. basal cell
    C. melanoma
    D. Kaposi sarcoma

If you had difficulty with this section, review pages 156-164.

BURNS

Circle the correct answer.

47. A first-degree burn (*will* or *will not*) blister.

48. A second-degree burn (*will* or *will not*) scar.

49. A third-degree burn (*will* or *will not*) cause pain immediately.

50. According to the "rule of nines," the body is divided into (*9* or *11*) areas of 9% each.

51. Destruction of the subcutaneous layer occurs in (*second-* or *third-*) degree burns.

If you had difficulty with this section, review pages 157-161.

UNSCRAMBLE THE WORDS

52. **PIDEEMIRS**

□□□◯◯◯□□□

53. **REKTAIN**

□◯□□◯□□

54. **AHIR**

◯□◯◯

55. **UGONAL**

□□□□◯□

56. **DRTONIDEHYA**

◯◯□□□□□□□□□

Take the circled letters, unscramble them, and fill in the solution.

What Amanda's mother gave her after every date.

57. □□□□□ □□□□□□

APPLYING WHAT YOU KNOW

58. Mr. Ziven was admitted to the hospital with second- and third-degree burns. Both arms, the anterior trunk, the right anterior leg, and the genital region were affected by the burns. The doctor quickly estimated that _____% of Mr. Ziven's body had been burned.

59. Mrs. James complained to her doctor that she had severe pain in her chest and feared that she was having a heart attack. An ECG revealed nothing unusual, but Mrs. James insisted that every time she took a breath she experienced pain. What might be the cause of Mrs. James' pain?

60. Mrs. Collins was born with a rare condition known as xeroderma pigmentosum. What activity should she avoid?

61. After investigating the scene of the crime, Officer Gorski announced that dermal papillae were found that would help solve the case. What did he mean?

62. Word Find

Find and circle 15 terms presented in this chapter. Words may be spelled top to bottom, bottom to top, right to left, left to right, or diagonally.

Apocrine   Lunula
Blister   Melanocyte
Cuticle   Mucus
Dehydration   Peritoneum
Depilatories Pleurisy
Epidermis   Serous
Follicle   Sudoriferous
Lanugo

```
S U D O R I F E R O U S V K R
E J U Q U E S T E C N O H Y U
I S J L M E L A N O C Y T E H
R I M U E N O T I R E P H S B
O M K N V A S T R L A N U G O
T R G U F G A U C E G O V W D
A E A L P R D I O N T F D R N
L D V A D M L C P D H S L Z F
I I N Y N L R L A M E N I R E
P P H Q O N E U X R R F E L G
E E Z F J U M Y O U U O C C B
D Z P E R J Y U V F C I I E O
G J S I W J S K C D T N O Z C
C O S M Z M F I B U G U X O J
X Y P M E I W E C V S U G B I
```

KNOW YOUR MEDICAL TERMS

Match the correct term with the literal translation below.

a. arrector   f. integ   k. sudo
b. kera   g. bursa   l. melan
c. append   h. sclero   m. stratum
d. lanugo   i. alb
e. sebum   j. dermis

63. _____ raiser

64. _____ down

65. _____ purse

66. _____ hang upon

67. _____ skin

68. _____ grease

69. _____ layer

70. _____ sweat

71. _____ on/cover

72. _____ white

73. _____ hard

74. _____ horn

75. _____ black

If you had difficulty with this section, review pages 145 and 166-167.

Chapter **7 Skin and Membranes**

DID YOU KNOW?

- Because the dead cells of the epidermis are constantly being worn and washed away, we get a new outer skin layer every 27 days.
- A large amount of the dust in your home is actually dead skin.
- Humans shed about 600,000 particles of skin every hour, or about 1.5 pounds a year. By age 70, an average person will have lost 105 pounds of skin!
- A fetus acquires fingerprints at the age of three months.

SKIN/BODY MEMBRANES

Fill in the crossword puzzle.

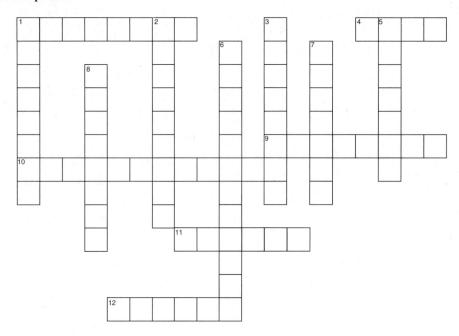

ACROSS

1. Inflammation of the serous membrane that lines the chest and covers the lungs
4. Cutaneous
9. Membrane that lines joint spaces
10. "Goose pimples" (two words)
11. Cushionlike sacs found between moving body parts
12. Deeper of the two primary skin layers

DOWN

1. Forms the lining of serous body cavities
2. Oil gland
3. Bluish-gray color of skin due to decreased oxygen
5. Tough waterproof substance that protects body from excess fluid loss
6. Sweat gland
7. Brown pigment
8. Covers the surface of organs found in serous body cavities

Multiple Choice

Circle the correct answer.

1. What type of serous membrane that covers organs is found in all body cavities?
   A. Visceral
   B. Pleural
   C. Parietal
   D. Synovial

2. Which of the following statements about synovial membranes is true?
   A. They are classified as epithelial
   B. They line joints
   C. They contain a parietal layer
   D. All of the above are true

3. Which of the following statements about hair follicles is true?
   A. Arrector pili muscles are associated with them
   B. Sudoriferous glands empty into them
   C. They arise directly from the epidermis layer of skin
   D. All of the above are true

4. Which of the following statements about apocrine glands is true?
   A. They can be classified as sudoriferous
   B. They are found primarily in armpit and genital regions
   C. They secrete a thick substance that has a strong odor associated with it
   D. All of the above are true

5. Which of the following, if any, is *not* found in the dermis layer of the skin?
   A. Nerves
   B. Melanin
   C. Blood vessels
   D. All of the above are found in the dermis

6. What characterizes second-degree burns?
   A. Blisters
   B. Swelling
   C. Severe pain
   D. All of the above

7. Blackheads can result from the blockage of which of the following glands?
   A. Lacrimal
   B. Sebaceous
   C. Ceruminous
   D. Sudoriferous

8. Keratin is found in which layer of the skin?
   A. Dermis
   B. Epidermis
   C. Subcutaneous
   D. Serous

9. What is the fold of skin that hides the root of a nail called?
   A. Lunula
   B. Body
   C. Cuticle
   D. Papillae

10. Which of the following is *not* an important function of the skin?
    A. Sense organ activity
    B. Absorption
    C. Protection
    D. Temperature regulation

Matching

Match each term in column A with its corresponding description in column B. (Only one answer is correct for each.)

Column A

_____ 11. Melanin

_____ 12. Epithelial membrane (serous)

_____ 13. Pacini corpuscle

_____ 14. Sebaceous

_____ 15. Waterproofing

_____ 16. Hair

_____ 17. Lunula

_____ 18. Connective tissue membrane

_____ 19. Dermal papillae

_____ 20. Sudoriferous

Column B

A. Fingerprint

B. Skin receptor

C. Brown pigment

D. Pleura

E. Synovial membrane

F. Perspiration

G. Oil

H. Follicle

I. Keratin

J. Little moon

Completion

Complete the following using the terms below. Write the corresponding letter in the answer blank.

A. Skin

B. Eccrine sweat glands

C. Peritonitis

D. Mucous

E. Epidermis

F. Fourth-degree burns

G. Pleurisy

H. Sebaceous

I. Hair follicles

J. Receptors

_____ 21. Which glands secrete oil or sebum for hair and skin?

_____ 22. The first line of defense for the body is the _____.

_____ 23. Which glands work throughout the body, helping to regulate body heat?

_____ 24. Which burn extends below the subcutaneous tissue to muscle or bone?

_____ 25. Hair growth requires epidermal tubelike structures called _____.

_____ 26. The outermost and thinnest primary layer of skin is _____.

_____ 27. A condition that involves inflammation of the serous membranes lining the chest cavity and covering the lungs is called _____.

_____ 28. Which membrane lines body surfaces that open directly to the exterior of the body and produces mucus?

_____ 29. Specialized nerve endings that make it possible for skin to act as a sense organ are called _____.

_____ 30. An inflammation of the serous membranes lining the abdominal cavity and abdominal organs is called _____.

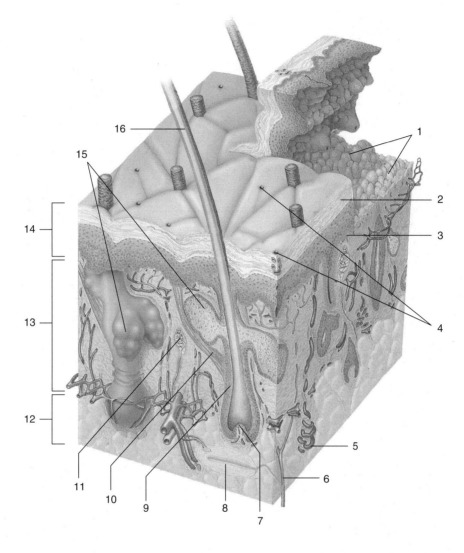

1. _____

2. _____

3. _____

4. _____

5. _____

6. _____

7. _____

8. _____

9. _____

10. _____

11. _____

12. _____

13. _____

14. _____

15. _____

16. _____

Chapter **7 Skin and Membranes**

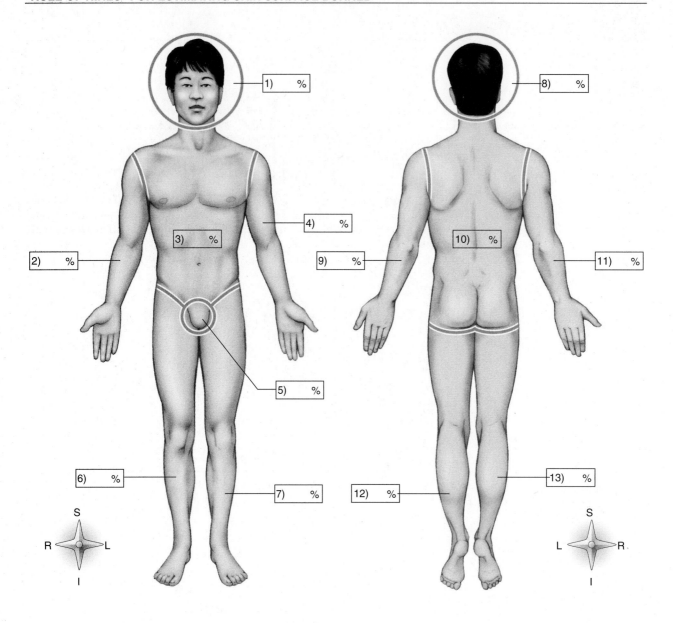

8 Skeletal System

How strange we would look without our skeleton! It is the skeleton that provides us with the rigid, supportive framework that gives shape to our bodies. But this is just the beginning, because the skeleton also protects the organs beneath it, maintains homeostasis of blood calcium, produces blood cells, and assists the muscular system in providing movement for us.

After reviewing the microscopic structure of bone and cartilage, you will understand how skeletal tissues are formed, their differences, and their importance in the human body. Your microscopic investigation will make the study of this system easier as you logically progress from this view to macroscopic bone formation and growth and visualize the structure of long bones.

The skeleton is divided into two main divisions: the axial skeleton and the appendicular skeleton. All of the 206 bones of the human body may be classified into one of these two areas. Although men and women have the same number and types of bones, subtle differences exist between a man's and a woman's skeleton. These structural differences provide us with insight into the functional differences between men and women.

Three types of joints exist in the body. They are classified according to the degree of movement they allow in the body. They are synarthroses, amphiarthroses, and diarthroses. It is important to have a knowledge of these joints to understand how movement is facilitated by articulations.

TOPICS FOR REVIEW

Before progressing to Chapter 9, you should familiarize yourself with the functions of the skeletal system, the structure and function of bone and cartilage, bone formation and growth, and the types of joints found in the body. Additionally, your understanding of the skeletal system should include identification of the two major subdivisions of the skeleton, the bones found in each area, and any differences that exist between a man's and a woman's skeleton. Your study should conclude with a review of the major skeletal disorders.

FUNCTIONS OF THE SKELETAL SYSTEM

GROSS STRUCTURE OF LONG BONES

Fill in the blanks.

1. There are _____ types of bones.

2. The _____ _____ is the hollow area inside the diaphysis of a bone.

3. A thin layer of cartilage covering each epiphysis is the _____ _____.

4. The _____ lines the medullary cavity of long bones.

5. _____ is used to describe the process of blood cell formation.

6. Blood cell formation is a vital process carried on in _____ _____ _____.

7. The _____ is a strong fibrous membrane that covers a long bone everywhere except at joint surfaces.

8. Bones may be classified by shape. Those shapes include _____, _____, _____, and _____.

9. Bones serve as a safety-deposit box for _____, a vital substance required for normal nerve and muscle function.

10. As muscles contract and shorten, they pull on bones and thereby _____ them.

If you had difficulty with this section, review pages 176-177.

69

Copyright © 2018, Elsevier Inc. All rights reserved.

Chapter **8 Skeletal System**

MICROSCOPIC STRUCTURE OF BONE AND CARTILAGE

Match each term on the left with its corresponding description on the right.

Group A

_____ 11. Trabeculae   A. Layer of cancellous bone on flat bones

_____ 12. Compact   B. Dense bone tissue

_____ 13. Spongy   C. Fibers embedded in a firm gel

_____ 14. Diploe   D. Needlelike threads of spongy bone

_____ 15. Cartilage   E. Cancellous bone

Group B

_____ 16. Osteocytes   A. Connect lacunae

_____ 17. Canaliculi   B. Cartilage cells

_____ 18. Lamellae   C. Structural unit of compact bone

_____ 19. Chondrocytes   D. Mature bone cells

_____ 20. Haversian system   E. Ring of bone

If you had difficulty with this section, review page 177.

BONE DEVELOPMENT

If the statement is true, write "T" in the answer blank. If the statement is false, correct the statement by circling the incorrect term and writing the correct term in the answer blank.

_____ 21. When the skeleton forms in a baby before birth, it consists of cartilage and fibrous structures.

_____ 22. The diaphyses are the ends of the bone.

_____ 23. Bone-forming cells are known as *osteoclasts*.

_____ 24. It is the combined action of osteoblasts and osteoclasts that sculpts bones into their adult shapes.

_____ 25. The soft spots, or fontanels, on a newborn baby's skull are areas of fibrous membrane that have not yet fully ossified.

_____ 26. The epiphyseal plate can be seen in both external and cutaway views of an adult long bone.

_____ 27. The shaft of a long bone is known as the *articulation*.

_____ 28. Cartilage in the newborn becomes bone when it is replaced with calcified bone matrix deposited by osteoblasts.

_____ 29. When epiphyseal cartilage becomes bone, growth begins.

_____ 30. The epiphyseal cartilage is visible, if present, on x-ray films.

If you had difficulty with this section, review page 179.

DIVISIONS OF SKELETON

Circle the correct answer.

31. Which of the following is/are not a part of the axial skeleton?
    A. Scapula
    B. Cranial bones
    C. Vertebra
    D. Ribs
    E. Sternum

32. Which one of the following is not a cranial bone?
    A. Frontal
    B. Parietal
    C. Occipital
    D. Lacrimal
    E. Sphenoid

33. Which of the following is *not* correct?
    A. A baby is born with a straight spine
    B. In the adult, the sacral and thoracic curves are convex
    C. The normal curves of the adult spine provide greater strength than a straight spine
    D. A curved structure has more strength than a straight one of the same size and materials

34. True ribs:
    A. attach to the cartilage of other ribs
    B. do not attach to the sternum
    C. attach directly to the sternum without cartilage
    D. attach directly to the sternum by means of cartilage

35. The bone that runs along the lateral side of your forearm is the:
    A. humerus
    B. ulna
    C. radius
    D. tibia

36. The shinbone is also known as the:
    A. fibula
    B. femur
    C. tibia
    D. ulna

37. The bones in the palm of the hand are called:
    A. metatarsals
    B. tarsals
    C. carpals
    D. metacarpals

38. Which one of the following is *not* a bone of the upper extremity?
    A. Radius
    B. Clavicle
    C. Humerus
    D. Ilium

39. The heel bone is known as the:
    A. calcaneus
    B. talus
    C. metatarsal
    D. phalanges

40. The mastoid process is part of which bone?
    A. Parietal
    B. Temporal
    C. Occipital
    D. Frontal

41. When a baby learns to walk, which area of the spine becomes concave?
    A. Lumbar
    B. Thoracic
    C. Cervical
    D. Coccyx

42. Which bone is the "funny" bone?
    A. Radius
    B. Ulna
    C. Humerus
    D. Carpal

43. There are how many pairs of true ribs?
    A. 14
    B. 7
    C. 5
    D. 3

44. The 27 bones in the wrist and the hand allow for more:
    A. strength
    B. dexterity
    C. protection
    D. red blood cell products

45. The longest bone in the body is the:
    A. tibia
    B. fibula
    C. femur
    D. humerus

46. Distally, the _____ articulates with the patella.
    A. femur
    B. fibula
    C. tibia
    D. humerus

47. Which bones form the cheek bones?
    A. Mandible
    B. Palatine
    C. Maxillary
    D. Zygomatic

48. In a child, there are five of these bones. In an adult, they are fused into one.
    A. Pelvic
    B. Lumbar vertebrae
    C. Sacrum
    D. Carpals

49. The spinal cord enters the cranium through a large hole (foramen magnum) in which bone?
    A. Temporal
    B. Parietal
    C. Occipital
    D. Sphenoid

Circle the word in each word group that does not belong.

50. Cervical	Thoracic	Coxal	Coccyx
51. Pelvic girdle	Ankle	Wrist	Axial
52. Frontal	Occipital	Maxilla	Sphenoid
53. Scapula	Pectoral girdle	Ribs	Clavicle
54. Malleus	Vomer	Incus	Stapes
55. Ulna	Ilium	Ischium	Pubis
56. Carpal	Phalanges	Metacarpal	Ethmoid
57. Ethmoid	Parietal	Occipital	Nasal
58. Anvil	Atlas	Axis	Cervical

If you had difficulty with this section, review pages 180-195.

SKELETAL VARIATIONS

Identify each skeletal structure as being typically male or female.

A. Male   B. Female

_____ 59. Funnel-shaped pelvis

_____ 60. Broader-shaped pelvis

_____ 61. Wider pubic angle

_____ 62. Larger coxal bones

_____ 63. Wider pelvic inlet

If you had difficulty with this section, review page 195.

BONE MARKINGS

From the choices given, match each bone with its identification marking. Answer choices may be used more than once.

A. Mastoid	H. Glenoid cavity	O. Medial malleolus
B. Pterygoid process	I. Olecranon process	P. Calcaneus
C. Foramen magnum	J. Ischium	Q. Acromion process
D. Sella turcica	K. Acetabulum	R. Frontal sinuses
E. Mental foramen	L. Symphysis pubis	S. Condyloid process
F. Conchae	M. Ilium	T. Tibial tuberosity
G. Xiphoid process	N. Greater trochanter	

_____ 64. Occipital

_____ 65. Sternum

_____ 66. Coxal

_____ 67. Femur

_____ 68. Ulna

_____ 69. Temporal

_____ 70. Tarsals

_____ 71. Sphenoid

_____ 72. Ethmoid

_____ 73. Scapula

_____ 74. Tibia

_____ 75. Frontal

_____ 76. Mandible

If you had difficulty with this section, review pages 183-194.

JOINTS (ARTICULATIONS)

Circle the correct answer.

77. Freely movable joints are (*amphiarthroses* or *diarthroses*).

78. The sutures in the skull are (*synarthrotic* or *amphiarthrotic*) joints.

79. All (*diarthrotic* or *amphiarthrotic*) joints have a joint capsule, a joint cavity, and a layer of cartilage over the ends of the two joining bones.

80. (*Ligaments* or *Tendons*) grow out of periosteum and attach two bones together.

81. The (*articular cartilage* or *epiphyseal cartilage*) absorbs jolts.

82. Gliding joints are the (*least movable* or *most movable*) of the diarthrotic joints.

83. The knee is the (*largest* or *smallest*) joint.

84. Hinge joints allow motion in (*2* or *4*) directions.

85. The saddle joint at the base of each of our thumbs allows for greater (*strength* or *mobility*).

86. When you rotate your head, you are using a (*gliding* or *pivot*) joint.

If you had difficulty with this section, review pages 196-206.

SKELETAL DISORDERS

Fill in the blanks.

87. _____ is an imaging technique that allows a physician to examine the internal structure of a joint without the use of extensive surgery.

88. One of the most common skeletal tumors and one of the most rapidly fatal is _____.

89. _____ is the name of a common disorder in which bones lose minerals and become less dense.

90. A metabolic disorder involving mineral loss in bones due to a lack of vitamin D is _____.

91. A metabolic disorder that is often asymptomatic and affects older adults is _____

_____.

92. The general name for bacterial infections of bone and marrow tissue is _____.

93. Closed fractures, also known as _____ _____, do not pierce the skin.

94. _____ _____ are breaks that produce many fragments.

95. The most common noninflammatory joint disease is _____ or _____

_____ _____.

96. Three major types of arthritis are _____, _____, and

_____.

97. One form of infectious arthritis, _____ _____, was identified in 1975 in Connecticut and has since spread across the continent.

If you had difficulty with this section, review pages 200-208.

UNSCRAMBLE THE BONES

98. E T V E R R B A E

⬭ ☐ ☐ ⬭ ⬭ ☐ ☐ ☐

99. B P S U I

⬭ ☐ ⬭ ☐

100. S C A L U P A

☐ ⬭ ☐ ☐ ⬭ ☐ ☐

101. I M D B A L N E

☐ ☐ ☐ ⬭⬭ ☐ ☐ ⬭

102. A P N H G A E L S

☐ ☐ ⬭ ☐ ⬭ ☐ ☐ ☐

Take the circled letters, unscramble them, and fill in the solution.

What the fat lady wore to the ball.

103. ☐☐☐☐☐   ☐☐☐☐☐☐☐

APPLYING WHAT YOU KNOW

104. Mrs. Perine had advanced cancer of the bone. As the disease progressed, Mrs. Perine required several blood transfusions throughout the time she was receiving therapy. She asked the doctor one day to explain the necessity for the transfusions. What explanation might the doctor give to Mrs. Perine?

105. Dr. Kennedy, an orthopedic surgeon, called the admissions office of the hospital and advised that he would be admitting a patient in the next hour with an epiphyseal fracture. Without any other information, the office assigned the patient to the pediatric ward. What prompted this assignment?

106. Mrs. Van Skiver, age 75, noticed when she went in for her physical examination that she was a half inch shorter than she was on her last visit. Dr. Veazey suggested she begin a regimen of dietary supplements of calcium, vitamin D, and a prescription for sex hormone therapy. What bone disease did Dr. Veazey suspect?

107. Mr. Ferber was moving and experienced severe sharp pain in his lower back while lifting some boxes. The pain was not relieved by traditional home remedies or pain medication. He finally sought the advice of a physician after being unable to relieve the pain for 48 hours. What might be a possible diagnosis?

108. Word Find

Find and circle 13 terms presented in this chapter. Words may be spelled top to bottom, bottom to top, right to left, left to right, or diagonally.

Amphiarthroses   Lacunae

Articulation   Osteoblasts

Axial   Osteoclasts

Canaliculi   Periosteum

Compact   Sinus

Fontanels   Trabeculae

Hematopoiesis

```
S A N A R T I C U L A T I O N
I O M P L T C A P M O C E S C
M H E P T T A M A S A I A T P
O E L F H T A E P N I F L E T
S M L A S I E I A O O P U O S
S A M O I L A L O N I E C B T
E T S U N X I R T R A T E L S
S O B T E C A A T N A E B A A
R P I E U T N E U H O O A S L
S O T L C E S C T A R S R T C
U I I R L O A O O O A O T S O
N E T S H L T A I R I I S A E
I S T H E U O A M R C X S E T
S I S T A I E T C R E S I A S
L S C A S H S T O I O P T S O
```

DID YOU KNOW?

- The bones of the hands and feet make up more than half of the total 206 bones of the body.
- You are taller in the morning. Throughout the day the cartilage between your bones is compressed, making you about 1 cm shorter by the end of the day.
- The bones of the middle ear are mature at birth.

KNOW YOUR MEDICAL TERMS

Identify the term and match it with its meaning.

109. _____ Key/little   A. Herniate

110. _____ Basin   B. Clavicle

111. _____ Flank   C. Palpable

112. _____ Hip   D. Pelvis

113. _____ Rupture/act of   E. Suture

114. _____ Seam   F. Coxal

115. _____ Touch gently/capable of   G. Ilium

If you had difficulty with this section, review pages 209-211.

SKELETAL SYSTEM

Fill in the crossword puzzle.

ACROSS

7. Space inside cranial bone
9. Division of skeleton
10. Bone cell
11. Type of bone
12. Bone-absorbing cells
13. Freely movable joints

DOWN

1. Spaces in bones where osteocytes are found
2. Joint
3. Suture joints
4. Ends of long bones
5. Covers long bone except at its joint surfaces
6. Process of blood cell formation
8. Chest

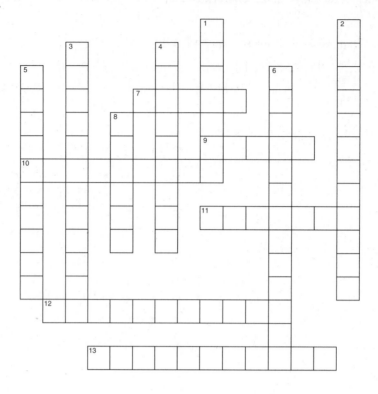

CHECK YOUR KNOWLEDGE

Multiple Choice

Circle the correct answer.

1. Which of the following statements concerning the ribs is true?
   A. The first seven pairs attach to the sternum by cartilage
   B. The last four pairs are called *floating ribs* because they are free in the front
   C. The eighth, ninth, and tenth pairs do not move because they are not attached to the sternum
   D. All of the above statements concerning the ribs are true

2. Which is the longest bone in the body?
   A. Humerus
   B. Ulna
   C. Femur
   D. Radius

3. Of what is yellow bone marrow primarily made?
   A. Fatty tissue
   B. Blood cells
   C. Epithelial tissue
   D. Fibrous tissue

4. Which of the following statements regarding the female pelvis is *not* true?
   A. Its shape can be described as more broad, shallow, and basinlike when compared with that of the male
   B. Its pelvic inlet, or brim, is usually wider than that of the male
   C. Its individual hipbones are usually larger and heavier than those of the male
   D. All of the above statements are true

5. Which of the following statements is/are true about the normal curves of the spine (two concave and two convex)?
   A. They are present at birth
   B. They extend from the skull to the bottom of the ribcage
   C. They give the spine strength to support the weight of the rest of the body
   D. All of the above are true

6. Which of the following statements regarding diarthrotic joints is *not* true?
   A. They contain a synovial membrane that secretes a lubricating fluid called *synovial fluid*
   B. Diarthrotic joints may permit flexion, extension, abduction, adduction, or rotation
   C. These joints make up the largest category of body joints
   D. All of the above statements are true

7. Which of the following bones are components of the axial skeletal system?
   A. Ilium, ethmoid, clavicle
   B. Ulna, palatine, occipital
   C. Sacrum, parietal, zygomatic
   D. Scapula, patella, fibula

8. Which of the following bones is not classified as a cranial bone?
   A. Sphenoid
   B. Parietal
   C. Palatine
   D. Temporal

9. Which of the following statements characterizes the skeleton of a growing child?
   A. Epiphyses are separated from diaphyses by a layer of cartilage
   B. Osteoblasts deposit calcium in the gel-like matrix of cartilage
   C. The periosteum is present
   D. All of the above statements characterize the skeleton of a growing child

10. What are the joints between the cranial bones called?
    A. Synarthroses
    B. Diarthroses
    C. Amphiarthroses
    D. All of the above

Matching

Match each term in column A with its corresponding description in column B. (Only one answer is correct for each.)

Column A

_____ 11. Diarthroses

_____ 12. Spongy bone

_____ 13. Synarthrosis

_____ 14. Foramen magnum

_____ 15. Calcaneus

_____ 16. Chondrocyte

_____ 17. Compact bone

_____ 18. Ethmoid

_____ 19. Coxal

_____ 20. Hematopoiesis

_____ 21. Diploe

Column B

A. Central canal

B. Trabeculae

C. Perpendicular plate

D. Flat bone

E. Tarsal

F. Ilium

G. Synovial fluid

H. Cartilage

I. Suture

J. Occipital bone

K. Red bone marrow

Fill in the Blanks

22. The "growth plate" is the _____ _____.

23. The four pairs of sinuses are the _____, _____, _____, and _____.

24. The bone that does not form a joint with any other bone is the _____.

25. An abnormal side-to-side curvature of the spine is _____.

LONGITUDINAL SECTION OF LONG BONE

1. _____

2. _____

3. _____

4. _____

5. _____

6. _____

7. _____

8. _____

9. _____

10. _____

11. _____

12. _____

ANTERIOR VIEW OF SKELETON

1. _____

2. _____

3. _____

4. _____

5. _____

6. _____

7. _____

8. _____

9. _____

10. _____

11. _____

12. _____

13. _____

14. _____

15. _____

16. _____

17. _____

18. _____

19. _____

20. _____

21. _____

22. _____

23. _____

24. _____

25. _____

26. _____

27. _____

28. _____

29. _____

30. _____

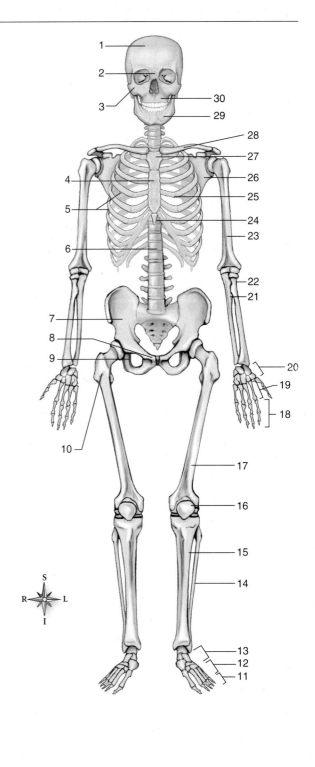

1. _____
2. _____
3. _____
4. _____
5. _____
6. _____
7. _____
8. _____
9. _____
10. _____
11. _____
12. _____
13. _____
14. _____
15. _____
16. _____
17. _____
18. _____
19. _____
20. _____
21. _____
22. _____
23. _____
24. _____
25. _____
26. _____
27. _____

1. _____

2. _____

3. _____

4. _____

5. _____

6. _____

7. _____

8. _____

9. _____

10. _____

11. _____

12. _____

13. _____

14. _____

15. _____

Chapter **8   Skeletal System**

1. _____

2. _____

3. _____

4. _____

5. _____

6. _____

7. _____

8. _____

9. _____

10. _____

11. _____

STRUCTURE OF A DIARTHROTIC JOINT

1. _____

2. _____

3. _____

4. _____

5. _____

6. _____

7. _____

8. _____

9. _____

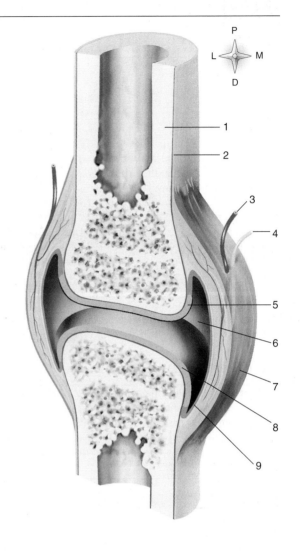

9 Muscular System

The muscular system is often referred to as the "power system," and rightfully so, because it is this system that provides the force necessary to move the body and perform many organ functions. Just as an automobile relies on the engine to provide motion, the body depends on the muscular system to perform both voluntary and involuntary movements. Walking, breathing, and the digestion of food are but a few examples of body functions that require the healthy performance of the muscular system.

Although this system has several functions, the primary purpose is to provide movement or power. Muscles produce power by contracting. The ability of a large muscle or muscle group to contract depends on the ability of microscopic muscle fibers to contract within the larger muscle. An understanding of these microscopic muscle fibers will assist you as you progress in your study to the larger muscles and muscle groups.

Muscle contractions may be one of several types: isotonic, isometric, twitch, or tetanic. When skeletal or voluntary muscles contract, they provide us with a variety of motions. Flexion, extension, abduction, adduction, and rotation are examples of these movements that provide us with both strength and agility.

Muscles are also used to keep the body healthy and in good condition. Scientific evidence keeps pointing to the fact that the proper use and exercise of muscles may prolong longevity. An understanding of the structure and function of the muscular system may, therefore, add quality and quantity to our lives.

TOPICS FOR REVIEW

Before progressing to Chapter 10, you should familiarize yourself with the structure and function of the three major types of muscle tissue. Your review should include the microscopic structure of skeletal muscle tissue, how a muscle is stimulated, the major types of skeletal muscle contractions, and the skeletal muscle groups. Your study should conclude with an understanding of the types of movements produced by skeletal muscle contractions and the major muscular disorders.

MUSCLE TISSUE

Match each descriptive word or phrase to its related muscle type and write the corresponding letter(s) in the answer blank.

A. Skeletal muscle   B. Cardiac muscle   C. Smooth muscle

_____ 1. Striated

_____ 2. Cells branch frequently

_____ 3. Moves food into the stomach

_____ 4. Nonstriated

_____ 5. Voluntary

_____ 6. Intercalated disks

_____ 7. Involuntary

_____ 8. Attaches to bone

_____ 9. Hollow internal organs

_____ 10. Visceral muscle

If you had difficulty with this section, review page 220.

STRUCTURE OF SKELETAL MUSCLES

Match each term on the left with its corresponding description on the right.

_____ 11. Origin   A. The muscle unit excluding the ends

_____ 12. Insertion   B. Attachment to the more movable bone

_____ 13. Body   C. Fluid-filled sacs

_____ 14. Tendons   D. Attachment to more stationary bone

_____ 15. Bursae   E. Anchor muscles to bones

MICROSCOPIC STRUCTURE

Match each term on the left with its corresponding description on the right.

_____ 16. Muscle fibers   A. Protein that forms thick myofilaments

_____ 17. Actin   B. Basic functional unit of skeletal muscle

_____ 18. Sarcomere   C. Protein that forms thin myofilaments

_____ 19. Myosin   D. Microscopic threadlike structures found in skeletal muscle fibers

_____ 20. Myofilaments   E. Elongated contractile cells of muscle tissue

If you had difficulty with this section, review pages 220-221.

FUNCTIONS OF SKELETAL MUSCLE

Fill in the blanks.

21. Muscles move bones by _____ on them.

22. As a rule, only the _____ bone moves.

23. The _____ bone moves toward the _____ bone.

24. Of all the muscles contracting simultaneously, the one mainly responsible for producing a particular movement is called the _____ _____ for that movement.

25. As prime movers contract, other muscles called _____ relax.

26. The biceps brachii is the prime mover during flexing, and the brachialis is its helper or _____ muscle.

27. We are able to maintain our body position because of a specialized type of skeletal muscle contraction called _____ _____ .

28. _____ _____ maintains body posture by counteracting the pull of gravity.

29. A decrease in temperature, a condition known as _____, will drastically affect cellular activity and normal body function.

30. Energy required to produce a muscle contraction is obtained from _____.

If you had difficulty with this section, review pages 223-224.

FATIGUE

INTEGRATION WITH OTHER BODY SYSTEMS

MOTOR UNIT

MUSCLE STIMULUS

If the statement is true, write "T" in the answer blank. If the statement is false, correct the statement by circling the incorrect term and writing the correct term in the answer blank.

_____ 31. The point of contact between the nerve ending and the muscle fiber is called a *motor neuron*.

_____ 32. A motor neuron together with the cells it innervates is called a *motor unit*.

_____ 33. If muscle cells are stimulated repeatedly without adequate periods of rest, the strength of the muscle contraction will decrease, resulting in fatigue.

_____ 34. The depletion of oxygen in muscle cells during vigorous and prolonged exercise is known as *fatigue*.

_____ 35. The type of neurotransmitter operating in each neuromuscular junction (NMJ) is called acetylcholine.

_____ 36. When oxygen supplies run low, muscle cells produce ATP and other waste products during contraction.

_____ 37. In a laboratory setting, a single muscle fiber can be isolated and subjected to stimuli of varying intensities so that it can be studied.

_____ 38. The minimal level of stimulation required to cause a fiber to contract is called the *threshold stimulus*.

_____ 39. Most smooth muscles bring about movements by pulling on bones across movable joints.

_____ 40. A nervous system disorder that shuts off impulses to certain skeletal muscles may result in paralysis.

TYPES OF SKELETAL MUSCLE CONTRACTION

Circle the correct answer.

41. When a muscle contracts and no movement results, the contraction is:
    A. isometric
    B. isotonic
    C. twitch
    D. tetanic

42. Walking is an example of which type of contraction?
    A. Isometric
    B. Isotonic
    C. Twitch
    D. Tetanic

43. Pushing against a wall is an example of which type of contraction?
    A. Isotonic
    B. Isometric
    C. Twitch
    D. Tetanic

44. Endurance training is also known as:
    A. isometrics
    B. hypertrophy
    C. aerobic training
    D. strength training

45. Benefits of regular exercise include all of the following *except*:
    A. improved lung functioning
    B. more efficient heart
    C. less fatigue
    D. atrophy

46. Twitch contractions easily can be seen:
    A. in isolated muscles prepared for research
    B. in a great deal of normal muscle activity
    C. during resting periods
    D. none of the above

47. Individual contractions "melt" together to produce a sustained contraction or:
    A. twitch
    B. tetanus
    C. isotonic response
    D. isometric response

48. In most cases, isotonic contraction of muscle produces movement at a/an:
    A. insertion
    B. beginning
    C. joint
    D. bursa

49. Prolonged inactivity causes muscles to shrink in mass, a condition called:
    A. hypertrophy
    B. disuse atrophy
    C. paralysis
    D. muscle fatigue

50. Muscle hypertrophy can be best enhanced by a program of:
    A. isotonic exercise
    B. better posture
    C. high-protein diet
    D. strength training

If you had difficulty with this section, review pages 224-228.

SKELETAL MUSCLE GROUPS

Match the function(s) to the muscles listed below and write the corresponding letter(s) in the answer blank. Multiple answers may apply.

A. Flexor
B. Extensor
C. Abductor
D. Adductor
E. Rotator
F. Dorsiflexor or plantar flexor

_____ 51. Deltoid

_____ 52. Tibialis anterior

_____ 53. Gastrocnemius

_____ 54. Biceps brachii

_____ 55. Gluteus medius

_____ 56. Soleus

_____ 57. Iliopsoas

_____ 58. Pectoralis major

_____ 59. Gluteus maximus

_____ 60. Triceps brachii

_____ 61. Sternocleidomastoid

_____ 62. Trapezius

_____ 63. Gracilis

If you had difficulty with this section, review pages 229-234.

MOVEMENTS PRODUCED BY MUSCLES

Circle the correct answer.

64. A movement that makes the angle between two bones smaller is:
    A. flexion
    B. extension
    C. abduction
    D. adduction

65. Moving a part toward the midline is:
    A. flexion
    B. extension
    C. abduction
    D. adduction

66. Moving a part away from the midline is:
    A. flexion
    B. extension
    C. abduction
    D. adduction

67. When you move your head from side to side as in shaking your head "no," you are _____ a muscle group.
    A. rotating
    B. pronating
    C. supinating
    D. abducting

68. _____ occurs when you turn the palm of your hand from an anterior to posterior position.
    A. Dorsiflexion
    B. Plantar flexion
    C. Supination
    D. Pronation

69. *Dorsiflexion* refers to:
    A. hand movements
    B. eye movements
    C. foot movements
    D. head movements

If you had difficulty with this section, review pages 228-229.

MUSCULAR DISORDERS

Circle the correct answer.

70. Muscle strains are characterized by (*myalgia* or *fibromyositis*).

71. Crush injuries can cause (*hemoglobin* or *myoglobin*) to accumulate in the blood and result in kidney failure.

72. A viral infection of the nerves that control skeletal muscle movement is known as (*poliomyelitis* or *muscular dystrophy*).

73. (*Muscular dystrophy* or *Myasthenia gravis*) is a group of genetic diseases characterized by atrophy of skeletal muscle tissues.

74. (*Muscular dystrophy* or *Myasthenia gravis*) is an autoimmune disease in which the immune system attacks muscle cells at the neuromuscular junction.

If you had difficulty with this section, review pages 235-237.

75. Casey noticed pain whenever she reached for anything in her cupboards. Her doctor told her that the small fluid-filled sacs in her shoulder were inflamed. What condition did Casey have?

76. The nurse was preparing an injection for Mrs. Tatakis. The amount to be given was 2 mL. What area of the body will the nurse most likely select for administering this injection?

77. Chris was playing football and pulled a band of fibrous connective tissue that attached a muscle to a bone. What is the common term for this tissue?

78. **Word Find**

Find and circle 25 muscle terms. Words may be spelled top to bottom, bottom to top, right to left, left to right, or diagonally.

```
G A S T R O C N E M I U S D U
M S G I O N O I S N E T X E U
U R N N T O M S R B S F D T T
S U I S C I B O N T P N E A R
C B R E U X V T O O E C L I A
L Q T R D E C O D A C M T R P
E T S T B L M N N V I E O T E
X F M I A F Y I E Y B N I S Z
S I A O V I E C T L S S D I I
S Y H N S S R O T A T O R G U
U A M G A R H P A I D J N R S
E H A T R O P H Y L N J T E B
L N O H T D E U G I T A F N T
O R I G I N O S N V S B Z Y L
S B V T O J C T R I C E P S S
```

Abductor	Flexion	Soleus
Atrophy	Gastrocnemius	Striated
Biceps	Hamstrings	Synergist
Bursa	Insertion	Tendon
Deltoid	Isometric	Tenosynovitis
Diaphragm	Isotonic	Trapezius
Dorsiflexion	Muscle	Triceps
Extension	Origin	
Fatigue	Rotator	

KNOW YOUR MEDICAL TERMS

Fill in the blanks.

79. mus _____   cle _____

80. myo _____   fila _____   ment _____

81. gastro _____   cnemius _____

82. pector _____   alis _____   major _____

83. posture _____

84. rigor _____   mortis _____

85. syn _____   erg _____   ist _____

If you had difficulty with this section, review pages 238-239.

DID YOU KNOW?

- If all of your muscles pulled in one direction, you would have the power to move 25 tons.
- When you take a step, you are using up to 200 muscles. Walking uses a great deal of muscle power and is good exercise.
- Compared to its size, the tongue is the strongest muscle in your body.
- Jaw muscles can provide about 200 pounds of force to bring the back teeth together for chewing.

UNSCRAMBLE THE WORDS

86. **N F O X L I E**

⬜⬜⬜Ⓞ⬜⬜⬜

87. **T N I C A**

⬜Ⓞ⬜Ⓞ⬜

88. **V R S N E I O E**

⬜⬜⬜⬜Ⓞ⬜⬜Ⓞ

89. **I O R N I G**

Ⓞ⬜⬜⬜Ⓞ⬜

90. **S E A R R E C M O**

⬜⬜⬜⬜⬜⬜Ⓞ⬜Ⓞ⬜

What Kevin requested for his IOU.

91.

⬜⬜⬜⬜⬜⬜⬜⬜⬜⬜

Fill in the crossword puzzle.

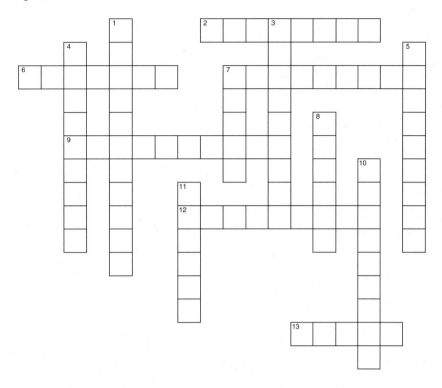

ACROSS

2. Shaking your head "no"
6. Muscle shrinkage
7. Toward the body's midline
9. Produces movement opposite to prime movers
12. Movement that makes joint angles larger
13. Small fluid-filled sac between tendons and bones

DOWN

1. Increase in size
3. Away from the body's midline
4. Turning your palm from an anterior to posterior position
5. Attachment to the more movable bone
7. Protein which composes myofilaments
8. Attachment to the more stationary bone
10. Assists prime movers with movement
11. Anchors muscles to bones

Multiple Choice

Circle the correct answer.

1. Which of the following statements about a motor unit is true?
   A. It consists of a muscle cell group and a motor neuron
   B. The point of contact between the nerve ending and the muscle fiber is called the *neuromuscular junction*
   C. Chemicals generate events within the muscle cell that result in contraction of the muscle cell
   D. All of the above are true

2. What is movement of a part away from the midline of the body called?
   A. Abduction
   B. Adduction
   C. Pronation
   D. Plantar flexion

3. According to the sliding filament theory of muscle contraction:
   A. muscle fibers contain thin myofilaments made of a protein called *myosin*
   B. muscle fibers contain thick myofilaments made up of a protein called *actin*
   C. thin and thick myofilaments move toward each other to cause muscle contraction
   D. all of the above are true

4. Which of the following statements is true of the hamstring group of muscles?
   A. It includes the rectus femoris
   B. It flexes the knee
   C. It originates on the pubis
   D. All of the above are true

5. Muscles that help other muscles in producing movement are called:
   A. prime movers
   B. synergists
   C. antagonists
   D. bursae

6. Which of the following statements about oxygen debt is true?
   A. It is caused when excess oxygen is present in the environment
   B. It causes lactic acid buildup and soreness in muscles
   C. It can be replaced by slow, shallow breathing
   D. All of the above are true

7. What is a quick, jerky response of a given muscle to a single stimulus called?
   A. Isometric
   B. Lockjaw
   C. Tetanus
   D. Twitch

8. Which of the following statements about muscle atrophy is true?
   A. It decreases the size of a muscle
   B. It increases the size of a muscle
   C. It has no effect on muscle size
   D. None of the above is true

9. Which of the following occurs during isometric exercises?
   A. Muscle length remains the same
   B. Muscle tension remains the same
   C. Muscle length shortens
   D. None of the above occurs

10. Which of the following statements about skeletal muscle contraction is true?
    A. Its attachment to the more stationary bone is called its *origin*
    B. Its attachment to the more movable bone is called its *insertion*
    C. Both A and B are true
    D. None of the above is true

True or False

If the statement is true, write "T" on the answer blank. If the statement is false, correct the statement by circling the incorrect term and writing the correct term in the answer blank.

_____ 11. When a part is moved toward the midline, it is called *adduction*.

_____ 12. In most cases, isotonic contraction of a muscle produces movement at a joint.

_____ 13. Dorsiflexion occurs when you turn the palm of your hand from an anterior to a posterior position.

_____ 14. Exercise may cause an increase in muscle size called *atrophy*.

_____ 15. Isotonic contraction is an example of a contraction used while walking.

_____ 16. If a muscle is overworked without sufficient rest, the result will be a decrease in muscle strength and fatigue.

_____ 17. A bone of insertion moves toward the bone of origin.

_____ 18. A condition in which the body temperature is drastically low is referred to as *hyperthermia*.

_____ 19. Tetanic contraction is caused by a series of rapid stimuli.

_____ 20. When the angle between two bones becomes smaller, it is called *extension*.

Fill in the Blanks

21. To supplement the oxygen carried to muscle fibers by the hemoglobin in the blood, muscle fibers contain

_____.

22. Tension during muscle lengthening is often called _____

_____.

23. Muscle cells are stimulated by a nerve fiber called a _____

_____.

24. _____ turns the ankle so that the bottom of the foot faces toward the midline of the body.

25. The _____ _____ is on the posterior or back surface of the arm.

1. _____

2. _____

3. _____

4. _____

5. _____

6. _____

7. _____

8. _____

9. _____

10. _____

11. _____

12. _____

13. _____

14. _____

15. _____

16. _____

17. _____

18. _____

Pectineus
Adductor longus
Gracilis
14

Vastus lateralis
Rectus femoris
Vastus medialis
7

MUSCLES—POSTERIOR VIEW

1. _____

2. _____

3. _____

4. _____

5. _____

6. _____

7. _____

8. _____

9. _____

10. _____

11. _____

12. _____

13. _____

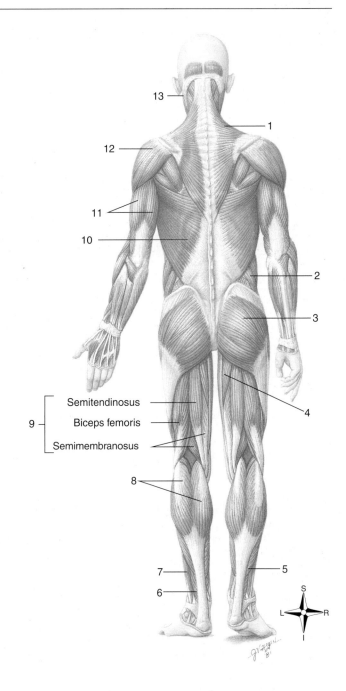

9 — Semitendinosus
    Biceps femoris
    Semimembranosus

10 Nervous System

The nervous system organizes and coordinates the millions of impulses received each day to make communication with and enjoyment of our environment possible. The functioning unit of the nervous system is the neuron. Three types of neurons exist—sensory, motor, and interneurons—which are classified according to the direction in which they transmit impulses. Nerve impulses travel over routes made up of neurons and provide the rapid communication necessary for maintaining life. The central nervous system is made up of the spinal cord and brain. The spinal cord provides access to and from the brain by means of ascending and descending tracts. In addition, the spinal cord functions as the primary reflex center of the body. The brain consists of the brainstem, cerebellum, diencephalon, and cerebrum. These areas provide the extraordinary network necessary to receive, interpret, and respond to the simplest or most complex impulses.

While you concentrate on this chapter, your body is performing a multitude of functions. Fortunately for us, the beating of the heart, the digestion of food, breathing, and most of our other day-to-day processes do not require our supervision or thought. They function automatically, and the division of the nervous system that regulates these functions is known as the *autonomic nervous system*. The autonomic nervous system consists of two divisions called the *sympathetic system* and the *parasympathetic system*. The sympathetic system functions as an emergency system and prepares us for "fight or flight." The parasympathetic system dominates control of many visceral effectors under normal everyday conditions. Together, these two divisions regulate the body's automatic functions in an effort to assist with the maintenance of homeostasis. Your understanding of this chapter will help you comprehend the complex functions of the nervous system and the "automatic pilot" of your body—the autonomic system.

TOPICS FOR REVIEW

Before progressing to Chapter 11, you should review the organs and divisions of the nervous system, the structure and function of the major types of cells in this system, the structure and function of a reflex arc, and the transmission of nerve impulses. Your study should include the anatomy and physiology of the brain and spinal cord and the nerves that extend from these two areas. Finally, an understanding of the autonomic nervous system, the specific functions of the subdivisions of this system, and the major disorders of the nervous system are necessary to complete the review of this chapter.

ORGANS AND DIVISIONS OF THE NERVOUS SYSTEM

CELLS OF THE NERVOUS SYSTEM

NERVES

Match each term on the left with the most appropriate description on the right.

Group A

_____ 1. Sense organ

_____ 2. Central nervous system

_____ 3. Peripheral nervous system

_____ 4. Autonomic nervous system

A. Subdivision of peripheral nervous system

B. Ear

C. Brain and spinal cord

D. Nerves that extend to the outlying parts of the body

Group B

_____ 5. Dendrite

_____ 6. Schwann cell

_____ 7. Motor neuron

_____ 8. Nodes of Ranvier

_____ 9. Fascicles

_____ 10. Epineurium

A. Indentations between adjacent Schwann cells

B. Branching projection of neuron

C. Also known as *efferent*

D. Forms myelin outside the CNS

E. Tough sheath that covers the whole nerve

F. Groups of wrapped axons

96

CELLS OF THE NERVOUS SYSTEM

NERVES AND TRACTS

Match each of the following words or phrases to its corresponding nervous system structure. Write the correct letter in the answer blank.

A. Neurons   B Neuroglia

_____ 11. Axon

_____ 12. Supporting cells

_____ 13. Astrocytes

_____ 14. Sensory

_____ 15. Conduct impulses

_____ 16. Form the myelin sheath around central nerve fibers

_____ 17. Phagocytosis

_____ 18. Efferent

_____ 19. Multiple sclerosis

_____ 20. Neurilemma

If you had difficulty with this section, review pages 249-252.

NERVE SIGNALS

REFLEX ARCS

Fill in the blanks.

21. The simplest kind of reflex arc is a _____ _____

_____.

22. Three-neuron arcs consist of all three kinds of neurons, _____,

_____, and _____.

23. Impulse conduction in a reflex arc normally starts in _____.

24. A _____ is the microscopic space that separates the axon of one neuron from the dendrites of another neuron.

25. A _____ is the response to impulse conduction over reflex arcs.

26. Contraction of a muscle that causes it to pull away from an irritating stimulus is known as the _____

_____.

27. A _____ is a group of nerve-cell bodies located in the peripheral nervous system.

28. All _____ lie entirely within the gray matter of the central nervous system.

29. In a patellar reflex, the nerve impulses that reach the quadriceps muscle (the effector) result in the classic _____ _____ response.

30. _____ _____ forms the H-shaped inner core of the spinal cord.

If you had difficulty with this section, review pages 253-254.

NERVE IMPULSES

THE SYNAPSE

Circle the correct answer.

31. Nerve impulses (*do* or *do not*) continually race along every nerve cell's surface.

32. When a stimulus acts on a neuron, it (*increases* or *decreases*) the permeability of the stimulated point of its membrane to sodium ions.

33. An inward movement of positive ions leaves a/an (*lack* or *excess*) of negative ions outside.

34. The plasma membrane of the (*presynaptic* or *postsynaptic*) neuron makes up a portion of the synapse.

35. A synaptic knob is a tiny bulge at the end of the (*presynaptic* or *postsynaptic*) neuron's axon.

36. Acetylcholine is an example of a (*neurotransmitter* or *protein molecule receptor*).

37. Neurotransmitters are chemicals that allow neurons to (*communicate* or *reproduce*) with one another.

38. Neurotransmitters are distributed (*randomly* or *specifically*) into groups of neurons.

39. Catecholamines may play a role in (*sleep* or *reproduction*).

40. Endorphins and enkephalins are neurotransmitters that inhibit conduction of (*fear* or *pain*) impulses.

If you had difficulty with this section, review pages 255-258.

CENTRAL NERVOUS SYSTEM

DIVISIONS OF THE BRAIN

Circle the correct answer.

41. The portion of the brainstem that joins the spinal cord to the brain is the:
    A. pons
    B. cerebellum
    C. diencephalon
    D. hypothalamus
    E. medulla

42. Which one of the following is *not* a function of the brainstem?
    A. Conducts sensory impulses from the spinal cord to the higher centers of the brain
    B. Conducts motor impulses from the cerebrum to the spinal cord
    C. Controls heart beat, respiration, and blood vessel diameter
    D. Contains centers for speech and memory

43. Which one of the following is *not* part of the diencephalon?
    A. Cerebrum
    B. Thalamus
    C. Pituitary gland
    D. Third-ventricle gray matter

44. ADH is produced by the:
    A. pituitary gland
    B. medulla
    C. mammillary bodies
    D. third ventricle
    E. hypothalamus

45. Which one of the following is *not* a function of the hypothalamus?
    A. It helps control the heart rate
    B. It helps control the constriction and dilation of blood vessels
    C. It helps control the contraction of the stomach and intestines
    D. It produces hormones that control the release of certain anterior pituitary hormones
    E. All of the above are functions of the hypothalamus

46. Which one of the following parts of the brain helps in the association of sensations with emotions, as well as aiding in the arousal or alerting mechanism?
    A. Pons
    B. Hypothalamus
    C. Cerebellum
    D. Thalamus
    E. None of the above is correct

47. Which of the following is *not* true of the cerebrum?
    A. Its lobes correspond to the bones that lie over them
    B. Its grooves are called *gyri*
    C. Most of its gray matter lies on the surface of the cerebrum
    D. Its outer region is called the cerebral cortex
    E. Its two hemispheres are connected by a structure called the *corpus callosum*

48. Which one of the following is *not* a function of the cerebrum?
    A. Willed movement
    B. Consciousness
    C. Memory
    D. Conscious awareness of sensations
    E. All of the above are functions of the cerebrum

49. The area of the cerebrum responsible for the perception of sound lies in the _____ lobe.
    A. frontal
    B. temporal
    C. occipital
    D. parietal

50. Visual perception is located in the _____ lobe.
    A. frontal
    B. temporal
    C. parietal
    D. occipital
    E. none of the above

51. Which one of the following is *not* a function of the cerebellum?
    A. Maintains equilibrium
    B. Helps produce smooth, coordinated movements
    C. Helps maintain normal postures
    D. Associates sensations with emotions

52. Within the interior of the cerebrum are a few islands of gray matter known as:
    A. fissures
    B. basal ganglia
    C. gyri
    D. myelin

53. A cerebrovascular accident is commonly referred to as (a):
    A. stroke
    B. Parkinson disease
    C. tumor
    D. multiple sclerosis

54. Parkinson disease is a disease of the:
    A. myelin
    B. axons
    C. neuroglia
    D. basal nuclei

55. The largest section of the brain is the:
    A. cerebellum
    B. pons
    C. cerebrum
    D. midbrain

If you had difficulty with this section, review pages 260-264.

BRAIN DISORDERS

Match each numbered description to the most appropriate term and write the corresponding letter in the answer blank.

A. Chronic traumatic encephalopathy (CTE)
B. Epilepsy
C. Concussion
D. Hemiplegia

E. Cerebral palsy
F. EEG
G. Huntington disease
H. CVA

I. Dementia
J. Paraplegia

_____ 56. Stroke

_____ 57. Paralysis of one side of the body

_____ 58. A crippling disease that involves permanent, nonprogressive damage to motor control areas of the brain

_____ 59. A type of traumatic brain injury

_____ 60. Paralysis of both legs

_____ 61. Accumulation of abnormal proteins in the brain with memory loss

_____ 62. Recurring or chronic seizure episodes

Copyright © 2018, Elsevier Inc. All rights reserved.

Chapter 10 Nervous System

_____ 63. Measurement of electrical activity of the brain

_____ 64. Characteristic of Alzheimer disease

_____ 65. Inherited disease characterized by chorea

If you had difficulty with this section, review pages 264-266.

SPINAL CORD

If the statement is true, write "T" in the answer blank. If the statement is false, correct the statement by circling the incorrect term and writing the correct term in the answer blank.

_____ 66. The spinal cord is approximately 24 to 25 inches long.

_____ 67. The spinal cord ends at the bottom of the sacrum.

_____ 68. The extension of the meninges beyond the cord is convenient for performing CAT scans without danger of injuring the spinal cord.

_____ 69. Bundles of myelinated nerve fibers—dendrites—make up the white outer columns of the spinal cord.

_____ 70. Ascending tracts conduct impulses up the cord to the brain, and descending tracts conduct impulses down the cord from the brain.

_____ 71. Tracts are functional organizations in that all of the axons that compose a tract serve several functions.

_____ 72. A loss of sensation caused by a spinal cord injury is called *paralysis*.

If you had difficulty with this section, review pages 266-272.

COVERINGS AND FLUID SPACES OF THE BRAIN AND SPINAL CORD

Circle the word in each word group that does not belong.

73. Meninges	Pia mater	Ventricles	Dura mater
74. Arachnoid	Middle layer	CSF	Cobweblike
75. CSF	Ventricles	Subarachnoid space	Pia mater
76. Tough	Outer layer	Dura mater	Choroid plexus
77. Brain tumor	Subarachnoid space	CSF	Fourth lumbar vertebra

CRANIAL NERVES

78. Fill in the missing areas on the chart below.

Nerve		Conduct Impulses	Function
I		From nose to brain	Sense of smell
II	Optic	From eye to brain	
III	Oculomotor		Eye movements
IV		From brain to external eye muscles	Eye movements
V	Trigeminal	From skin and mucous membrane of head and from teeth to brain; also from brain to chewing muscles	
VI	Abducens		Eye movements
VII	Facial	From taste buds of tongue to brain; from brain to face muscles	
VIII		From ear to brain	Hearing; sense of balance
IX	Glossopharyngeal		Sensations of throat, taste, swallowing movements, secretion of saliva
X		From throat, larynx, and organs in thoracic and abdominal cavities to brain; also from brain to muscles of throat and abdominal cavities	Sensations of throat, larynx, and thoracic and abdominal organs; swallowing, voice production, slowing of heart beat, acceleration of peristalsis (gut movements)
XI	Accessory	From brain to certain shoulder and neck muscles	
XII		From brain to muscles of tongue	Tongue movements

If you had difficulty with this section, review pages 268-271.

CRANIAL NERVES

SPINAL NERVES

Match each of the numbered words with cranial or spinal nerves as appropriate and write the corresponding letter in the answer blank.

A. Cranial nerves   B. Spinal nerves

_____ 79. 12 pairs

_____ 80. Dermatome

_____ 81. Vagus

_____ 82. Shingles

_____ 83. 31 pairs

_____ 84. Optic

_____ 85. C1

_____ 86. Plexus

If you had difficulty with this section, review pages 267-273.

AUTONOMIC NERVOUS SYSTEM

Match each term on the left with the appropriate description on the right.

_____ 87. Autonomic nervous system   A. Divisions of ANS

_____ 88. Autonomic neurons   B. Tissues to which autonomic neurons conduct impulses

_____ 89. Preganglionic neurons   C. Voluntary actions

_____ 90. Visceral effectors   D. Regulates body's involuntary functions

_____ 91. Sympathetic division   E. Motor neurons that make up the ANS

_____ 92. Somatic nervous system   F. Conduct impulses between the spinal cord and a ganglion

SYMPATHETIC NERVOUS DIVISION

PARASYMPATHETIC NERVOUS DIVISION

Circle the correct answer.

93. Dendrites and cell bodies of sympathetic pregangli-onic neurons are located in the:
    A. brainstem and sacral portion of the spinal cord
    B. sympathetic ganglia
    C. gray matter of the thoracic and upper lumbar segments of the spinal cord
    D. ganglia close to effectors

94. Which of the following is *not* correct?
    A. Sympathetic preganglionic neurons have their cell bodies located in the lateral gray column of certain parts of the spinal cord
    B. Sympathetic preganglionic axons pass along the dorsal root of certain spinal nerves
    C. There are synapses within sympathetic ganglia
    D. Sympathetic responses are usually widespread, involving many organs

95. Another name for the parasympathetic nervous division is:
    A. thoracolumbar
    B. craniosacral
    C. visceral
    D. ANS
    E. cholinergic

96. Which statement is *not* correct?
    A. Sympathetic postganglionic neurons have their dendrites and cell bodies in sympathetic ganglia or collateral ganglia
    B. Sympathetic ganglia are located in front of and at each side of the spinal column
    C. Separate autonomic nerves distribute many sympathetic postganglionic axons to various internal organs
    D. Very few sympathetic preganglionic axons synapse with postganglionic neurons

97. Sympathetic stimulation usually results in a/an:
    A. response by numerous organs
    B. response by only one organ
    C. increase in peristalsis
    D. constriction of pupils

98. Parasympathetic stimulation frequently results in a/an:
    A. response by only one organ
    B. response by numerous organs
    C. fight-or-flight syndrome
    D. increase in heart beat

Match each numbered description to its related nervous control system and write the corresponding letter in the answer blank.

A. Sympathetic control   B. Parasympathetic control

_____ 99. Constricts pupils

_____ 100. "Goose pimples"

_____ 101. Increases sweat secretion

_____ 102. Increases secretion of digestive juices

_____ 103. Constricts blood vessels

_____ 104. Slows heart beat

102

_____ 105. Relaxes bladder

_____ 106. Increases epinephrine secretion

_____ 107. Increases peristalsis

_____ 108. Stimulates lens for near vision

If you had difficulty with this section, review pages 275-277.

AUTONOMIC NEUROTRANSMITTERS

AUTONOMIC NERVOUS SYSTEM AS A WHOLE

Fill in the blanks.

109. Sympathetic preganglionic axons release the neurotransmitter _____.

110. Axons that release norepinephrine are classified as _____

_____.

111. Axons that release acetylcholine are classified as _____

_____.

112. The function of the autonomic nervous system is to regulate the body's involuntary functions in ways that maintain or restore _____.

113. Your _____ _____ is determined by the combined forces of the sympathetic and parasympathetic nervous systems.

114. According to some physiologists, meditation leads to _____ sympathetic activity and changes opposite to those of the fight-or-flight response.

115. _____ is a malignant tumor of the sympathetic nervous system.

If you had difficulty with this section, review pages 278-279.

UNSCRAMBLE THE WORDS

116. **R O N N E S U**

☐☐☐☐☐☐◯

117. **A P S Y E N S**

☐◯☐◯◯☐☐

118. **C I A T U N O M O**

☐☐◯☐☐☐◯◯☐

119. **S H T O M O   U L M S E C**

☐☐☐☐◯◯☐   ☐☐☐◯☐◯☐

Take the circled letters, unscramble
them, and fill in the solution.

**What the man hoped the IRS agent
would be during his audit.**

120. ☐☐☐☐☐☐☐☐☐☐☐☐☐

APPLYING WHAT YOU KNOW

121. Mr. Hemstreet suffered a cerebrovascular accident, and it was determined that the resulting damage affected the left side of his cerebrum. On which side of his body will he most likely notice any paralysis?

122. Baby Dania was born with an excessive accumulation of cerebrospinal fluid in the ventricles. A catheter was placed in the ventricle, and the fluid was drained by means of a shunt into the circulatory bloodstream. What condition does this medical history describe?

123. Mrs. Muhlenkamp looked out her window to see a man trapped under the wheel of a car. Although slightly built, Mrs. Muhlenkamp rushed to the car, lifted it, and saved the man. What division of the autonomic nervous system made this seemingly impossible task possible?

124. Lynn's heart raced and her palms became clammy as she watched the monster at the local theater. When the movie was over, however, she told her friends that she was not afraid at all. She appeared to be as calm as before the movie. What division of the autonomic nervous system made this possible?

125. Bill is scheduled to meet with his boss for his annual evaluation. He is planning to ask for a raise and hopes the evaluation will be good. Which subdivision of the autonomic nervous system will be active during this conference? Should he have a large meal before his appointment? Support your answer with facts from the chapter.

126. WORD FIND

Find and circle 14 terms presented in this chapter. Words may be spelled top to bottom, bottom to top, right to left, left to right, or diagonally.

Axon
Catecholamines
Dopamine
Endorphins
Ganglion
Glia
Microglia

Myelin
Oligodendroglia
Receptors
Serotonin
Synapse
Synaptic cleft
Tract

```
M  C  C  D  Q  S  Y  N  A  P  S  E  Q  G  O
E  N  A  Q  D  W  H  N  W  E  J  N  A  L  W
S  R  O  T  P  E  C  E  R  Y  Z  N  I  S  M
I  D  S  X  E  K  N  O  K  X  G  G  C  Y  Y
J  O  T  R  A  C  T  D  F  L  O  N  E  N  A
R  P  W  E  K  O  H  X  I  D  A  L  H  A  M
F  A  L  O  N  A  Y  O  E  I  I  I  X  P  C
C  M  Z  I  F  D  N  N  L  N  G  Z  U  T  Z
S  I  N  V  C  G  D  G  Z  A  N  A  K  I  P
G  N  A  T  Z  R  O  W  V  A  M  Y  T  C  O
K  E  N  D  O  R  P  H  I  N  S  I  L  C  X
C  P  Q  G  C  J  X  F  J  D  Q  S  N  L  F
X  U  L  I  H  I  G  Q  A  N  S  W  O  E  U
A  I  M  H  Q  E  X  K  D  B  W  Y  T  F  S
A  A  D  A  X  O  C  K  G  B  F  H  B  T  K
```

KNOW YOUR MEDICAL TERMS

True or False. Indicate in the blank space if the literal translation is true or false for the medical term.

_____ 127. astrocyte   star shaped/cell

_____ 128. axon   pole

_____ 129. efferent   away/carry/relating to

_____ 130. glia   glue

_____ 131. myelin   yellow/relating to

_____ 132. reflex arc   back/bend/curve

_____ 133. synapse   same/join/current

_____ 134. corpus callosum   body/callous

_____ 135. plexus   braid or network

If you had difficulty with this section, review pages 280-281.

DID YOU KNOW?

- Although all pain is felt and interpreted in the brain, the brain itself has no pain sensation—even when cut!
- The smarter you are, the more you dream. Some people even believe that they are smarter in their dreams than when they are awake.
- The brain has huge oxygen needs. It requires 20% of the oxygen and calories that your body needs—even though it makes up only 2% of your total body weight.

Fill in the crossword puzzle.

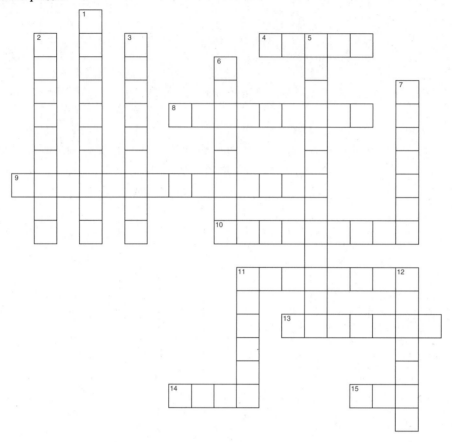

ACROSS

4. Bundle of axons located within the CNS
8. Transmits impulses toward the cell body
9. Neurons that conduct impulses from a ganglion
10. Astrocytes
11. Pia mater
13. Nerve cells
14. Transmits impulses away from the cell body
15. Peripheral nervous system (abbreviation)

DOWN

1. Neuroglia
2. Peripheral beginning of a sensory neuron's dendrite
3. Two-neuron arc (two words)
5. Neurotransmitter
6. Cluster of nerve cell bodies outside the central nervous system
7. Area of brainstem

11. Fatty substance found around some nerve fibers
12. Where impulses are transmitted from one neuron to another

Multiple Choice
Circle the correct answer.

1. What are the neurons called that pick up sensations from receptors and carry them into the brain or spinal cord?
   A. Motor neurons
   B. Central neurons
   C. Interneurons
   D. Sensory neurons

2. What are the brain cavities called that are filled with cerebrospinal fluid?
   A. Hydrocephalics
   B. Ventricles
   C. Mater
   D. Meninges

3. What is the innermost layer of connective tissue that surrounds the brain and spinal cord?
   A. Pia mater
   B. Dura mater
   C. Arachnoid mater
   D. Pons mater

4. A nurse is caring for a patient with a tumor of the cerebellum. In view of the functions of this part of the brain, which of the following symptoms should the nurse expect to observe?
   A. Irregular heart beat and increased blood pressure
   B. Inability to coordinate body movements
   C. Loss of speech
   D. Inability to control emotions

5. What occurs as a result of stimulation of the sympathetic nervous system?
   A. Accelerated heart rate
   B. Constriction of blood vessels in skeletal muscles
   C. Increased peristalsis
   D. All of the above

6. The autonomic neurotransmitter called *acetylcholine* is released by the:
   A. sympathetic preganglionic axon
   B. parasympathetic preganglionic axon
   C. parasympathetic postganglionic axon
   D. all of the above

7. Which of the following statements about Schwann cells is true?
   A. They are found in the PNS
   B. They produce myelin
   C. They are separated by nodes of Ranvier
   D. All of the above are true

8. What are areas of the neuron called that secrete neurotransmitters?
   A. Synapses
   B. Synaptic clefts
   C. Synaptic knobs
   D. Gliomas

9. Which of the following statements about the neural tissues called *tracts* is true?
   A. They are located outside of the central nervous system
   B. They appear gray
   C. When carrying messages upward they are called *ascending*, and when carrying messages downward they are called *descending*
   D. All of the above are true

10. Which of the following statements about the autonomic division of the nervous system is true?
    A. It is composed of two divisions: the sympathetic and parasympathetic
    B. Autonomic neurotransmitters assist the system in its effort to elicit responses
    C. The system regulates the body's involuntary functions
    D. All of the above are true

Matching

Match each term in column A with its corresponding description in column B. (Only one answer is correct for each.)

Column A

_____ 11. Tract

_____ 12. Axon

_____ 13. Brainstem

_____ 14. Neurotransmitter

_____ 15. Central neuron

_____ 16. Skin map

_____ 17. Brain tumor

_____ 18. Diencephalon

_____ 19. Vagus

_____ 20. Limbic system

Column B

A. Transmits away from the cell body

B. Interneuron

C. White matter

D. Cranial nerve

E. Thalamus

F. Glioma

G. Emotional brain

H. Acetylcholine

I. Dermatome

J. Medulla oblongata

Fill in the Blanks

21. The most common primary disease of the CNS is a myelin disorder called _____.

22. A _____ is a group of peripheral nerve fibers (axons) bundled together like strands of a cable.

23. A basic type of neuron pathway that allows impulse conduction in only one direction is called a _____

_____.

24. If a traveling impulse encounters a section of membrane covered with insulating myelin, it "jumps" around the myelin from one gap to the next. This is called _____ _____.

25. The neurotransmitter _____ _____ is

important in regulating smooth muscles in the blood vessels of the penis to allow for penile erection. The drug Viagra promotes the same response as this neurotransmitter.

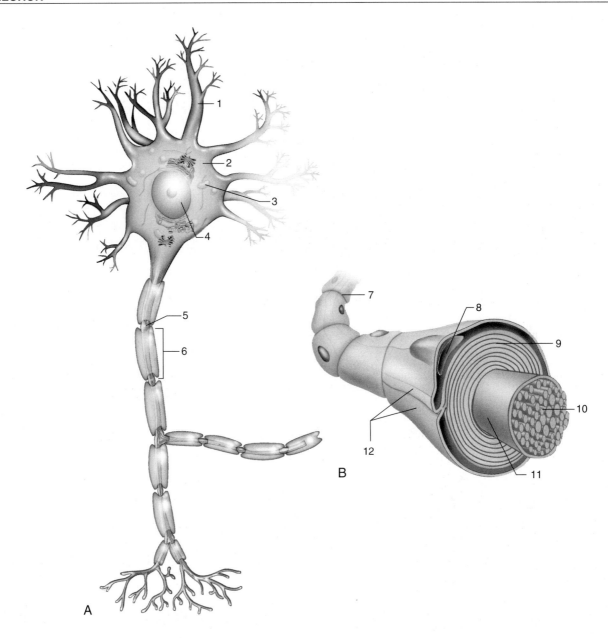

A

B

1. _____

2. _____

3. _____

4. _____

5. _____

6. _____

7. _____

8. _____

9. _____

10. _____

11. _____

12. _____

1. _____

2. _____

3. _____

4. _____

5. _____

6. _____

7. _____

8. _____

9. _____

10. _____

11. _____

12. _____

SAGITTAL SECTION OF THE CENTRAL NERVOUS SYSTEM

1. _____

2. _____

3. _____

4. _____

5. _____

6. _____

7. _____

8. _____

9. _____

10. _____

11. _____

12. _____

13. _____

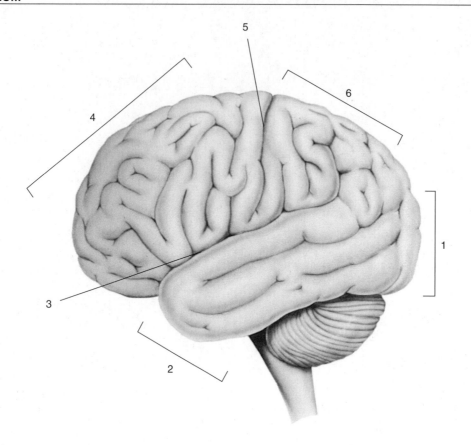

1. _____

2. _____

3. _____

4. _____

5. _____

6. _____

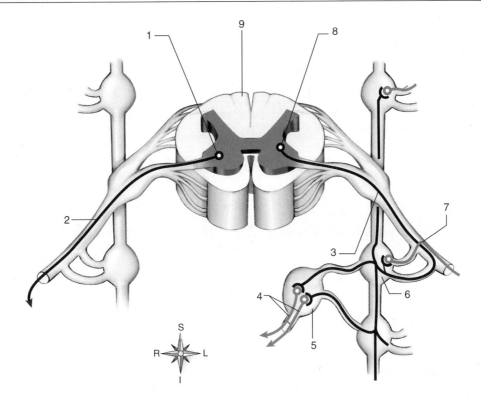

1. _____

2. _____

3. _____

4. _____

5. _____

6. _____

7. _____

8. _____

9. _____

11 Senses

Consider this scene for a moment. You are walking along a beautiful beach while watching the sunset. You notice the various hues and are amazed at the multitude of shades that cover the sky. The waves are melodious as they splash along the shore, and you wiggle your feet with delight as you sense the warm, soft sand trickling between your toes. You sip on a soda and then inhale the fresh salt air as you continue your stroll along the shore. It is a memorable scene, but it is one that would not be possible without the assistance of your sense organs. The sense organs pick up messages that are sent over nerve pathways to specialized areas in the brain for interpretation. They make communication with and enjoyment of the environment possible. The visual, auditory, tactile, olfactory, and gustatory sense organs not only protect us from danger but also add an important dimension to our daily pleasures of life.

Your study of this chapter will give you an understanding of another one of the systems necessary for homeostasis and survival.

TOPICS FOR REVIEW

Before progressing to Chapter 12, you should review the classification of sense organs and the process for converting a stimulus into a sensation. Your study should also include an understanding of the special sense organs and the general sense organs.

CLASSIFICATION OF SENSES

GENERAL SENSES

Match each term on the left with the corresponding description on the right.

_____ 1. Special sense organ

_____ 2. General sense organ

_____ 3. Nose

_____ 4. Bulboid (Krause) corpuscle

_____ 5. Taste

A. Olfactory cells

B. Detects stimuli such as pain or touch

C. Gustatory cells

D. Eye

E. Touch and possibly cold

If you had difficulty with this section, review pages 291-293 and Tables 11-1 and 11-2.

SPECIAL SENSES

Vision

Circle the correct answer.

6. The "white" of the eye is more commonly called the:
   A. choroid
   B. cornea
   C. sclera
   D. retina
   E. none of the above is correct

7. The "colored" part of the eye is known as the:
   A. retina
   B. cornea
   C. pupil
   D. sclera
   E. iris

8. The transparent portion of the sclera, referred to as the "window" of the eye, is the:
   A. retina
   B. cornea
   C. pupil
   D. iris

9. The mucous membrane that covers the front of the eye is called the:
   A. cornea
   B. choroid
   C. conjunctiva
   D. ciliary body
   E. none of the above is correct

10. The structure that can contract or dilate to allow more or less light to enter the eye is the:
    A. lens
    B. choroid
    C. retina
    D. cornea
    E. iris

11. When the eye is looking at objects far in the distance, the lens is _____ and the ciliary muscle is _____.
    A. rounded, contracted
    B. rounded, relaxed
    C. slightly rounded, contracted
    D. slightly curved, relaxed
    E. none of the above is correct

12. The lens of the eye is held in place by the:
    A. ciliary muscle
    B. aqueous humor
    C. vitreous body
    D. cornea

13. The fluid in front of the lens that is constantly being formed, drained, and replaced in the anterior cavity is the:
    A. vitreous body
    B. protoplasm
    C. aqueous humor
    D. conjunctiva

14. If drainage of the aqueous humor is blocked, the internal pressure within the eye will increase, and a condition known as _____ could occur.
    A. presbyopia
    B. glaucoma
    C. color blindness
    D. cataracts

15. The rods and cones are the visual receptors and are located on the:
    A. sclera
    B. cornea
    C. choroid
    D. retina

16. Photoreception is the sense of:
    A. vision
    B. smell
    C. taste
    D. balance

17. The "blind spot" may also be referred to as the:
    A. fovea centralis
    B. macula lutea
    C. retinal artery
    D. optic disc

If you had difficulty with this section, review pages 295-297.

Disorders of Vision
Match the following terms with the numbered descriptions and write the corresponding letter in the answer blank.

A. Strabismus
B. Retinopathy
C. Myopia
D. Glaucoma

E. Astigmatism
F. Conjunctivitis
G. Nyctalopia
H. Hyperopia

I. Scotoma
J. Cataracts
K. Presbyopia

_____ 18. "Oldsightedness"

_____ 19. Nearsightedness

_____ 20. An irregularity in the cornea

_____ 21. "Pink-eye"

_____ 22. "Cross-eye"

_____ 23. Cloudy spots in the eye's lens

_____ 24. Often caused by diabetes mellitus

_____ 25. Farsightedness

_____ 26. "Night blindness"

_____ 27. Loss of only the center of the visual field

_____ 28. Excessive intraocular pressure caused by abnormal accumulation of aqueous humor

If you had difficulty with this section, review pages 299-302.

Hearing and Equilibrium

Match the divisions of the ear with the numbered terms and write the corresponding letter in the answer blank.

A. External ear   B. Middle ear   C. Inner ear

_____ 29. Malleus

_____ 30. Perilymph

_____ 31. Incus

_____ 32. Ceruminous glands

_____ 33. Cochlea

_____ 34. Acoustic canal

_____ 35. Semicircular canals

_____ 36. Stapes

_____ 37. Tympanic membrane

_____ 38. Organ of Corti

Fill in the blanks.

39. The external ear has two parts: the _____ and the _____

    _____ _____.

40. Another name for the tympanic membrane is the _____.

41. The bones of the middle ear are collectively referred to as _____.

42. The stapes presses against a membrane that covers a small opening called the _____.

43. A middle ear infection is called _____ _____.

44. The _____ is located adjacent to the oval window between the semicircular canals and the cochlea.

45. Located within the semicircular canals and the vestibule are _____ for balance and equilibrium.

46. The sensory cells in the _____ _____ are stimulated when movement of the head causes the endolymph to move.

If you had difficulty with this section, review pages 302-304.

Hearing and Equilibrium Disorders

Match the terms with the numbered descriptions and write the corresponding letter in the answer blank.

A. Tinnitus
B. Presbycusis
C. Otosclerosis

D. Otitis media
E. Mastoiditis
F. Ménière disease

_____ 47. Inherited bone disorder that impairs conduction by causing structural irregularities in the stapes

_____ 48. "Ringing in the ear"

_____ 49. Middle ear infection

_____ 50. Untreated otitis media can lead to this condition

_____ 51. Progressive hearing loss associated with aging

_____ 52. Chronic inner ear disease characterized by progressive nerve deafness and vertigo

If you had difficulty with this section, review page 307.

TASTE RECEPTORS

SMELL RECEPTORS

Circle the correct answer.

53. Structures known as (*papillae* or *olfactory cells*) are found on the tongue.

54. Nerve impulses generated by stimulation of taste buds travel primarily through two (*cranial* or *spinal*) nerves.

55. To be detected by olfactory receptors, chemicals must be dissolved in the watery (*mucus* or *plasma*) that lines the nasal cavity.

56. The pathways taken by olfactory nerve impulses and the areas where these impulses are interpreted are closely associated with areas of the brain important in (*hearing* or *memory*).

57. Receptors responsible for the sense of smell are known as (*chemoreceptors* or *mechanoreceptors*).

If you had difficulty with this section, review pages 307-309.

UNSCRAMBLE THE WORDS

58. **C A L R I E U**

[ ][⃝][ ][ ][ ][ ]

59. **R A E C L S**

[⃝][ ][⃝][ ][ ][ ]

60. **L A P I L A E P**

[⃝][ ][⃝][ ][ ][ ][ ][ ]

61. **C T V N U C N O I A J**

[ ][ ][ ][ ][ ][ ][ ][ ][⃝][ ][ ]

Take the circled letters, unscramble
them, and fill in the solution.

What Mr. Tuttle liked best about his classroom.

62. [ ][ ][ ][ ][ ][ ]

APPLYING WHAT YOU KNOW

63. Mr. Nay was an avid swimmer and competed regularly in his age group. He had to withdraw from the last competition because of an infection of his ear. Antibiotics and analgesics were prescribed by the doctor. What is the medical term for his condition?

64. Mrs. Metheny loved the outdoors and spent a great deal of her spare time basking in the sun on the beach. Her physician suggested that she begin wearing sunglasses regularly when he noticed milky spots beginning to appear on Mrs. Metheny's lenses. What condition was Mrs. Metheny's physician trying to prevent from occurring?

65. Amanda repeatedly became ill with throat infections during her first few years of school. Lately, however, she has noticed that whenever she has a throat infection, her ears become very sore also. What might be the cause of this additional problem?

66. Richard was hit in the nose with a baseball during practice. His sense of smell was temporarily gone. What nerve receptors were damaged during the injury?

67. Word Find

Find and circle 19 terms presented in this chapter. Words may be spelled top to bottom, bottom to top, right to left, left to right, or diagonally.

Cataracts   Mechanoreceptor
Cerumen   Olfactory
Cochlea   Papillae
Cones   Photopigment
Conjunctiva   Presbyopia
Eustachian   Receptors
Eye   Refraction
Gustatory   Rods
Hyperopia   Senses
Incus

```
M E C H A N O R E C E P T O R
H R A T B Q I R T B N H M A E
P F T Y R O T C A F L O X R C
G U A Y I N A I H C A T S U E
G P R A C E R U M E N O P X P
I E A I P O Y B S E R P K D T
W L C P L Y N E Y K E I T O O
C Q T O I B R J B S F G L M R
Z U S R C L E O U J R M N N S
F D M E O H L Q T N A E Y I S
H I D P N D L A M A C N X S Z
A M L Y E S S E E D T T M Z H
D D M H S F E X A Y I S I I A
J C G N J T I S L P O G U V J
P H G Y A K H S U C N I S G A
```

KNOW YOUR MEDICAL TERMS

Use the following terms to construct medical terms from the given literal definitions.

chor   chemo   ulla
os   vestibule   on
gangli   crista   iris
aris   lymph   recept
endo   or   icle
ampu   oid   stapes

68. skin/like _____

69. within/water _____

70. knot/unit _____

71. chemical/receive/agent _____

72. ridge/flask/little/relating to _____

73. rainbow _____

74. bone/little _____

75. stirrup _____

76. entrance hall _____

If you had difficulty with this section, review pages 291-311.

- Glaucoma is the leading cause of blindness among African Americans.
- It is possible for your nose to identify and remember more than 50,000 scents.
- Your hearing decreases when you overeat! Overeating actually reduces your ability to hear.
- Every person has a unique tongue print.

THE SENSES

Fill in the crossword puzzle.

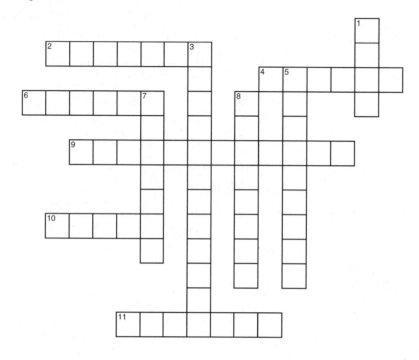

ACROSS

2. Organ of Corti located here
4. Innermost layer of the eye
6. White of the eye
9. Located in posterior cavity (two words)
10. Hole in the center of the iris
11. Front part of this coat is the ciliary muscle and iris

DOWN

1. Transparent body behind pupil
3. Located in anterior cavity in front of lens (two words)
5. Membranous labyrinth filled with this fluid
7. External ear
8. Bones of the middle ear

CHECK YOUR KNOWLEDGE

Multiple Choice

Circle the correct answer.

1. Where are the specialized mechanoreceptors of hearing and balance located?
   A. Inner ear
   B. Malleus
   C. Helix
   D. All of the above

2. The organ of Corti is the organ of what sense?
   A. Sight
   B. Hearing
   C. Pressure
   D. Taste

3. Where are taste sensations interpreted?
   A. Cerebral cortex
   B. Area of stimulation
   C. Nasal cavity
   D. None of the above

4. General sensory receptors found near the point of junction between the tendons and muscles and others found deep within the skeletal muscle tissue are called:
   A. mechanoreceptors
   B. chemoreceptors
   C. proprioceptors
   D. olfactory receptors

5. Which of the following statements about the cornea is true?
   A. It is a mucous membrane
   B. It is called the "window of the eye"
   C. It lies behind the iris
   D. All of the above are true

6. Which of the following are general sense organs?
   A. Gustatory receptors
   B. Pacini corpuscles
   C. Olfactory receptors
   D. All of the above

7. The retina contains microscopic receptor cells called:
   A. mechanoreceptors
   B. chemoreceptors
   C. olfactory receptors
   D. rods and cones

8. Which two involuntary muscles make up the front part of the eye?
   A. Malleus and incus
   B. Iris and ciliary muscle
   C. Retina and Pacinian muscle
   D. Sclera and iris

9. Which of the following statements about gustatory sense organs is true?
   A. They are called *taste buds*
   B. They are innervated by cranial nerves VII and IX
   C. They work together with the olfactory senses
   D. All of the above are true

10. The external ear consists of the:
    A. auricle and acoustic canal
    B. labyrinth
    C. corti and cochlea
    D. none of the above

True or False

If the statement is true, write "T" in the answer blank. If the statement is false, correct the statement by circling the incorrect term and writing the correct term in the answer blank.

_____ 11. The tympanic membrane separates the middle ear from the external ear.

_____ 12. Glaucoma may result from a blockage of flow of the vitreous body.

_____ 13. With the condition of presbyopia, the eye lens loses its elasticity.

_____ 14. The bones of the middle ear are the malleus, incus, and ossicles.

_____ 15. Myopia occurs when images are focused in front of the retina rather than on it.

_____ 16. Light enters through the pupil, and the size of the pupil is regulated by the iris.

_____ 17. The retina is the innermost layer of the eye. It contains the structures called *rods*.

_____ 18. A commonly used name for the "white of the eye" is the sclera.

_____ 19. The olfactory receptors are chemical receptors.

_____ 20. The organ of Corti contains mechanoreceptors.

Fill in the Blanks

21. Sensory receptor cells that are sensitive to physical injury are called _____ .

22. The conjunctiva is kept moist by tears secreted by _____ .

23. Light enters the eye through the pupil and is _____ or bent, so that it is focused on the retina.

24. The glands that are located in the acoustic canal are known as the _____ glands.

25. The bony labyrinth is filled with a watery fluid called _____ .

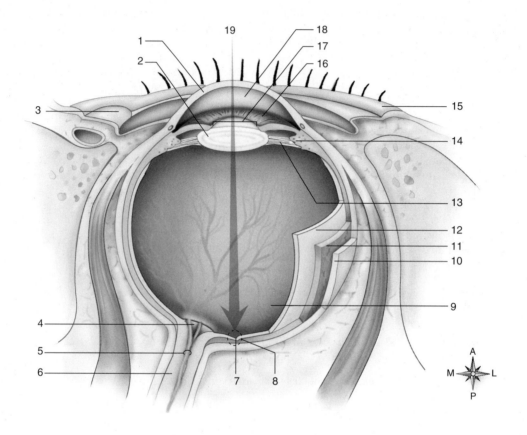

1. _____   11. _____

2. _____   12. _____

3. _____   13. _____

4. _____   14. _____

5. _____   15. _____

6. _____   16. _____

7. _____   17. _____

8. _____   18. _____

9. _____   19. _____

10. _____

1. _____

2. _____

3. _____

4. _____

5. _____

6. _____

7. _____

8. _____

9. _____

10. _____

11. _____

12. _____

13. _____

14. _____

12 Endocrine System

The endocrine system is often compared to a fine concert symphony. When all instruments are playing properly, the sound is melodious. If one instrument plays too loudly or too softly, however, it affects the overall quality of the entire performance.

The endocrine system is a ductless system that releases hormones into the bloodstream to help regulate body functions. The pituitary gland may be considered the conductor of the orchestra, because it stimulates many of the endocrine glands to secrete their powerful hormones. All hormones, whether stimulated in this manner or by other control mechanisms, are interdependent. A change in the level of one hormone may affect the level of many other hormones.

In addition to the endocrine glands, prostaglandins, or "tissue hormones," are powerful substances similar to hormones that have been found in a variety of body tissues. These hormones are often produced in a tissue and diffuse only a short distance to act on cells within that area. Prostaglandins influence respiration, blood pressure, gastrointestinal secretions, and the reproductive system and may someday play an important role in the treatment of diseases such as hypertension, asthma, and ulcers.

The endocrine system is a system of communication and control. It differs from the nervous system in that hormones provide a slower, longer-lasting effect than do nerve stimuli and responses. Your understanding of the "system of hormones" will give you a new awareness of the mechanism of our emotions, response to stress, growth, chemical balances, and many other body functions.

TOPICS FOR REVIEW

Before progressing to Chapter 13, you should be able to identify and locate the primary endocrine glands of the body. Your understanding should include the hormones that are produced by these glands and the method by which these secretions are regulated. Your study will conclude with the pathological conditions that result from the malfunction of this system.

ENDOCRINE GLANDS

MECHANISMS OF HORMONE ACTION

REGULATION OF HORMONE SECRETION

MECHANISMS OF ENDOCRINE DISEASE

PROSTAGLANDINS

Match each term on the left with the corresponding word or phrase on the right.

Group A

_____ 1. Pituitary   A. Pelvic cavity

_____ 2. Parathyroids   B. Mediastinum

_____ 3. Adrenals   C. Neck

_____ 4. Ovaries   D. Cranial cavity

_____ 5. Thymus   E. Abdominal cavity

Group B

_____ 6. Negative feedback   A. Result from hyposecretion or hypersecretion of several hormones

_____ 7. Tissue hormones   B. Respond to a particular hormone

_____ 8. Polyendocrine disorders   C. Prostaglandins

_____ 9. Exocrine glands   D. Discharge secretions into ducts

_____ 10. Target cells   E. Specialized homeostatic mechanism that regulates release of hormones

124

Fill in the blanks.

Nonsteroid hormones work according to the (11) _____ _____

_____ mechanism. According to this concept, a (12) _____

hormone acts as a (13) _____ _____,

providing communication between endocrine glands and (14) _____ _____

_____. A second messenger, such as (15) _____ _____

_____, provides communication within a hormone's (16) _____

_____ _____. (17) _____ _____

_____ disrupts the normal negative feedback control of hormones throughout the body

and may result in tissue damage, sterility, mental imbalance, and a host of life-threatening metabolic problems.

If you had difficulty with this section, review pages 320-321, and 325.

PITUITARY GLAND

HYPOTHALAMUS

Circle the correct answer.

18. The pituitary gland lies in the _____ bone.
    A. ethmoid
    B. sphenoid
    C. temporal
    D. frontal
    E. occipital

19. Which one of the following structures would *not* be stimulated by a tropic hormone from the anterior pituitary?
    A. Ovaries
    B. Testes
    C. Thyroid
    D. Adrenals
    E. Uterus

20. Which one of the following is *not* a function of FSH?
    A. Stimulates the growth of follicles
    B. Stimulates the secretion of estrogens
    C. Stimulates the growth of seminiferous tubules
    D. Stimulates the interstitial cells of the testes

21. Which one of the following is *not* a function of LH?
    A. Stimulates maturation of a developing follicle
    B. Stimulates the secretion of estrogens
    C. Stimulates the development of a corpus luteum
    D. Stimulates sperm cells to mature in the male
    E. Causes ovulation to occur

22. Which one of the following is *not* a function of GH?
    A. Increases glucose catabolism
    B. Increases fat catabolism
    C. Speeds up the movement of amino acids into cells from the bloodstream
    D. Has opposing effect of insulin on blood glucose

23. Which one of the following hormones is *not* released by the anterior pituitary gland?
    A. ACTH
    B. TSH
    C. ADH
    D. FSH
    E. LH

24. Which one of the following is *not* a function of prolactin?
    A. Stimulates breast development during pregnancy
    B. Stimulates milk secretion after delivery
    C. Causes the release of milk from glandular cells of the breast
    D. All of the above are functions of prolactin

25. The anterior pituitary gland secretes:
    A. eight major hormones
    B. tropic hormones that stimulate other endocrine glands to grow and secrete
    C. ADH
    D. oxytocin

26. TSH acts on the:
    A. thyroid
    B. thymus
    C. pineal gland
    D. testes

27. ACTH stimulates the:
    A. adrenal cortex
    B. adrenal medulla
    C. hypothalamus
    D. ovaries

125

28. Which hormone is secreted by the posterior pituitary gland?
   A. MSH
   B. LH
   C. GH
   D. ADH

29. ADH serves the body by:
   A. initiating labor
   B. accelerating water reabsorption from urine into the blood
   C. stimulating the pineal gland
   D. regulating the calcium/phosphorus levels in the blood

30. The disease caused by hyposecretion of ADH is:
   A. diabetes insipidus
   B. diabetes mellitus
   C. acromegaly
   D. myxedema

31. The actual production of ADH and oxytocin takes place in which area?
   A. Anterior pituitary
   B. Posterior pituitary
   C. Hypothalamus
   D. Pineal gland

32. Inhibiting hormones are produced by the:
   A. anterior pituitary
   B. posterior pituitary
   C. hypothalamus
   D. pineal gland

Match one of the glands listed with each numbered term and write the corresponding letter in the answer blank.

A. Anterior pituitary   B. Posterior pituitary   C. Hypothalamus

_____ 33. Adenohypophysis

_____ 34. Neurohypophysis

_____ 35. Induced labor

_____ 36. Appetite

_____ 37. Acromegaly

_____ 38. Body temperature

_____ 39. Sex hormones

_____ 40. Tropic hormones

_____ 41. Gigantism

_____ 42. Releasing hormones

If you had difficulty with this section, review pages 322-329 and Table 12-1.

THYROID GLAND

PARATHYROID GLANDS

Circle the correct answer.

43. The thyroid gland lies (*above* or *below*) the larynx.

44. The thyroid gland secretes (*calcitonin* or *glucagon*).

45. For thyroxine to be produced in adequate amounts, the diet must contain sufficient (*calcium* or *iodine*).

46. Most endocrine glands (*do* or *do not*) store their hormones.

47. Colloid is a storage medium for the (*thyroid* or *parathyroid*) hormone.

48. Calcitonin (*increases* or *decreases*) the concentration of calcium in the blood.

49. A goiter results from (*hyperthyroidism* or *hypothyroidism*).

50. Hyposecretion of thyroid hormones during the formative years leads to (*cretinism* or *myxedema*).

51. The parathyroid glands secrete the hormone (*PTH* or *PTA*).

52. Parathyroid hormone tends to (*increase* or *decrease*) the concentration of calcium in the blood.

If you had difficulty with this section, review pages 329-331.

ADRENAL GLANDS

Fill in the blanks.

53. The adrenal gland is actually two separate endocrine glands, the _____ ____ _____ and the _____ _____ _____.

54. Hormones secreted by the adrenal cortex are known as _____.

55. The outer zone of the adrenal cortex, the zona glomerulosa, secretes _____.

56. The middle zone, the zona fasciculata, secretes _____.

57. The innermost zone, the zona reticularis, secretes _____ _____ _____.

58. Glucocorticoids act in several ways to increase _____.

59. Glucocorticoids also play an essential part in maintaining _____ _____ _____.

60. The adrenal medulla secretes the hormones _____ and _____ _____.

61. The adrenal glands may help the body resist _____.

62. A _____ tumor of the adrenal cortex causes masculinizing symptoms to appear in a woman.

Match each numbered term with the related adrenal structure and write the corresponding letter in the answer blank.

A. Adrenal cortex   B. Adrenal medulla

_____ 63. Addison disease

_____ 64. Anti-immunity

_____ 65. Adrenaline

_____ 66. Cushing syndrome

_____ 67. Fight-or-flight syndrome

_____ 68. Aldosterone

_____ 69. Androgens

If you had difficulty with this section, review pages 331-334.

PANCREATIC ISLETS _____

SEX GLANDS _____

THYMUS _____

PLACENTA _____

PINEAL GLAND _____

Circle the word in each word group that does not belong.

70. Alpha cells	Glucagon	Beta cells	Glycogenolysis
71. Insulin	Glucagon	Beta cells	Diabetes mellitus
72. Estrogens	Progesterone	Corpus luteum	Thymosin
73. Chorion	Interstitial cells	Testosterone	Semen
74. Immune system	Mediastinum	Aldosterone	Thymosin
75. Pregnancy	ACTH	Estrogen	Chorion
76. Melatonin	Sleep cycle	"Third eye"	Semen

Match each term on the left with the corresponding hormone on the right.

Group A

_____ 77. Alpha cells   A. Estrogen

_____ 78. Beta cells   B. Progesterone

_____ 79. Corpus luteum   C. Insulin

_____ 80. Interstitial cells   D. Testosterone

_____ 81. Ovarian follicles   E. Glucagon

Group B

_____ 82. Placenta   A. Melatonin

_____ 83. Pineal gland   B. ANH

_____ 84. Heart atria   C. Testosterone

_____ 85. Testes   D. Thymosin

_____ 86. Thymus   E. Chorionic gonadotropin

If you had difficulty with this section, review pages 334-339.

UNSCRAMBLE THE WORDS

87. **R O O D I I T S C C**

☐☐☐☐☐☐☐☐◯

88. **S I U I S E R D**

☐☐☐☐◯◯☐☐

89. **U O O O T D C S I I L R C C G**

☐☐☐☐☐☐◯☐☐☐☐☐☐

90. **R I O D S T E S**

◯☐☐◯☐☐☐

Take the circled letters, unscramble them, and fill in the solution.

Why Billy didn't like to take exams.

91. ☐☐☐☐☐☐

APPLYING WHAT YOU KNOW

92. Mrs. Tips made a routine visit to her physician last week. When the laboratory results came back, the report indicated a high level of chorionic gonadotropin in her urine. What did this mean to Mrs. Tips?

93. Mrs. Wilcox noticed that her daughter was beginning to take on the secondary sex characteristics of a male. The pediatrician diagnosed the condition as a tumor of an endocrine gland. Where specifically was the tumor located?

94. Mrs. Liddy was pregnant and was 2 weeks past her due date. Her doctor suggested that she enter the hospital and he would induce labor. What hormone will he give Mrs. Liddy?

95. Word Find

Find and circle 16 terms presented in this chapter. Words may be spelled top to bottom, bottom to top, right to left, left to right, or diagonally.

Corticoids Hormone
Cretinism   Hypercalcemia
Diabetes   Hypoglycemia
Diuresis   Luteinization
Endocrine   Myxedema
Exocrine   Prostaglandins
Glucagon   Steroids
Goiter   Stress

```
S S I S E R U I D M E S I T W
N D N X E B A M E D E X Y M I
I I G O N R S G X T I I Y V B
D O M S I N I T E R C C U Q D
N C X S R T N B O T V M Y O M
A I M E C L A C R E P Y H I X
L T Y R O I E Z Q R T J V K F
G R E T D P S N I L D J M X N
A O O S N I D K I N K S P P O
T C P R E T I O G R I F M X G
S L M H Y P O G L Y C E M I A
O A J L H O R M O N E O T G C
R C E L T S E L C N P N X U U
P I O S W R T X C G U L O E L
G G V Y H M S H Y K A K N Q G
```

KNOW YOUR MEDICAL TERMS

Fill in the term from its literal meaning.

96. Inward or within/secrete/acorn _____

97. Sweet/lead or bring _____

98. Island/substance _____

99. Sharp or quick/birth/substance _____

100. Before/milk/substance _____

101. Saddle/Turkish _____

102. Extremities/great/state _____

103. Something tiny/condition _____

104. Under or below/sweet/blood condition _____

105. Medicine or poison/study of words/activity _____

If you had difficulty with this section, review pages 339-341.

DID YOU KNOW?

- The total daily output of the pituitary gland is less than 1/1,000,000 of a gram, yet this small amount is responsible for stimulating the majority of all endocrine functions. It weighs little more than a small paper clip.
- People with dwarfism very often have normal-sized children even if both parents have dwarfism.
- As of January 2011, 25.8 million children and adults in the United States—8.3% of the population—have diabetes. Another 79 million are considered prediabetic.

THE ENDOCRINE SYSTEM

Fill in the crossword puzzle.

ACROSS

2. Antagonist to diuresis
4. Hypersecretion of insulin
7. Hormone thought to initiate labor
8. Gland thought to regulate the onset of puberty
9. Hyposecretion of islets of Langerhans (one word)
11. Estrogens

DOWN

1. Hyposecretion of thyroid
2. Adrenal cortex
3. Adrenal medulla
5. Increases calcium concentration
6. Converts amino acids to glucose
10. Secreted by cells in the walls of the heart's atria

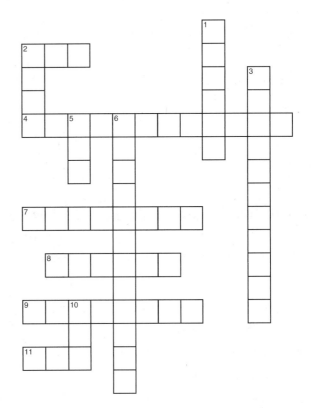

CHECK YOUR KNOWLEDGE

Multiple Choice

Circle the correct answer.

1. What does the outer zone of the adrenal cortex secrete?
   A. Mineralocorticoids
   B. Sex hormones
   C. Glucocorticoids
   D. Epinephrine

2. From what condition does diabetes insipidus result?
   A. Low insulin levels
   B. High glucagon levels
   C. Low antidiuretic hormone levels
   D. High steroid levels

3. Which of the following statements is true regarding a young child whose growth is stunted, metabolism is low, sexual development is delayed, and mental development is retarded?
   A. The child suffers from cretinism
   B. The child has an underactive thyroid
   C. The child could suffer from a pituitary disorder
   D. All of the above are true

4. What can result when too much growth hormone is produced by the pituitary gland?
   A. Hyperglycemia
   B. A pituitary giant
   C. Both A and B
   D. None of the above

5. Which of the following glands is *not* regulated by the pituitary?
   A. Thyroid
   B. Ovaries
   C. Adrenals
   D. Thymus

6. Which of the following statements about the antidiuretic hormone is true?
   A. It is released by the posterior lobe of the pituitary
   B. It causes diabetes insipidus when produced in insufficient amounts
   C. It decreases urine volume
   D. All of the above are true

131

7. What controls the development of the body's immune system?
   A. Pituitary
   B. Thymus
   C. Pineal body
   D. Thyroid

8. Administration of what would best treat a person suffering from severe allergies?
   A. Gonadocorticoids
   B. Glucagon
   C. Mineralocorticoids
   D. Glucocorticoids

9. What endocrine gland is composed of cell clusters called the *islets of Langerhans*?
   A. Adrenals
   B. Thyroid
   C. Pituitary
   D. Pancreas

10. Which of the following statements concerning prostaglandins is true?
    A. They control activities of widely separated organs
    B. They can be called *tissue hormones*
    C. They diffuse over long distances to act on cells
    D. All of the above are true

Matching

Match each term in column A with the corresponding hormone in column B. (Only one answer is correct for each.)

Column A

_____ 11. Goiter

_____ 12. Ovulation

_____ 13. Diabetes mellitus

_____ 14. Lactation

_____ 15. Retention of water by kidneys

_____ 16. Chorionic gonadotropins

_____ 17. Cushing syndrome

_____ 18. Labor

_____ 19. Acromegaly

_____ 20. Hypercalcemia

Column B

A. Glucocorticoid hormones

B. Antidiuretic hormone

C. Calcitonin

D. Oxytocin

E. Growth hormone

F. Placenta

G. Luteinizing hormone

H. Insulin

I. Prolactin

J. Thyroid hormones

True or False

21. _____ Cyclic AMP is only one of several second messengers that have been discovered.

22. _____ Steroid hormone responses are typically rapid compared with responses triggered by nonsteroid hormones.

23. _____ Positive feedback mechanisms amplify changes rather than reverse them.

24. _____ Prostaglandins, leukotrienes, and thromboxane are sometimes called polyendocrine agents.

25. _____ The anterior pituitary is also known as the neurohypophysis.

ENDOCRINE GLANDS

1. _____

2. _____

3. _____

4. _____

5. _____

6. _____

7. _____

8. _____

9. _____

10. _____

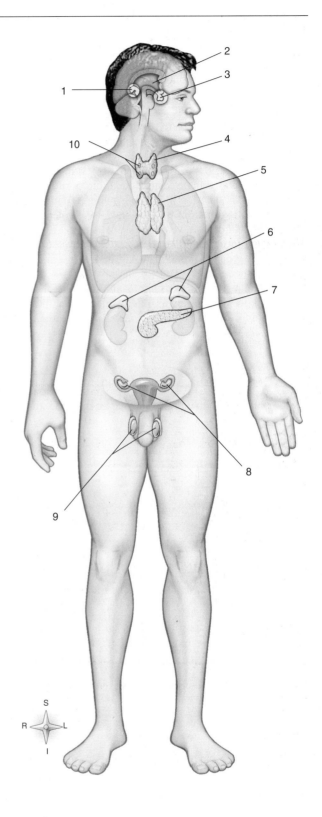

13 Blood

Blood, the river of life, is the body's primary means of internal transportation. Although it is the respiratory system that provides oxygen for the body, the digestive system that provides nutrients, and the urinary system that eliminates wastes, none of these functions could be provided for the individual cells without blood. In less than 1 minute, a drop of blood will complete a trip through the entire body, distributing nutrients and collecting the wastes of metabolism.

Blood is divided into plasma (the liquid portion of blood) and the formed elements (the blood cells). There are three types of blood cells: red blood cells, white blood cells, and platelets. Together these cells and plasma provide a means of transportation that delivers the body's daily necessities.

Although all of us have red blood cells that are similar in shape, we have different blood types. Blood types are identified by the presence of certain antigens on the surface of red blood cells. Every person's blood belongs to one of four main blood groups: Type A, B, AB, or O. Any one of the four groups or "types" may or may not have the Rh factor present on the red blood cells. If an individual has a specific antigen called the Rh factor present on his or her blood, the blood is Rh positive. If this factor is missing, the blood is Rh negative. Approximately 85% of the population has the Rh factor (Rh positive), whereas 15% does not have the Rh factor (Rh negative).

Your understanding of this chapter will be necessary to prepare a proper foundation for learning about the circulatory system.

TOPICS FOR REVIEW

Before progressing to Chapter 14, you should have an understanding of the structure and function of blood plasma and cells. Your review should also include an understanding of blood types and Rh factors.

BLOOD COMPOSITION

MECHANISMS OF BLOOD DISEASE

Circle the correct answer.

1. Which one of the following substances is *not* a part of the plasma?
   A. Water
   B. Proteins
   C. Nutrients
   D. Waste products
   E. Leukocytes

2. The normal volume of blood in an adult is approximately:
   A. 2 to 3 pints
   B. 2 to 3 quarts
   C. 2 to 3 gallons
   D. 4 to 6 liters

3. Blood is normally:
   A. very acidic
   B. slightly acidic
   C. neutral
   D. slightly alkaline

4. Which is *not* a formed element?
   A. Leukocytes
   B. Erythrocytes
   C. Globulins
   D. Platelets

5. The liquid (extracellular) part of blood is the:
   A. monocytes
   B. plasma
   C. basophils
   D. lymphocytes

6. Myeloid tissue is _____ tissue.
   A. epithelial
   B. connective
   C. muscle
   D. nervous

7. A platelet may also be referred to as a/an:
   A. neutrophil
   B. eosinophil
   C. thrombocyte
   D. erythrocyte

8. An example of an agranular leukocyte is a/an:
   A. platelet
   B. erythrocyte
   C. eosinophil
   D. monocyte

134

9. Myeloid tissue is found in all of the following locations *except*:
   A. sternum
   B. ribs
   C. wrist bones
   D. hip bones
   E. cranial bones

10. Lymphatic tissue is found in which of the following locations?
    A. Lymph nodes
    B. Thymus
    C. Spleen
    D. All of the above contain lymphatic tissue

11. If bone marrow failure is suspected, a procedure that allows for examination of the tissue is a/an:
    A. aspiration biopsy cytology procedure
    B. transplantation
    C. stem cell smear
    D. hematopoietic injection technique

12. The failure of blood-producing tissues to form blood cells properly may be due to:
    A. radiation
    B. inherited defects
    C. viral infections
    D. all of the above

RED BLOOD CELLS

13. A red blood cell has:
    A. a biconcave disk shape that provides greater surface area for the exchange of dissolved gases and solutes
    B. a large nucleus for rapid reproduction
    C. a life span of 6 months
    D. several cytoplasmic organelles that maintain the homeostasis of the cell

14. The "buffy coat" layer that appears in the hematocrit tube contains:
    A. red blood cells and platelets
    B. plasma only
    C. platelets only
    D. white blood cells and platelets
    E. none of the above is correct

15. Any additional intracellular space that becomes available in a red blood cell is filled with:
    A. iron
    B. nutrients
    C. hemoglobin
    D. ATP

16. The hematocrit value for red blood cells is

    _____ %.
    A. 75
    B. 60
    C. 50
    D. 45
    E. 35

17. A critical component of hemoglobin is:
    A. potassium
    B. calcium
    C. vitamin K
    D. iron

18. One of the most useful and frequently performed clinical blood tests is called the:
    A. WBC
    B. CBC
    C. RBC
    D. hematocrit

If you had difficulty with this section, review pages 350-354.

BLOOD TYPES

19.   Fill in the blank areas.

Blood Type	Antigen Present in RBC	Antibody Present in Plasma
A		Anti-B
B	B	
AB		None
O	None	

Fill in the blanks.

20. An _____ is a substance that can stimulate the body to make antibodies.

21. An _____ is a substance made by the body in response to stimulation by an antigen.

22. Many antibodies react with their antigens to clump or _____ them.

23. If a baby is born to an Rh-negative mother and Rh-positive father, it may develop the disease _____

_____ _____.

24. The term "Rh" is used because the antigen was first discovered in the blood of a _____

_____ _____.

25. The universal donor blood is _____.

26. The universal recipient blood is _____.

If you had difficulty with this section, review pages 355-357.

RED BLOOD CELL DISORDERS

Matching

Match each term in column A with the corresponding description in column B.

27. _____ Pernicious anemia

28. _____ Polycythemia

29. _____ Sickle cell anemia

30. _____ Aplastic anemia

31. _____ Hemolytic anemia

32. _____ Thalassemia

33. _____ Erythroblastosis fetalis

34. _____ Iron-deficiency anemia

35. _____ Anemia

A. Dramatic increase in red blood cell numbers

B. Rh factor incompatibility

C. Production of abnormal type of hemoglobin

D. Low oxygen-carrying capacity of the blood

E. Decreased red blood cell life span

F. Lack of vitamin B_{12}

G. Abnormally low red blood cells and destruction of bone marrow

H. Ferrous sulfate is often used to treat this disorder

I. Inherited hemolytic anemia

If you had difficulty with this section, review pages 358-360.

WHITE BLOOD CELLS

Multiple Choice

Circle the correct answer.

36. Another name for white blood cells is:
    A. erythrocytes
    B. leukocytes
    C. thrombocytes
    D. platelets

37. Which one of the following types of cells is *not* a granular leukocyte?
    A. Neutrophil
    B. Monocyte
    C. Basophil
    D. Eosinophil

38. An unusually low white blood cell count would be termed:
    A. leukemia
    B. leukopenia
    C. leukocytosis
    D. anemia
    E. none of the above is correct

39. The most numerous of the phagocytes are the

    _____.
    A. lymphocytes
    B. neutrophils
    C. basophils
    D. eosinophils
    E. monocytes

40. Which one of the following types of cells is *not* phagocytic?
    A. Neutrophils
    B. Eosinophils
    C. Lymphocytes
    D. Monocytes
    E. All of the above are phagocytic cells

41. Which of the following cell types functions in the immune process?
    A. Neutrophils
    B. Lymphocytes
    C. Monocytes
    D. Basophils
    E. Reticuloendothelial cells

42. A special type of white blood cell count used as a diagnostic tool is known as a/an:
    A. leukopenia
    B. granulocyte count
    C. differential WBC count
    D. CBC

If you had difficulty with this section, review pages 353, 361-362.

WHITE BLOOD CELL DISORDERS

Matching

Match each term in column A with the corresponding description in column B.

Column A

43. _____ Multiple myeloma

44. _____ Leukemia

45. _____ Acute lymphocytic leukemia

46. _____ Chronic myeloid leukemia

47. _____ Acute myeloid leukemia

48. _____ Infectious mononucleosis

49. _____ Lymphoid neoplasms

50. _____ Chronic lymphocytic leukemia

Column B

A. Most common form of blood cancer in children between 3 to 7 years of age

B. Results from cancerous transformation of granulocytic precursor cells in the bone marrow

C. Most common blood cancer in people over 65 years of age

D. Arises from lymphoid precursor cells that normally produce B lymphocytes, T lymphocytes, or their descendant cell types

E. General classification for a number of blood cancers affecting white blood cells

F. Malignant precursor B lymphocytes are produced in large numbers.

G. Usually caused by the Epstein-Barr virus (EBV)

H. Prognosis is poor, with only 50% of children and 30% of adults achieving long-term survival.

If you had difficulty with this section, review pages 363-364.

BLOOD CLOTTING DISORDERS

Circle the correct answer.

51. Vitamin K stimulates liver cells to increase the synthesis of:
    A. prothrombin
    B. thrombin
    C. platelets
    D. heparin
    E. calcium

52. Thrombocytes:
    A. are tiny cell fragments
    B. are filled with chemicals necessary to initiate blood clotting
    C. are formed elements
    D. all of the above

53. If part of a clot dislodges and circulates through the bloodstream, the dislodged part is called a/an:
    A. thrombus
    B. thrombosis
    C. anticoagulant
    D. clotting factor
    E. embolus

54. Which of the following is *not* a critical component of coagulation?
    A. Thrombin
    B. Fibrinolysis
    C. Fibrinogen
    D. Fibrin

55. Which of the following does *not* hasten clotting?
    A. A rough spot in the endothelium
    B. Abnormally slow blood flow
    C. Heparin
    D. All of the above hasten clotting

Circle the correct response.

56. Tissue plasminogen activator (TPA) is used to dissolve (*heart* or *hemorrhagic stroke*) clots.

57. An International Normalized Ratio (INR) of (*0.8* or *2.5*) is normal.

58. The disease that results from a failure to form blood clotting factor VIII is (*thrombocytopenia* or *hemophilia*).

59. Reduced platelet count is common in diseases such as (*thrombosis* or *HIV/AIDS*).

60. Hemophilia involves avoiding such common drugs as (*aspirin* or *antihistamines*).

If you had difficulty with this section, review pages 365-368.

UNSCRAMBLE THE WORDS

61. **H G A P O Y C E T**

⬚⬚⬚⬚⬚⬚⬚⬚ (with circles on positions 1 and 6)

62. **N T H I R B M O**

⬚⬚⬚⬚⬚⬚⬚⬚ (with circles on positions 1 and 8)

63. **A T N I G N E**

⬚⬚⬚⬚⬚⬚⬚ (with circle on position 5)

64. **B R N I F I**

⬚⬚⬚⬚⬚⬚ (with circle on position 2)

Take the circled letters, unscramble them, and fill in the solution.

What Shelley thought was the most difficult task to learn on her new computer.

65. ⬚⬚⬚⬚⬚⬚⬚

APPLYING WHAT YOU KNOW

66. Mrs. Florez's blood type is O positive. Her husband's type is O negative. Her newborn baby's blood type is O negative. Is there any need for concern with this combination?

67. After Mrs. Freund's baby was born, the doctor applied a gauze dressing for a short time on the umbilical cord. He also gave the baby a dose of vitamin K. Why did the doctor perform these two procedures?

68. Valerie is a teenager with a picky appetite. She loves junk food and seldom eats properly. She complains of being tired all the time. A visit to her doctor reveals a hemoglobin of 10 and RBCs that are classified as hypochromic. What condition does Valerie have?

69. Jack was prescribed a daily dose of Coumadin since his diagnosis of atrial fibrillation. He was advised that he must be monitored monthly with a lab test to regulate his dosage. What is the name of that lab test? Describe how the test is performed and the information that it provides for the doctor.

70. Word Find

Find and circle 24 terms presented in this chapter. Words may be spelled top to bottom, bottom to top, right to left, left to right, or diagonally.

```
H S H K L S U L O B M E A E S
K E E V M Z H E P A R I N D N
D T M F A C T O R Y E T I Q P
O Y A O H N B A T Q Y A R A R
N C T J G W E H N P N L B U D
O O O S Q L R M E T I S I P M
R K C E M O O N I H I Q F W W
H U R T C N I B P A S G Z T G
E E I Y O B O O I V E W E T X
S L T C M D S E C N R T U N R
U E Y O Y A I M E K U E L Y S
S T R G B S T H R O M B U S Q
E H Z A M S A L P N D Z P O N
T E N H F P D A P M E E I B W
E W B P H K B O N C K W X V J
```

AIDS	Factor	Phagocytes
Anemia	Fibrin	Plasma
Antibody	Hematocrit	Recipient
Antigen	Hemoglobin	Rhesus
Basophil	Heparin	Serum
Donor	Leukemia	Thrombin
Embolus	Leukocytes	Thrombus
Erythrocytes	Monocyte	Type

KNOW YOUR MEDICAL TERMS

Select the literal translations for the medical terms.

71. _____ Leukocyte		A. red/cell
72. _____ Platelet		B. clot/substance
73. _____ Macrophage		C. neither/love
74. _____ Hematocrit		D. flat/small
75. _____ Heparin		E. white/cell
76. _____ Agglutinate		F. blood/separate
77. _____ Neutrophil		G. large/eat
78. _____ Erythrocyte		H. glue/process
79. _____ Purpura		I. liver/substance
80. _____ Thrombin		J. purple

If you had difficulty with this section, review pages 349, 368-370.

BLOOD

Fill in the crossword puzzle.

ACROSS

1. Abnormally high WBC count
4. Final stage of clotting process
6. Oxygen-carrying mechanism of blood
9. To engulf and digest microbes
10. Stationary blood clot
12. RBC
13. Circulating blood clot
14. Liquid portion of blood

DOWN

2. Type O (two words)
3. Substances that stimulate the body to make antibodies
5. Type of leukocyte
7. Platelets
8. Prevents clotting of blood
11. Inability of the blood to carry sufficient oxygen

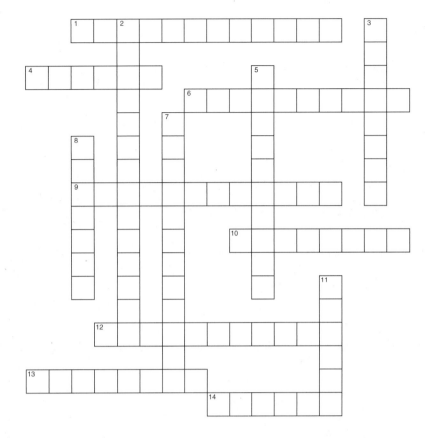

DID YOU KNOW?

■ Blood products are good for approximately 3 to 6 weeks, but fresh frozen plasma is good for at least 6 months.
■ In the second it takes to turn the page of a book, you will lose about 3 million red blood cells. During that same second, your bone marrow will have produced the same number of new ones.
■ There is enough iron in a human to make a small nail.
■ Statistics show that 25% or more of us will require blood at least once in our lifetime.
■ The most common blood type in the world is Type O. The rarest, Type A-H, has been found in less than a dozen people since the type was discovered.

CHECK YOUR KNOWLEDGE

Multiple Choice

Circle the correct answer.

1. Which of the following statements is false?
   A. Sickle cell anemia is caused by a genetic defect
   B. Leukemia is characterized by a low number of WBCs
   C. Polycythemia is characterized by an abnormally high number of erythrocytes
   D. Pernicious anemia is caused by a lack of vitamin B_{12}

2. Deficiency in the number or function of erythrocytes is called:
   A. leukemia
   B. anemia
   C. polycythemia
   D. leukopenia

3. Which of the following statements does *not* describe a characteristic of leukocytes?
   A. They are disk-shaped cells that do not contain a nucleus
   B. They have the ability to fight infection
   C. They provide defense against certain parasites
   D. They provide immune defense

4. Red bone marrow forms all of the following blood cells *except*:
   A. platelets and basophils
   B. lymphocytes
   C. red blood cells
   D. neutrophils and eosinophils

5. Which of the following substances is *not* found in blood plasma?
   A. Albumins
   B. Gases
   C. Waste products
   D. All of the above substances are found in blood plasma

6. An allergic reaction may increase the number of:
   A. eosinophils
   B. neutrophils
   C. lymphocytes
   D. monocytes

7. What is a blood clot that is moving through the body called?
   A. Embolism
   B. Fibrosis
   C. Heparin
   D. Thrombosis

8. When could difficulty with the Rh blood factor arise?
   A. When an Rh-negative man and woman produce a child
   B. When an Rh-positive man and woman produce a child
   C. When an Rh-positive woman and an Rh-negative man produce a child
   D. When an Rh-negative woman and an Rh-positive man produce a child

9. What is the primary function of hemoglobin?
   A. To fight infection
   B. To make blood clots
   C. To carry oxygen
   D. To transport hormones

10. Which of the following steps is *not* involved in blood clot formation?
    A. A blood vessel is injured, and platelet factors are formed
    B. Thrombin is converted into prothrombin
    C. Fibrinogen is converted into fibrin
    D. All of the above are involved in blood clot formation

Matching

Match each term in column A with its corresponding term or description in column B. (Only one answer is correct for each.)

Column A

_____ 11. Lymphocytes

_____ 12. Erythrocytes

_____ 13. Type AB

_____ 14. Basophils

_____ 15. Leukemia

_____ 16. Platelets

_____ 17. Type O

_____ 18. Rh factor

_____ 19. Red bone marrow

_____ 20. Neutrophils

Column B

A. Heparin

B. Contains anti-A and anti-B antibodies

C. Clotting

D. Immunity

E. Erythroblastosis fetalis

F. Anemia

G. Cancer

H. Contains A and B antigens

I. Myeloid tissue

J. Phagocytosis

MATCHING

Match each numbered descriptive term with the related formed element and write the corresponding letter in the answer blank.

A. Red blood cells   B. White blood cells   C. Platelets

21. _____ Rh factor

22. _____ Agranulocytes

23. _____ Macrophages

24. _____ Thrombocytes

25. _____ Hemophilia

26. _____ Prothrombin time

27. _____ Hemoglobin

28. _____ Blood types

29. _____ Hematocrit

30. _____ Eosinophils

HUMAN BLOOD CELLS

Fill in the missing areas of the table.

BODY CELL	FUNCTION

BLOOD TYPING

Using the key below the table shown, draw the appropriate reaction with the donor's blood in the circles provided.

Recipient's blood		Reactions with donor's blood			
RBC antigens	Plasma antibodies	Donor type O	Donor type A	Donor type B	Donor type AB
None (Type O)	Anti-A Anti-B	◯	◯	◯	◯
A (Type A)	Anti-B	◯	◯	◯	◯
B (Type B)	Anti-A	◯	◯	◯	◯
AB (Type AB)	(None)	◯	◯	◯	◯

 Normal blood

 Agglutinated blood

14 Heart

The heart is actually two pumps—one moves blood to the lungs, and the other pushes it out into the body. These two functions seem rather elementary in comparison to the complex and numerous functions performed by most of the other body organs, and yet if this pump stops, within a few short minutes all life ceases.

The heart is divided into two upper compartments called *atria*, or receiving chambers, and two lower compartments, or discharging chambers, called *ventricles*. By age 45, approximately 300,000 tons of blood will have passed through these chambers to be circulated to the blood vessels. This closed system of circulation provides distribution of blood to the entire body (systemic circulation) and to specific regions, such as the pulmonary circulation or coronary circulation.

The beating of the heart must be coordinated in a rhythmic manner if the heart is to pump effectively. This is achieved by electrical impulses that are stimulated by specialized structures embedded in the walls of the heart. The sinoatrial node, atrioventricular node, bundle of His, and Purkinje fibers combine efforts to conduct the tiny electrical currents necessary to contract the heart. Any interruption or failure of this system may result in serious pathology or death.

A healthy heart is necessary to pump sufficient blood throughout the body to nourish and oxygenate cells continuously. Your review of this chapter will provide you with an understanding of this vital organ that is necessary for survival.

TOPICS FOR REVIEW

Before progressing to Chapter 15, you should have an understanding of the structure and function of the heart. Your review should include a study of the coronary circulation and the conduction system of the heart. Your study should conclude with an understanding of the major coronary diseases and disorders.

FUNCTIONAL ANATOMY OF THE HEART

Fill in the blanks.

1. The system that supplies our cells' transportation needs is the _____ _____.

2. The _____ or blunt point at the lower edge of the heart lies on the diaphragm, pointing to the left.

3. The _____ _____ divides the heart into right and left sides between the atria.

4. The _____ are the two upper chambers of the heart.

5. The _____ are the two lower chambers of the heart.

6. The cardiac muscle tissue is referred to as the _____.

7. Inflammation of the heart lining is _____.

8. The two AV valves are _____ and _____.

9. The inner layer of the pericardium is called the _____ _____ _____ or _____.

10. The outer layer of pericardium is called _____ _____ _____.

11. If the pericardium becomes inflamed, a condition called _____ results.

12. The _____ _____ are located between the two ventricular chambers and the large arteries that carry blood away from the heart when contraction occurs.

146

13. A _____ _____ _____

_____ is a condition caused when the flaps of this valve extend back into the left atrium, causing

the valve to leak.

14. _____ _____ _____

_____ is cardiac damage resulting from a delayed inflammatory response to a streptococcal infection

that occurs most often in children.

If you had difficulty with this section, review pages 379-383.

HEART SOUNDS

BLOOD FLOW THROUGH THE HEART

BLOOD SUPPLY TO THE HEART MUSCLE

Select the term that best matches each of the numbered descriptions. Write the corresponding letter in the answer blank.

_____ 15. Movement of blood from the left ventricle through the body

_____ 16. Blood clot

_____ 17. Myocardial infarction

_____ 18. Abnormal heart sound often caused by disorders of the valves

_____ 19. Movement of blood from the right ventricle to the lungs

_____ 20. Hardening of the arteries

_____ 21. Severe chest pain

_____ 22. High blood pressure

_____ 23. Structures through which blood returns to the left atrium

_____ 24. Treatment for certain coronary disorders

A. Heart murmur

B. Pulmonary circulation

C. Embolism

D. Heart attack

E. Angina pectoris

F. Systemic circulation

G. Atherosclerosis

H. Hypertension

I. Coronary bypass

J. Pulmonary veins

If you had difficulty with this section, review pages 384-386.

CARDIAC CYCLE

ELECTRICAL ACTIVITY OF THE HEART

CARDIAC OUTPUT

HEART FAILURE

Circle the correct answer.

25. The heart beats at an average rate of _____ beats per minute.
   A. 50
   B. 72
   C. 100
   D. 120

26. Each complete beat of the heart is called:
   A. cardiac output
   B. stroke volume
   C. a cardiac cycle
   D. a contraction

147

27. The pacemaker of the heart is also known as the:
   A. SA node
   B. AV node
   C. AV bundle
   D. Purkinje fibers

28. A rapid heart rhythm, over 100 beats per minutes, is referred to as:
   A. bradycardia
   B. sinus arrhythmia
   C. tachycardia
   D. premature contractions

29. The term _____ describes the electrical activity that triggers contraction of the heart muscle.
   A. depolarization
   B. repolarization
   C. AV node block
   D. cardiac arrhythmia

30. A diagnostic tool that uses ultrasound to detect valve and heart disorders is known as a/an:
   A. electrocardiogram
   B. pacemaker
   C. TPA
   D. echocardiogram

31. Frequent premature contractions can lead to:
   A. extra systoles
   B. bradycardia
   C. fibrillation
   D. heart failure

32. A drug that slows and increases the strength of cardiac contractions is:
   A. digitalis
   B. nitroglycerin
   C. calcium-channel blocker
   D. anticoagulant

33. Congestive heart failure inevitably causes:
   A. extra systole
   B. pulmonary edema
   C. fibrillation
   D. bradycardia

34. Failure of the right side of the heart due to blockage of pulmonary blood flow is called:
   A. cardiomyopathy
   B. ventricular fibrillation
   C. cor pulmonale
   D. TPA

35. A nonmedical rescuer can defibrillate a victim in ventricular fibrillation with the use of a/an:
   A. AED
   B. beta blocker
   C. demand pacemaker
   D. ECG

36. Coumadin and dicumarol are examples of commonly used oral:
   A. beta blockers
   B. nitroglycerines
   C. calcium-channel blockers
   D. anticoagulants

True or False

If the statement is true, write "T" in the answer blank. If the statement is false, correct the statement by circling the incorrect term(s) and writing the correct term(s) in the answer blank.

37. _____ Most of the atrial blood moves into the ventricles before the atria have a chance to contract.

38. _____ Cardiac muscle fibers are unable to contract rhythmically on their own.

39. _____ The four structures embedded in the wall of the heart that make up the conduction system of the heart are the SA node, the pacemaker, the AV bundle, and the bundle of His.

40. _____ A special type of radiography used to visualize arteries is known as angiography.

41. _____ The T wave on an ECG results from the electrical activity generated by repolarization of the ventricles.

42. _____ Heart block may be treated by implanting an artificial pacemaker.

43. _____ Atrial ablation treats atrial fibrillation by dilating the pathway of abnormal electrical signals.

44. _____ Cardiac output (CO) is the volume of blood pumped by one atrium per minute.

45. _____ The sympathetic division of the ANS decreases the heart rate.

46. _____ Stroke volume (SV) refers to the volume of blood ejected from the ventricles during each beat.

47. _____ Stroke volume may be decreased due to several causes such as ion imbalances, valve disorders, coronary artery blockages, or myocardial infarctions.

If you had difficulty with this section, review pages 384-395.

UNSCRAMBLE THE WORDS

48. **C T S S Y M E I**

□ Ⓞ □ Ⓞ □ □ □

49. **L M T R I A**

Ⓞ □ □ □ □ □

50. **T H R E A**

Ⓞ □ □ Ⓞ □

51. **S B T U M H O R**

□ Ⓞ □ □ □ □ □ □

Take the circled letters, unscramble them, and fill in the solution.

What Tom lacked on the dance floor.

52. □ □ □ □ □ □

APPLYING WHAT YOU KNOW

53. Else was experiencing angina pectoris. Her doctor suggests a surgical procedure that would require the removal of a vein from another region of her body, which would then be used to bypass a partial blockage in her coronary arteries. What is this procedure called?

54. Phil has a heart block. His electrical impulses are being blocked and prevented from reaching the ventricles. An electrical device that causes ventricular contractions at a rate necessary to maintain circulation is being considered as possible treatment for his condition. What is this device?

55. Mrs. Haygood was diagnosed with an acute case of endocarditis. What is the real danger of this diagnosis?

56. Jeanne's homework assignment was to demonstrate knowledge of the path of blood flow through the heart. Can you help her?

Trace the blood flow through the heart by numbering the following structures in the correct sequence. Start with number 1, the vena cava, where blood enters the heart, and proceed until you have numbered all 12 structures.

_____ Tricuspid valve   _____ Pulmonary veins

_____ Pulmonary arteries   _____ Pulmonary semilunar valve

_____ Bicuspid valve   _____ Left ventricle

_____ Vena cava   _____ Right atrium

_____ Right ventricle   _____ Left atrium

_____ Aorta   _____ Aortic semilunar valve

57. Word Find

Find and circle 12 terms presented in this chapter. Words may be spelled top to bottom, bottom to top, right to left, left to right, or diagonally.

```
P W S T L W G V F V W Q U S Y
U T X U L Q L V M J W O U J D
R E S P E B S W Z W K N X Q Y
K V Y T E V E N T R I C L E S
I F K U O E L O T S Y S X V R
N G Z O A R G A Y C M X F K H
J B B C U J T R V K P Y P W Y
E V L A V R A N U L I M E S T
F D T I Z N H I Y A A D U T H
I T B D O D S H Y P U R W I M
B P E R I C A R D I U M T D I
E M O A B R A D Y C A R D I A
R C U C E N D O C A R D I U M
S A I D R A C Y H C A T B Y P
```

Bradycardia   Endocardium   Semilunar valve
Cardiac output   Mitral valve   Systole
Coronary sinus   Pericardium   Tachycardia
Dysrhythmia   Purkinje fibers   Ventricle

KNOW YOUR MEDICAL TERMS

Fill in the blank with the proper medical term.

58. entrance or courtyard _____

59. string or cord/pulled tight _____

60. contraction _____

61. strangling/breast/relating to _____

62. heart/muscle/disease/state _____

63. electricity/heart/drawing _____

64. within/heart/thing _____

65. slow/heart/condition _____

66. plug/condition _____

67. fiber/little/process _____

If you had difficulty with this section, review pages 379, 395-397.

DID YOU KNOW?

- Your heart pumps more than 5 quarts of blood every minute—that's 2,000 gallons a day!
- People who have an optimistic attitude as opposed to a pessimistic attitude suffer fewer strokes and heart attacks and have a 55% less chance of suffering cardiovascular diseases.
- A kitchen faucet would need to be turned on all the way for at least 45 years to equal the amount of blood pumped by the heart in an average lifetime.
- German surgeon Werner Forssmann (1904–1979) examined the inside of his own heart in 1929 by threading a catheter into his arm vein and pushing it 20 inches into his heart, inventing cardiac catheterization—a now common procedure.

HEART AND HEART DISEASE

Fill in the crossword puzzle.

ACROSS

1. Inflammation of the pericardium
3. A condition in which muscle fibers contract out of step with each other
6. Disease of the myocardial tissue
8. Also known as the *visceral pericardium*
9. Relaxation of the heart
10. Upper chambers of the heart

DOWN

2. Heart specialist
4. Also known as the *sinoatrial node*
5. Complex that occurs as a result of depolarization of the ventricles
7. Also known as the *mitral valve*
8. Graphic record of the heart's electrical activity

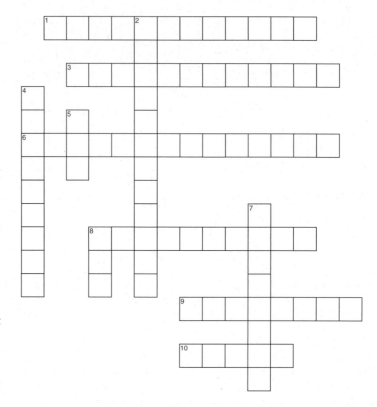

CHECK YOUR KNOWLEDGE

Multiple Choice
Circle the correct answer.

1. The superior vena cava carries blood to the:
   A. left ventricle
   B. coronary arteries
   C. right atrium
   D. pulmonary veins

2. Which of the following events, if any, does *not* precede ventricular contraction?
   A. P wave
   B. Atrial depolarization
   C. Ventricular depolarization
   D. All of these events precede contraction

3. Which of the following pairs is mismatched?
   A. Angina pectoris—chest pain
   B. Congestive heart failure—left-sided heart failure
   C. Tachycardia—slow heart rhythm
   D. Dysrhythmia—heart block

4. Which of the following statements is *not* true regarding pericarditis?
   A. It may be caused by infection or trauma
   B. It often causes severe chest pain
   C. It may result in impairment of the pumping action of the heart
   D. All of the above statements are true

5. The outside covering that surrounds and protects the heart is called the:
   A. endocardium
   B. myocardium
   C. pericardium
   D. ectocardium

6. Thin-walled upper heart cavities that receive blood from veins are called:
   A. chordae tendineae
   B. atria
   C. pericardia
   D. ventricles

7. A valve that permits blood to flow from the right ventricle into the pulmonary artery is called:
   A. tricuspid
   B. mitral
   C. aortic semilunar
   D. pulmonary semilunar

8. Ventricular contraction of the heart occurs *immediately after* depolarization of the:
   A. Purkinje fibers
   B. atrioventricular node
   C. sinoatrial node
   D. bundle of His

9. A variation in heart rate during the breathing cycle is called:
   A. mitral valve prolapse
   B. fibrillation
   C. sinus dysrhythmia
   D. none of the above

10. Heart implants:
   A. allow patients to move around freely without external pumps
   B. are artificial hearts that are made of biologically inert synthetic materials
   C. still have limited use
   D. all of the above are true

Matching

Match each term in column A with its corresponding term in column B. (Only one answer is correct for each.)

Column A

_____ 11. Heart attack

_____ 12. QRS complex

_____ 13. Systole

_____ 14. Pulmonary circulation

_____ 15. Bicuspid

_____ 16. Heart compression

_____ 17. Heart muscle

_____ 18. Pacemaker

_____ 19. T wave

_____ 20. Chest pain

Column B

A. Sinoatrial node

B. Cardiac tamponade

C. Myocardium

D. Ventricular repolarization

E. Angina pectoris

F. Myocardial infarction

G. Ventricular depolarization

H. Ventricular contraction

I. Lungs

J. Mitral

Fill in the Blanks

21. The _____ _____ attach edges of the leaflets of the AV valves to fingerlike projections of cardiac muscle in the wall of the ventricles.

22. _____ _____ are valves that are narrower than normal, which causes a slower blood flow from a heart chamber.

23. Blood flows into the heart muscle by way of two small vessels—the right and left _____ _____ _____.

24. A common treatment for heart block is the surgical implantation of an _____ _____.

25. Cardiac output is determined mainly by the heart rate and _____ _____.

1. _____

2. _____

3. _____

4. _____

5. _____

6. _____

7. _____

8. _____

9. _____

10. _____

11. _____

12. _____

13. _____

14. _____

15. _____

16. _____

17. _____

18. _____

19. _____

1. _____   8. _____

2. _____   9. _____

3. _____   10. _____

4. _____   11. _____

5. _____   12. _____

6. _____   13. _____

7. _____

1. _____

2. _____

3. _____

15 Circulation of the Blood

One hundred thousand miles of blood vessels make up the elaborate transportation system that circulates materials needed for energy, growth, and repair and that also eliminates wastes from your body. These vessels, called *arteries*, *veins*, and *capillaries*, serve different functions. Arteries carry blood from the heart, veins carry blood to the heart, and capillaries are exchange vessels, or connecting links, between the arteries and veins. The pumping action of the heart keeps blood moving, or circulating, through this closed system of vessels. This system provides distribution of blood to the entire body (systemic circulation) and to specific regions such as the pulmonary circulation or hepatic portal circulation.

Blood pressure is the force of blood in the vessels. This force is highest in the arteries and lowest in the veins. Normal blood pressure varies among individuals and depends on the volume of blood in the arteries. The larger the volume of blood in the arteries, the more pressure is exerted on the walls of the arteries, and the higher the arterial pressure. Conversely, the less blood in the arteries, the lower the blood pressure.

A functional cardiovascular system is vital for survival because without circulation, tissues would lack a supply of oxygen and nutrients. Waste products would begin to accumulate and could become toxic. Your review of this system will provide you with an understanding of the complex transportation mechanism of the body necessary for survival.

TOPICS FOR REVIEW

Before progressing to Chapter 16, you should have an understanding of the structure and function of the blood vessels. Your review should include a study of systemic, pulmonary, hepatic portal, and fetal circulation and should conclude with a thorough understanding of blood pressure, pulse, and circulatory shock.

BLOOD VESSELS

Match each term on the left with its corresponding description on the right.

_____ 1. Arteries   A. Smooth muscle cells that guard the entrance to capillaries

_____ 2. Veins   B. Carry blood to the heart

_____ 3. Capillaries   C. Function as exchange vessels

_____ 4. Tunica externa   D. Carry blood away from the heart

_____ 5. Precapillary sphincters   E. Largest vein

_____ 6. Superior vena cava   F. Carries blood out of the left ventricle

_____ 7. Aorta   G. Outermost layer of arteries and veins

If you had difficulty with this section, review pages 404-406.

DISORDERS OF BLOOD VESSELS

Match each definition on the left with its corresponding term on the right.

_____ 8. Hardening of the arteries

_____ 9. Decreased blood supply to a tissue

_____ 10. Tissue death

_____ 11. Necrosis that has progressed to decay

_____ 12. A type of arteriosclerosis caused by lipids

_____ 13. A section of an artery that has become abnormally widened

_____ 14. Varicose veins in the rectum

_____ 15. Vein inflammation

_____ 16. Clot formation

_____ 17. Cerebral vascular accident

A. Atherosclerosis

B. Ischemia

C. Aneurysm

D. Necrosis

E. Gangrene

F. Hemorrhoids

G. Phlebitis

H. Stroke

I. Arteriosclerosis

J. Thrombus

If you had difficulty with this section, review pages 406-408.

ROUTES OF CIRCULATION

Circle the correct answer.

18. The aorta carries blood out of the:
    A. right atrium
    B. left atrium
    C. right ventricle
    D. left ventricle
    E. none of the above

19. The superior vena cava returns blood to the:
    A. left atrium
    B. left ventricle
    C. right atrium
    D. right ventricle
    E. none of the above

20. The _____ function as exchange vessels.
    A. venules
    B. capillaries
    C. arteries
    D. arterioles
    E. veins

21. Blood returns from the lungs during pulmonary circulation via the:
    A. pulmonary artery
    B. pulmonary veins
    C. aorta
    D. inferior vena cava

22. The hepatic portal circulation serves the body by:
    A. removing excess glucose and storing it in the liver as glycogen
    B. detoxifying blood
    C. assisting the body to maintain proper blood glucose balance
    D. all of the above

23. The structure used to bypass the liver in the fetal circulation is the:
    A. foramen ovale
    B. ductus venosus
    C. ductus arteriosus
    D. umbilical vein

24. The foramen ovale serves the fetal circulation by:
    A. connecting the aorta and the pulmonary artery
    B. shunting blood from the right atrium directly into the left atrium
    C. bypassing the liver
    D. bypassing the lungs

25. The structure used to connect the aorta and pulmonary artery in the fetal circulation is the:
    A. ductus arteriosus
    B. ductus venosus
    C. aorta
    D. foramen ovale

26. Which of the following is *not* an artery?
    A. Femoral
    B. Popliteal
    C. Coronary
    D. Inferior vena cava

If you had difficulty with this section, review pages 408-413.

HEMODYNAMICS

BLOOD PRESSURE

PULSE

True or False

If the statement is true, write "T" in the answer blank. If the statement is false, correct the statement by circling the incorrect term and writing the correct term in the answer blank.

_____ 27. Blood pressure is highest in the veins and lowest in the arteries.

_____ 28. The difference between two blood pressures is referred to as *blood pressure deficit*.

_____ 29. If the blood pressure in the arteries were to decrease so that it became equal to the average pressure in the arterioles, circulation would increase.

_____ 30. A stroke is often the result of low blood pressure.

_____ 31. Massive hemorrhage increases blood pressure.

_____ 32. Blood pressure is the volume of blood in the vessels.

_____ 33. Both the strength and the rate of heartbeat affect cardiac output and blood pressure.

_____ 34. The diameter of the arterioles helps determine how much blood drains out of arteries into arterioles.

_____ 35. A stronger heartbeat tends to decrease blood pressure, and a weaker heartbeat tends to increase it.

_____ 36. The systolic pressure is the maximum arterial pressure during each cardiac cycle.

_____ 37. If blood becomes less viscous than normal, blood pressure increases.

_____ 38. A device called a *sphygmomanometer* is used to measure blood pressures in clinical situations.

_____ 39. Loud, tapping Korotkoff sounds suddenly begin when the cuff pressure measured by the mercury column equals the systolic pressure.

_____ 40. The venous blood pressure within the left atrium is called the *central venous pressure*.

_____ 41. The pulse is a vein expanding and then recoiling.

_____ 42. The radial artery is located at the wrist.

_____ 43. The common carotid artery is located in the neck along the front edge of the sternocleido-mastoid muscle.

_____ 44. The artery located at the bend of the elbow that is used for locating the pulse is the dorsalis pedis.

If you had difficulty with this section, review pages 414-419.

Fill in the blanks.

45. Complications of septicemia may result in _____ _____

_____.

46. _____ _____ results from any type of heart failure.

47. An acute type of allergic reaction called _____ results in _____

_____ _____.

48. _____ _____ results from widespread dilation of blood vessels caused by an imbalance in autonomic stimulation of smooth muscles in vessel walls.

49. *Hypovolemia* means "_____ _____

_____."

50. A type of septic shock that results from staphylococcal infections that begin in the vagina of menstruating women and spread to the blood is _____ _____

_____.

If you had difficulty with this section, review page 421.

UNSCRAMBLE THE WORDS

51. **STMESYCI**

⬜◯⬜◯⬜⬜⬜⬜

52. **NULVEE**

◯⬜⬜⬜◯⬜

53. **RYTREA**

⬜⬜⬜◯⬜⬜

54. **USLEP**

⬜⬜◯⬜⬜

Take the circled letters, unscramble them, and fill in the solution.

How Noah survived the flood.

55. ⬜⬜⬜⬜⬜⬜⬜

56. Caryl is enjoying a picnic lunch when a bee suddenly flies down and stings her. Within seconds, Caryl begins to experience difficulty breathing, tachycardia, a decrease in blood pressure, and cyanosis. What is Caryl experiencing?

57. Wilson is scheduled to undergo extensive surgery. His surgeon, Dr. Berger, requests that 2 units of blood be available for Wilson should he require them. What complication of surgery is Dr. Berger hoping to avoid?

58. Rochelle is a hairstylist who works long hours. Lately she has noticed that her feet are sore and edematous. What might be the cause of these symptoms? What advice could offer Rochelle some relief from these symptoms?

59. Rubin returned from surgery in stable condition. The nurse noted that each time she took Rubin's pulse and blood pressure, the pulse was higher and the blood pressure lower than the last time. What might be the cause?

60. Word Find

Find and circle 15 terms presented in this chapter. Words may be spelled top to bottom, bottom to top, right to left, left to right, or diagonally.

Angina pectoris	Pulse
Apex	Semilunar
Atrium	Systemic
Depolarization	Thrombosis
Diastolic	Tricuspid
ECG	Umbilical
Endocardium	Venule
Hepatic portal	

```
Y  H  Y  S  I  S  O  B  M  O  R  H  T  A  R
L  A  C  I  L  I  B  M  U  O  A  Y  N  I  Y
E  E  S  Y  S  T  E  M  I  C  C  G  D  E  U
M  V  E  N  U  L  E  D  D  C  I  X  M  D  I
E  Y  M  U  I  R  T  A  R  N  L  E  C  G  Y
N  O  I  T  A  Z  I  R  A  L  O  P  E  D  N
U  D  L  A  T  R  O  P  C  I  T  A  P  E  H
S  I  U  K  M  U  E  T  O  E  S  L  U  P  U
R  P  N  F  Y  C  B  E  D  R  A  L  Z  P  J
D  S  A  H  T  I  T  V  N  L  I  I  B  D  W
Q  U  R  O  I  V  A  Q  E  O  D  A  K  R  K
K  C  R  M  P  G  A  I  G  N  D  D  Z  Y  J
Y  I  Y  R  I  N  E  A  F  Z  L  Q  S  P  X
S  R  M  I  C  C  Q  O  A  W  U  N  H  O  K
P  T  A  V  H  H  Z  L  H  I  J  J  X  K  Z
```

True or False

Indicate in the blank space if the literal translation is true or false for the medical term.

61. _____ Placenta means "flat cake."

62. _____ Tunica intima means "innermost coat."

63. _____ Aneurysm means "rupture."

64. _____ Gangrene means "black stump."

65. _____ Hemorrhoid means "vessel tightening."

66. _____ Necrosis means "death condition."

67. _____ Phlebitis means "vein inflammation."

68. _____ Sphygmomanometer means "a thin pulse measure."

69. _____ Varices means "swollen arteries."

70. _____ Septic shock means "relating to a putrid jolt."

If you had difficulty with this section, review pages 422-423.

DID YOU KNOW?

- Every pound of excess fat contains 200 miles of additional capillaries.
- If laid out in a straight line, the average adult's circulatory system would be nearly 60,000 miles long—enough to circle the earth 2.5 times!

CIRCULATION OF THE BLOOD

Fill in the crossword puzzle.

ACROSS

2. Inflammation of the lining of the heart
3. Bicuspid valve (two words)
5. Inner layer of pericardium
7. Cardiopulmonary resuscitation (abbreviation)
10. Carries blood away from the heart
11. Upper chamber of the heart
12. Lower chambers of the heart
13. SA node

DOWN

1. Unique blood circulation through the liver (two words)
3. Muscular layer of the heart
4. Carries blood to the heart
6. Tiny artery
8. Heart rate
9. Carries blood from arterioles into venules

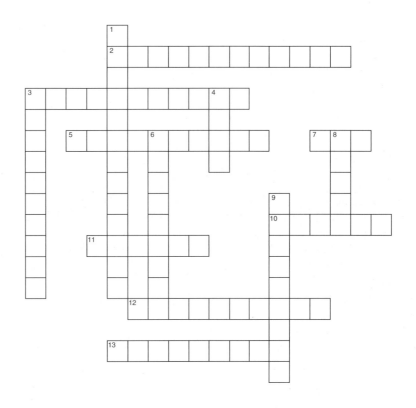

CHECK YOUR KNOWLEDGE

Multiple Choice
Circle the correct answer.

1. The medical term for high blood pressure is:
   A. arteriosclerosis
   B. cyanosis
   C. hypertension
   D. central venous pressure

2. Septic shock is caused by:
   A. complications of toxins in the blood
   B. a nerve condition
   C. a drop in blood pressure
   D. blood vessel dilation

3. Hypovolemic shock is caused by:
   A. heart failure
   B. dilated blood vessels
   C. a drop in blood volume
   D. a severe allergic reaction

4. Which vessels collect blood from the capillaries and return it to the heart?
   A. Arteries
   B. Sinuses
   C. Veins
   D. Arterioles

5. The innermost coat of an artery that comes into direct contact with blood is called the:
   A. lumen
   B. tunica externa
   C. tunica intima
   D. tunica media

6. Hemorrhoids can best be described as:
   A. varicose veins
   B. varicose veins in the rectum
   C. thrombophlebitis of the rectum
   D. clot formation in the rectum

7. In the fetal circulation:
   A. the ductus venosus allows most blood from the placenta to bypass the fetal liver
   B. the umbilical vein carries oxygen-poor blood
   C. the foramen ovale connects the aorta and the pulmonary artery
   D. none of the above is true

8. Which of the following events, if any, would *not* cause the blood pressure to increase?
   A. Hemorrhaging
   B. Increasing the viscosity of the blood
   C. Increasing the strength of the heartbeat
   D. All of the above

9. Arteriosclerosis is a disorder of the:
   A. heart
   B. veins
   C. capillaries
   D. arteries

10. A common type of vascular disease that occludes arteries by lipids and other matter is:
    A. arteriosclerotic plaque
    B. atherosclerosis
    C. varicose veins
    D. thrombophlebitis

Matching

Match each description in column A with its corresponding term in column B. (There is only one correct answer for each item.)

Column A

_____ 11. Main artery

_____ 12. Decreased blood supply

_____ 13. Leg vein

_____ 14. Fetal circulation

_____ 15. Arterial procedure

_____ 16. Vein inflammation

_____ 17. Lung circulation

_____ 18. Weakened artery

_____ 19. Largest vein

_____ 20. Myocardial infarction

Column B

A. Ischemia

B. Phlebitis

C. Foramen ovale

D. Aneurysm

E. Vena cava

F. Angioplasty

G. Aorta

H. Pulmonary

I. Great saphenous vein

J. Cardiogenic shock

Fill in the Blanks

21. The term _____ refers to the set of processes that influence the flow of blood.

22. The largest veins, often called _____, are the superior vena cava and the inferior vena cava.

23. There are two small umbilical _____ and a single, much larger umbilical

    _____.

24. The minimum arterial pressure during each cardiac cycle is known as the _____

    _____ _____.

25. Blood pressure is highest in the _____ and lowest in the _____

    _____.

FETAL CIRCULATION

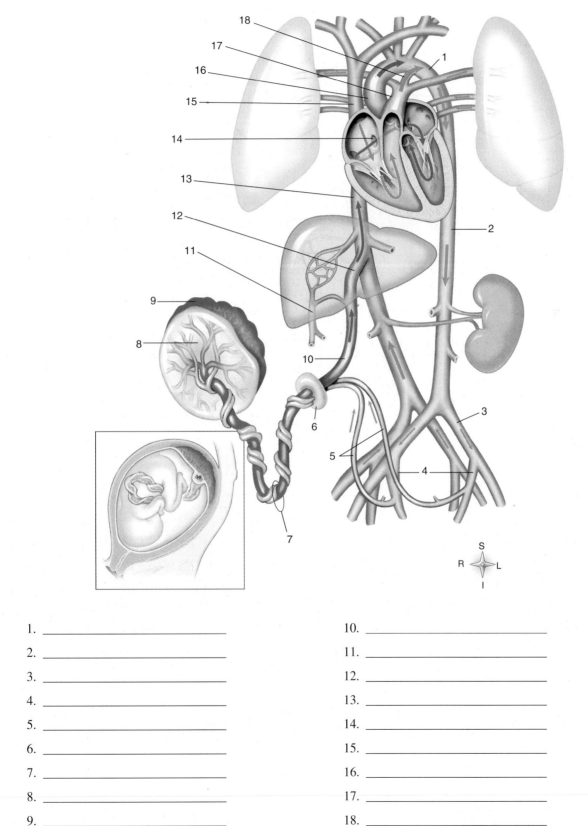

1. _____

2. _____

3. _____

4. _____

5. _____

6. _____

7. _____

8. _____

9. _____

10. _____

11. _____

12. _____

13. _____

14. _____

15. _____

16. _____

17. _____

18. _____

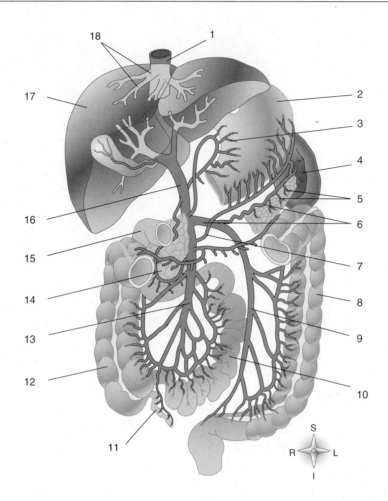

1. _____

2. _____

3. _____

4. _____

5. _____

6. _____

7. _____

8. _____

9. _____

10. _____

11. _____

12. _____

13. _____

14. _____

15. _____

16. _____

17. _____

18. _____

PRINCIPAL ARTERIES OF THE BODY

1. _____
2. _____
3. _____
4. _____
5. _____
6. _____
7. _____
8. _____
9. _____
10. _____
11. _____
12. _____
13. _____
14. _____
15. _____
16. _____
17. _____
18. _____
19. _____
20. _____
21. _____
22. _____
23. _____
24. _____
25. _____
26. _____
27. _____
28. _____
29. _____
30. _____

PRINCIPAL VEINS OF THE BODY

1. _____
2. _____
3. _____
4. _____
5. _____
6. _____
7. _____
8. _____
9. _____
10. _____
11. _____
12. _____
13. _____
14. _____
15. _____
16. _____
17. _____
18. _____
19. _____
20. _____
21. _____
22. _____
23. _____
24. _____
25. _____
26. _____
27. _____
28. _____
29. _____
30. _____
31. _____
32. _____
33. _____
34. _____
35. _____
36. _____
37. _____
38. _____

16 Lymphatic System and Immunity

The lymphatic system is similar to the circulatory system. Lymph, like blood, flows through an elaborate route of vessels. In addition to lymphatic vessels, the lymphatic system consists of lymph nodes, lymph, the thymus, tonsils, and the spleen. Unlike the circulatory system, the lymphatic vessels do not form a closed circuit. Lymph flows only once through the vessels before draining into the general blood circulation. This system is a filtering mechanism for microorganisms and serves as a protective device against foreign invaders such as cancer.

The immune system is the armed forces division of the body. Ready to attack at a moment's notice, the immune system defends us against the major enemies of the body: microorganisms, foreign transplanted tissue cells, and our own cells that have turned malignant.

The most numerous cells of the immune system are the lymphocytes. These cells circulate in the body's fluids, seeking invading organisms and destroying them with powerful lymphotoxins, lymphokines, or antibodies.

Phagocytes, another large group of immune system cells, assist with the destruction of foreign invaders by a process known as *phagocytosis*. Neutrophils, monocytes, and connective tissue cells called *macrophages* use this process to surround unwanted microorganisms and ingest and digest them, rendering them harmless to the body.

Another weapon that the immune system possesses is complement. Normally a group of inactive enzymes present in the blood, complement can be activated to kill invading cells by drilling holes in their cytoplasmic membranes, which allows fluid to enter the cell until it bursts.

Your review of this chapter will give you an understanding of how the body defends itself from the daily invasion of destructive substances.

TOPICS FOR REVIEW

Before progressing to Chapter 17, you should familiarize yourself with the functions of the lymphatic system, the immune system, and the major structures that make up these systems. Your review should include knowledge of lymphatic vessels, lymph nodes, lymph, lymphatic organs and tissues, antibodies, complement, and the development of B and T cells. Your study should also include the differences in humoral and cell-mediated immunity. Finally, an understanding of the excessive responses of the immune system and immune system deficiencies is necessary to complete your review of this chapter.

THE LYMPHATIC SYSTEM

Fill in the blanks.

1. _____ is a specialized fluid formed in the tissue spaces that will be transported by way of specialized vessels to eventually reenter the circulatory system.

2. Blood plasma that has filtered out of capillaries into microscopic spaces between cells is called _____

   _____ _____.

3. Tiny blind-ended tubes distributed in the tissue spaces are called _____

   _____.

4. Lymph eventually empties into two terminal vessels called the _____

   _____ _____ and the _____

   _____ _____.

5. The thoracic duct has an enlarged pouchlike structure called the _____ _____

   _____.

6. Lymph is filtered by moving through _____ _____

   _____, which are located in clusters along the pathway of lymphatic vessels.

7. Lymph enters the node through one or more _____ lymph vessels.

169

8. Lymph exits the node through one or more _____ lymph vessels.

9. An abnormal condition in which tissues exhibit edema because of the accumulation of lymph is _____ _____.

10. Swelling and tenderness of the lymph nodes is known as _____.

If you had difficulty with this section, review pages 430-433.

THYMUS _____

TONSILS _____

SPLEEN _____

Match each numbered description to one of the lymphatic system structures. Write the corresponding letter in the answer blank.

A. Thymus   B. Tonsils   C. Spleen

_____ 11. Palatine, pharyngeal, and lingual are examples

_____ 12. The largest lymphoid organ in the body

_____ 13. Destroys worn-out red blood cells

_____ 14. Located in the mediastinum

_____ 15. Serves as a reservoir for blood

_____ 16. T lymphocytes

_____ 17. Largest at puberty

If you had difficulty with this section, review pages 434-435.

THE IMMUNE SYSTEM _____

Match each term on the left with its corresponding description on the right.

_____ 18. Nonspecific immunity   A. Innate immunity

_____ 19. Phagocytes   B. Acquired immunity

_____ 20. Specific immunity   C. General protection

_____ 21. Lymphocytes   D. Artificial active immunity

_____ 22. Immunization   E. Memory

IMMUNE SYSTEM MOLECULES

Match each description with its related term. Write the corresponding letter in the answer blank.

_____ 23. A type of very specific antibody produced from a population of identical cells

_____ 24. Protein compounds normally present in the body

_____ 25. Also known as *antibody-mediated immunity*

_____ 26. Combines with antibody to produce humoral immunity

_____ 27. Antibody

_____ 28. The process of changing antibody molecule shape slightly to expose binding sites

_____ 29. Chemicals released from cells to act as direct agents of innate, nonspecific immunity

_____ 30. Inactive proteins in blood

A. Antibodies

B. Antigen

C. Monoclonal

D. Complement cascade

E. Complement

F. Humoral

G. Combining site

H. Cytokines

If you had difficulty with this section, review pages 436-440.

IMMUNE SYSTEM CELLS

Circle the correct answer.

31. The most numerous cells of the immune system are the:
    A. monocytes
    B. eosinophils
    C. neutrophils
    D. lymphocytes
    E. complement

32. The second stage of B-cell development changes a mature inactive B cell into a/an:
    A. plasma cell
    B. stem cell
    C. antibody
    D. activated B cell
    E. immature B cell

33. Which one of the following is activated last in the immune process?
    A. Plasma cells
    B. Stem cells
    C. Antibodies
    D. Activated B cells
    E. Immature B cells

34. Which one of the following is part of the cell membrane of B cells?
    A. Complement
    B. Antigens
    C. Antibodies
    D. Epitopes
    E. None of the above

35. Immature B cells have:
    A. four types of defense mechanisms on their cell membrane
    B. several kinds of defense mechanisms on their cell membrane
    C. one specific kind of defense mechanism on their cell membrane
    D. no defense mechanisms on their cell membrane

36. Development of an active B cell depends on the B cell coming in contact with:
    A. complement
    B. antibodies
    C. lymphotoxins
    D. lymphokines
    E. antigens

37. The kind of cell that produces large numbers of antibodies is the:
    A. B cell
    B. stem cell
    C. T cell
    D. memory cell
    E. plasma cell

38. Just one of these short-lived cells that make antibodies can produce _____ of them per second.
    A. 20
    B. 200
    C. 2,000
    D. 20,000

39. Which of the following statements is *not* true of memory cells?
A. They can secrete antibodies
B. They are found in lymph nodes
C. They develop into plasma cells
D. They can react with antigens
E. All of the above are true of memory cells

40. T-cell development begins in the:
A. lymph nodes
B. liver
C. pancreas
D. spleen
E. thymus

41. B cells function indirectly to produce:
A. humoral immunity
B. cell-mediated immunity
C. lymphotoxins
D. lymphokines

42. T cells function to produce:
A. humoral immunity
B. cell-mediated immunity
C. antibodies
D. memory cells

If you had difficulty with this section, review pages 441-443.

HYPERSENSITIVITY OF THE IMMUNE SYSTEM

Circle the correct answer.

43. The term *allergy* is used to describe (*hypersensitivity* or *hyposensitivity*) of the immune system to relatively harmless environmental antigens.

44. Antigens that trigger an allergic response are often called (*antibodies* or *allergens*).

45. (*Anaphylactic shock* or *Urticaria*) is a life-threatening condition.

46. A common autoimmune disease is (*lupus* or *SCID*).

47. Erythroblastosis fetalis is an example of (*isoimmunity* or *autoimmunity*).

48. The antigens most commonly involved in transplant rejection are called (*SCIDs* or *HLAs*).

If you had difficulty with this section, review pages 445-447.

IMMUNE DEFICIENCY

Match each condition with its origin. Write the corresponding letter in the answer blank.

A. Congenital   B. Acquired (after birth)

_____ 49. AIDS

_____ 50. SCID

_____ 51. Improper B-cell development

_____ 52. Viral infection

_____ 53. Genetic defect

If you had difficulty with this section, review pages 447-448.

UNSCRAMBLE THE WORDS

54. **N T C M P E O L E M**

▢⚪▢⚪▢⚪▢▢

55. **M T M Y I U N I**

▢⚪▢▢▢▢⚪▢

56. **O E N C L S**

⚪⚪▢▢▢⚪

57. **F N R O E R T E N I**

▢▢▢▢⚪▢⚪▢▢⚪

Take the circled letters, unscramble them, and fill in the solution.

What the student was praying for the night before exams.

58. ▢▢▢▢▢▢   ▢▢▢▢▢

APPLYING WHAT YOU KNOW

59. Two-year-old baby Metcalfe was exposed to chickenpox and subsequently developed the disease. What type of immunity will be developed as a result of this?

60. Marcia was an intravenous drug user. She has developed a type of skin cancer known as Kaposi sarcoma. What is Marcia's probable primary diagnosis?

61. Baby Wilson is born without a thymus gland. Immediate plans are made for a transplant to be performed. In the meantime, baby Wilson is placed in strict isolation. For what reason is he placed in isolation?

62. Word Find

Find and circle 14 terms presented in this chapter. Words may be spelled top to bottom, bottom to top, right to left, left to right, or diagonally.

Acquired	Lymphocytes
Antigen	Macrophage
Humoral	Monoclonal
Immunity	Proteins
Inflammatory	Spleen
Interferon	Thymus
Lymph	Tonsils

```
I N F L A M M A T O R Y F C G
Q N L O Y Z O C C P A O F S X
M W T A A M N J X Q K R N P H
U R L E R M P X B R U I A L C
C M A C R O P H A G E I E D Z
X M N D K F M N O T U C R N M
A E O R E Z E U O C F B Y E B
Y P L E B G G R H T Y T S E D
Y S C R I S P J O E I T M L A
Z M O T J X E T O N A E E P X
T O N S I L S S U M Y H T S Y
W A O C J N I M W K O Z E N D
D W M K W R M O I P S H Y B G
F H W U J I Z F V D Z L Y T X
```

KNOW YOUR MEDICAL TERMS

Provide the literal translation for the following words.

63. Cisterna chyli _____

64. Clone _____

65. Efferent _____

66. Lacteal _____

67. Thymus _____

68. Adenoid _____

69. Hypersensitivity _____

70. Lymphedema _____

71. Vaccine _____

72. Tonsillitis _____

If you had difficulty with this section, review pages 449-450.

DID YOU KNOW?

■ In the United States, the HIV infection rate is increasing 4 times faster in women than in men. Women tend to underestimate their risk.
■ Ten percent of all HIV/AIDS cases are individuals 50 years of age and older.
■ Every square inch of the human body has an average of 32 million bacteria on it.

Fill in the crossword puzzle.

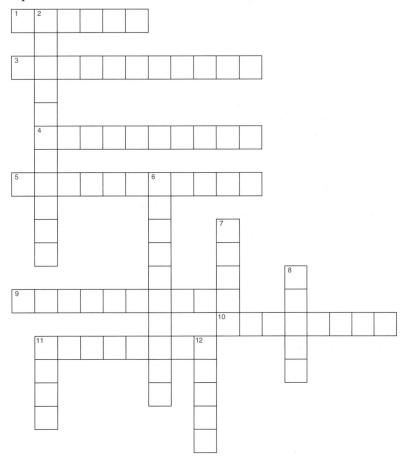

ACROSS

1. Largest lymphoid organ in the body
3. Connective tissue cells that are phagocytes
4. Protein compounds normally present in the body
5. Remain in reserve, then turn into plasma cells when needed (two words)
9. Synthetically produced to fight certain diseases
10. Lymph exits the node through this lymph vessel

11. Lymph enters the node through these lymph vessels

DOWN

2. Secretes a copious amount of antibodies into the blood (two words)
6. Inactive proteins
7. Family of identical cells descended from one cell
8. Type of lymphocyte (humoral immunity—two words)
11. Immune deficiency disorder

12. Type of lymphocyte (cell-mediated immunity—two words)

Multiple Choice

Circle the correct answer.

1. T cells do which of the following?
   A. Develop in the thymus
   B. Form memory cells
   C. Form plasma cells
   D. All of the above

2. Lymph does which of the following?
   A. Forms as blood plasma filters out of capillaries
   B. Empties into the heart
   C. Flows through lymphatic arteries
   D. All of the above

3. Acquired immune deficiency syndrome is characterized by which of the following?
   A. Caused by a retrovirus
   B. Causes inadequate T-cell formation
   C. Can result in death from cancer or infection
   D. All of the above

4. Interferon is:
   A. produced by B cells
   B. a protein compound that protects other cells by interfering with the ability of a virus to reproduce
   C. a group of inactive enzyme proteins normally present in blood
   D. all of the above

5. B cells do which of the following?
   A. Develop into plasma cells and memory cells
   B. Establish humoral immunity
   C. Develop from primitive cells in bone marrow called *stem cells*
   D. All of the above

6. Which of the following functions to kill invading cells by drilling a hole in the plasma membrane?
   A. Interferon
   B. Complement cascade
   C. Antibody
   D. Memory cell

7. Which of the following cell types function in the immune system?
   A. Macrophages
   B. Lymphocytes
   C. T cells
   D. All of the above

8. Which of the following is an example of phagocytes?
   A. Dendritic cells
   B. Neutrophils
   C. Macrophages
   D. All of the above

9. What is a rapidly growing population of identical cells that produce large quantities of specific antibodies called?
   A. Complementary
   B. Lymphotoxic
   C. Chemotactic
   D. Monoclonal

10. Which of the following is a form of passive natural immunity?
    A. A child develops measles and acquires an immunity to subsequent infection
    B. Antibodies are injected into an infected individual
    C. An infant receives protection through its mother's milk
    D. Vaccinations are given against smallpox

Matching

Match each of the terms in column A with its corresponding description in column B. (Only one answer is correct for each.)

Column A	Column B
_____ 11. Adenoids	A. Thoracic duct
_____ 12. B cell	B. Lymph node
_____ 13. Clone	C. Artificial immunity
_____ 14. HIV virus	D. Humoral immunity
_____ 15. Complement	E. Pharyngeal tonsils
_____ 16. Filtration	F. Shaped to combine with an antibody
_____ 17. Cisterna chyli	G. Inactive proteins
_____ 18. T cell	H. AIDS
_____ 19. Vaccination	I. Identical cells
_____ 20. Antigen	J. Cell-mediated immunity

Fill in the Blanks

21. _____ is caused by small parasitic worms that infest the lymphatic vessels and cause severe swelling.

22. Lymph exits lymph nodes through _____ lymphatic vessels.

23. A group of hormones, secreted by the thymus, that influence the development of T cells are _____ _____.

24. Abnormal spleen enlargement is _____.

25. Innate immunity is also sometimes called _____.

PRINCIPAL ORGANS OF THE LYMPHATIC SYSTEM

1. _____

2. _____

3. _____

4. _____

5. _____

6. _____

7. _____

8. _____

9. _____

10. _____

11. _____

12. _____

13. _____

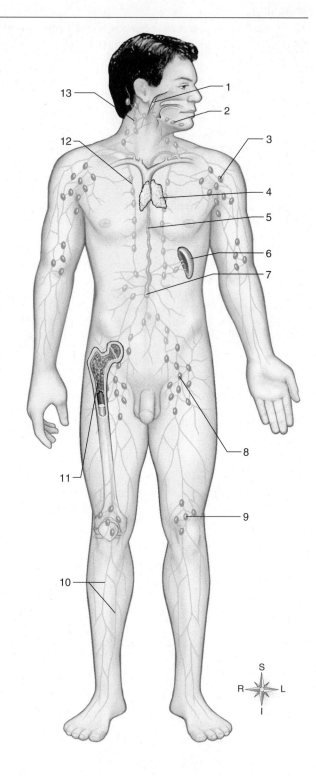

17 Respiratory System

As you sit reviewing this system, your body needs 16 quarts of air per minute. Walking requires 24 quarts of air, and running requires 50 quarts per minute. The respiratory system provides the air necessary for you to perform your daily activities and eliminates the waste gases from the air that you breathe. Take a deep breath, and think of the air as entering some 250 million tiny air sacs similar in appearance to clusters of grapes. These microscopic air sacs expand to let air in and contract to force it out. These tiny sacs, or alveoli, are the functioning units of the respiratory system. They provide the necessary volume of oxygen and eliminate carbon dioxide 24 hours a day.

Air enters either through the mouth or the nasal cavity. It next passes through the pharynx and past the epiglottis, and then through the glottis and the rest of the larynx. It then continues down the trachea, into the bronchi to the bronchioles, and finally through the alveoli. The reverse occurs for expelled air.

The exchange of gases between air in the lungs and in the blood is known as *external respiration*. The exchange of gases that occurs between the blood and the cells of the body is known as *internal respiration*. By constantly supplying adequate oxygen and removing carbon dioxide as it forms, the respiratory system helps maintain an environment conducive to maximum cell efficiency.

Your review of this system is necessary to provide you with an understanding of this essential homeostatic mechanism that supplies oxygen to our cells.

TOPICS FOR REVIEW

Before progressing to Chapter 18, you should have an understanding of the structure and function of the organs of the respiratory system. Your review should include knowledge of the mechanisms responsible for both internal and external respiration. Your study should conclude with a knowledge of the volumes of air exchanged in pulmonary ventilation, an understanding of how respiration is regulated, and the common disorders of the respiratory tract.

STRUCTURAL PLAN

RESPIRATORY TRACT

RESPIRATORY MUCOSA

Match each term with its definition. Write the corresponding letter in the answer blank.

_____	1. Function of respiratory system	A. Diffusion
_____	2. Pharynx	B. URI
_____	3. Passive transport process responsible for actual exchange of gases	C. Alveoli
_____	4. Assists with the movement of mucus toward the pharynx	D. Capillaries
_____	5. Head cold	E. Respiration
_____	6. Lines the tubes of the respiratory tree	F. Respiratory mucosa
_____	7. Terminal air sacs	G. Upper respiratory tract
_____	8. Trachea	H. Lower respiratory tract
_____	9. Surround alveoli	I. Cilia
_____	10. Homeostatic mechanism	J. Air distributor

Fill in the blanks.

The organs of the respiratory system are designed to perform two basic functions. They serve as an

(11) _____ _____ and as a (12) _____

_____ _____. In addition to the functions given

above, the respiratory system (13) _____, (14) _____

_____, and (15) _____ the air we breathe. Respiratory organs include the

(16) _____, (17) _____, (18) _____

_____, (19) _____, (20) _____

_____, and the (21) _____. The respiratory system ends in millions of

tiny, thin-walled sacs called (22) _____. (23) _____

_____ of gases takes place in these sacs. Two aspects of the structure of these sacs assist them in the exchange of

gases. First, an extremely thin tissue, the (24) _____ _____

_____, lines the alveoli where gas exchange takes place and allows for easy exchange. Second, the large

number of (25) _____ make an enormous surface area.

If you had difficulty with this section, review pages 459-461.

UPPER RESPIRATORY TRACT

NOSE

PHARYNX

LARYNX

DISORDERS OF UPPER RESPIRATORY TRACT

Circle the term in each word group that does not belong.

26. Nares	Septum	Oropharynx	Conchae
27. Conchae	Frontal	Maxillary	Sphenoidal
28. Oropharynx	Throat	5 inches	Epiglottis
29. Pharyngeal	Adenoids	Uvula	Nasopharynx
30. Middle ear	Tubes	Nasopharynx	Larynx
31. Voice box	Thyroid cartilage	Tonsils	Vocal cords
32. Palatine	Eustachian tube	Tonsils	Oropharynx
33. Pharynx	Epiglottis	Adam's apple	Voice box

Match each numbered term or phrase with the corresponding respiratory structure.

A. Nose   B. Pharynx   C. Larynx

_____ 34. Warms and humidifies air   _____ 40. Middle ear infections

_____ 35. Air and food pass through here   _____ 41. Epiglottis

_____ 36. Sinuses   _____ 42. Rhinitis

_____ 37. Conchae   _____ 43. Sore throat

_____ 38. Septum   _____ 44. Epistaxis

_____ 39. Tonsils

If you had difficulty with this section, review pages 462-466.

LOWER RESPIRATORY TRACT

TRACHEA

BRONCHI, BRONCHIOLES, AND ALVEOLI

LUNGS AND PLEURA

Fill in the blanks.

45. The windpipe is more properly referred to as the _____.

46. _____ ensure that the framework of the trachea is almost noncollapsible.

47. A life-saving technique designed to free the trachea of ingested food or foreign objects is the _____ _____ _____ _____.

48. The first branch or division of the trachea leading to the lungs is the _____ _____.

49. Each alveolar duct ends in several _____ _____.

50. The narrow part of each lung, up under the collarbone, is its _____.

51. The _____ covers the outer surface of the lungs and lines the inner surface of the rib cage.

52. Inflammation of the lining of the thoracic cavity is _____.

53. The presence of air in the pleural space on one side of the chest is a _____.

If you had difficulty with this section, review pages 466-470.

DISORDERS OF THE LOWER RESPIRATORY TRACT

Fill in the blanks.

54. _____ is an acute inflammation of the lungs in which the alveoli and bronchi become plugged with thick fluid.

55. _____ is still a major cause of death in many poor, densely populated regions of the world. It has recently reemerged as an important health problem in some major U.S. cities.

56. _____ may result from the progression of chronic bronchitis or other conditions as air becomes trapped within alveoli, causing them to enlarge and eventually rupture.

57. _____ is an obstructive disorder characterized by recurring spasms of the smooth muscle in the walls of the bronchial air passages.

If you had difficulty with this section, review pages 470-472.

RESPIRATION

True or False

If the statement is true, write "T" in the answer blank. If the statement is false, correct the statement by circling the incorrect term and writing the correct term in the answer blank.

_____ 58. Diffusion is the process that moves air into and out of the lungs.

_____ 59. For inspiration to take place, the diaphragm and other respiratory muscles must relax.

_____ 60. Diffusion is a passive process that results in movement up a concentration gradient.

_____ 61. The exchange of gases that occurs between blood in tissue capillaries and the body cells is external respiration.

_____ 62. Many different pulmonary volumes can be measured by having a person breathe into a spirometer.

_____ 63. Ordinarily we take about 2 pints of air into our lungs with each breath.

_____ 64. The amount of air normally breathed in and out with each breath is called *tidal volume*.

_____ 65. The largest amount of air that one can breathe out in one expiration is called *residual volume*.

_____ 66. The inspiratory reserve volume is the amount of air that can be forcibly inhaled after a normal inspiration.

If you had difficulty with this section, review pages 473-475.

Circle the correct answer.

67. The term that means the same thing as breathing is:
    A. gas exchange
    B. respiration
    C. inspiration
    D. expiration
    E. pulmonary ventilation

68. Carbaminohemoglobin is formed when _____ bind(s) to hemoglobin.
    A. oxygen
    B. amino acids
    C. carbon dioxide
    D. nitrogen
    E. none of the above

69. Most of the oxygen transported by the blood is:
    A. dissolved into white blood cells
    B. bound to white blood cells
    C. bound to hemoglobin
    D. bound to carbaminohemoglobin
    E. none of the above

70. Which of the following does *not* occur during inspiration?
    A. Elevation of the ribs
    B. Elevation of the diaphragm
    C. Contraction of the diaphragm
    D. Elongation of the chest cavity from top to bottom

71. A young adult male would have a vital capacity of about _____ mL.
    A. 500
    B. 1,200
    C. 3,300
    D. 4,800
    E. 6,200

72. The amount of air that can be forcibly exhaled after expiring the tidal volume is known as the:
    A. total lung capacity
    B. vital capacity
    C. inspiratory reserve volume
    D. expiratory reserve volume
    E. none of the above

73. Which one of the following formulas is correct?
    A. VC = TV − IRV + ERV
    B. VC = TV + IRV − ERV
    C. VC = TV + IRV × ERV
    D. VC = TV + IRV + ERV
    E. None of the above

If you had difficulty with this section, review pages 473-475, and 481.

REGULATION OF RESPIRATION

BREATHING PATTERNS

Match each term on the left with the corresponding description on the right.

_____ 74. Respiratory control centers

_____ 75. Chemoreceptors

_____ 76. Pulmonary stretch receptors

_____ 77. Dyspnea

_____ 78. Respiratory arrest

_____ 79. Eupnea

_____ 80. Hypoventilation

A. Difficult breathing

B. Located in carotid bodies

C. Slow and shallow respirations

D. Normal respiratory rate

E. Located in the brainstem

F. Failure to resume breathing after a period of apnea

G. Located throughout pulmonary airways and in the alveoli

If you had difficulty with this section, review pages 475-478.

182

UNSCRAMBLE THE WORDS

81. **S P U E L I R Y**

   ☐☐☐☐☐☐☐ (with circles on positions 1, 4, 5)

82. **C R N B O S I T H I**

   ☐☐☐☐☐☐☐☐☐ (with circles on positions 3, 4, 6)

83. **S E S X P T I A I**

   ☐☐☐☐☐☐☐☐☐ (with circles on positions 4, 5, 7)

84. **D D N E A O I S**

   ☐☐☐☐☐☐☐ (with circles on positions 1, 3)

Take the circled letters, unscramble them, and fill in the solution.

What Mona Lisa was to DaVinci.

85. ☐☐☐☐☐☐☐☐☐☐☐☐☐

APPLYING WHAT YOU KNOW

86. Mr. Gorski is a heavy smoker. Recently he has noticed that when he gets up in the morning, he has a bothersome cough that brings up a large accumulation of mucus. This cough persists for several minutes and then leaves until the next morning. What is an explanation for this problem?

87. Penny is 5 years old and is a mouth breather. She has had repeated episodes of tonsillitis, and her pediatrician, Dr. Smith, has suggested removal of her tonsils and adenoids. He further suggests that the surgery will probably cure her mouth breathing problem. Why is this a possibility?

88. Mrs. McCue developed emphysema. This disease reduces the capacity of the lungs to recoil elastically. Which respiratory air volumes will this condition affect? Why?

DID YOU KNOW?

- If the alveoli in our lungs were flattened out, they would cover one-half of a tennis court.
- Eighty percent of lung cancer cases are due to cigarette smoking.
- Only about 10% of the air in the lungs is actually changed with each cycle of inhaling and exhaling when a person at rest is breathing. However, up to 80% can be exchanged during deep breathing or strenuous exercise.
- A person's nose and ears continue to grow throughout his or her life.

89. Word Find

Find and circle 14 terms presented in this chapter. Words may be spelled top to bottom, bottom to top, right to left, left to right, or diagonally.

Adenoids	Inspiration
Carotid body	Oxyhemoglobin
Cilia	Pulmonary
Diffusion	Residual volume
Dyspnea	Surfactant
Epiglottis	URI
Hypoventilation	Vital capacity

```
N  K  S  A  Q  B  I  L  V  A  D  T  I  X  D
O  X  O  O  B  F  I  F  G  I  M  N  R  G  Y
I  G  N  X  W  D  E  E  F  L  B  A  U  T  S
T  B  K  Y  N  H  E  F  O  I  U  T  I  R  P
A  T  M  H  E  O  U  T  R  C  C  C  P  V  N
L  L  A  E  P  S  I  R  I  Z  A  A  N  F  E
I  P  T  M  I  H  G  T  I  P  R  F  P  C  A
T  U  B  O  G  Q  E  V  A  Q  O  R  V  N  W
N  L  N  G  L  R  J  C  C  R  T  U  P  D  C
E  M  U  L  O  V  L  A  U  D  I  S  E  R  E
V  O  V  O  T  A  N  G  J  E  D  P  Z  U  U
O  N  K  B  T  C  N  U  U  E  B  O  S  J  S
P  A  L  I  I  K  E  U  C  N  O  Z  K  N  A
Y  R  V  N  S  D  I  O  N  E  D  A  M  F  I
H  Y  O  M  L  O  A  Z  D  T  Y  M  N  L  K
```

KNOW YOUR MEDICAL TERMS

Matching

Select the medical term with matching literal translation.

90. _____ Alveolus

91. _____ Diffusion

92. _____ Olfaction

93. _____ Apnea

94. _____ Epiglottis

95. _____ Asthma

96. _____ Sinus

97. _____ Pleura

98. _____ Epistaxis

99. _____ Rhinitis

100. _____ Emphysema

A. Upon/mouth of windpipe

B. Hollow

C. Spread out/process

D. Side of body

E. Panting

F. Hollow/little

G. Not/breathe/condition

H. Upon/drip

I. Smell/condition

J. Nose/inflammation

K. In/blowing or puffing up

If you had difficulty with this section, review pages 482-484.

RESPIRATORY SYSTEM

Fill in the crossword puzzle.

ACROSS

1. Device used to measure the amount of air exchanged in breathing
6. Expiratory reserve volume (abbreviation)
7. Sphenoidal (two words)
8. Terminal air sacs
9. Shelflike structures that protrude into the nasal cavity
11. Inflammation of pleura
12. Respirations stop

DOWN

2. Surgical procedure to remove tonsils
3. Doctor who developed life-saving technique
4. Windpipe
5. Trachea branches into right and left structures
10. Voice box

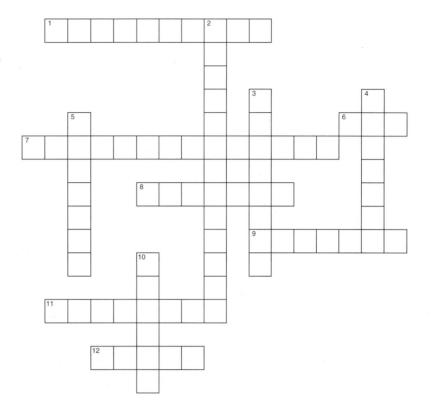

CHECK YOUR KNOWLEDGE

Multiple Choice

Circle the correct answer.

1. Chemoreceptors in the carotid and aortic bodies are characterized by which of the following?
   A. Sensitive to increases in blood carbon dioxide level
   B. Found in the brain
   C. Sensitive to increases in blood oxygen level
   D. Send impulses to the heart

2. What is the lowest segment of the pharynx called?
   A. Oropharynx
   B. Laryngopharynx
   C. Nasopharynx
   D. Hypopharynx

3. What is the narrow upper portion of a lung called?
   A. Base
   B. Notch
   C. Costal surface
   D. Apex

4. What is the largest amount of air that a person can breathe in and out in one inspiration and expiration called?
   A. Tidal volume
   B. Vital capacity
   C. Residual volume
   D. Inspiratory reserve volume

5. Which of the following statements, if any, is *not* characteristic of human lungs?
   A. Both right and left lungs are composed of three lobes
   B. Bronchi subdivide to form bronchioles
   C. Capillary supply is abundant to facilitate gas exchange
   D. All of the above statements are characteristic of human lungs

6. Which body function is made possible by the existence of fibrous bands stretched across the larynx?
   A. Swallowing
   B. Breathing
   C. Diffusion
   D. Speech

7. The trachea is almost noncollapsible because of the presence of which of the following?
   A. Rings of cartilage
   B. Thyroid cartilage
   C. Epiglottis
   D. Vocal cords

8. Which of the following is true of the exchange of respiratory gases between lungs and blood?
   A. It takes place by diffusion
   B. It is called *external respiration*
   C. Both A and B are true
   D. None of the above is true

9. When the diaphragm contracts, which phase of ventilation is taking place?
   A. External respiration
   B. Expiration
   C. Internal respiration
   D. Inspiration

10. Which of the following is *not* characteristic of the nasal cavities?
    A. They contain many blood vessels that warm incoming air
    B. They contain the adenoids
    C. They are lined with mucous membranes
    D. They are separated by a partition called the *nasal septum*

Matching

Match each term in column A with its corresponding term in column B. (Only one answer is correct for each.)

Column A	Column B
_____ 11. Vocal cords	A. Serous membrane
_____ 12. Pulmonary ventilation	B. Pharynx
_____ 13. Pleura	C. Paranasal sinus
_____ 14. Atelectasis	D. LVRS
_____ 15. Emphysema	E. Larynx
_____ 16. Throat	F. Diffusion
_____ 17. Ethmoidal	G. Collapsed lung
_____ 18. Windpipe	H. Trachea
_____ 19. Alveoli	I. Breathing
_____ 20. Surfactant	J. IRDS

Fill in the Blanks

21. The nasal conchae are sometimes called _____.

22. IRDS is a very serious, life-threatening condition that often affects newborns. It is caused by a lack of _____ _____.

23. The surgical removal of a lung is a _____.

24. Nerve impulses passing through both _____ nerves stimulate the diaphragm to contract.

25. _____ (RV) is simply the air that remains in the lungs after the most forceful expiration.

SAGITTAL VIEW OF FACE AND NECK

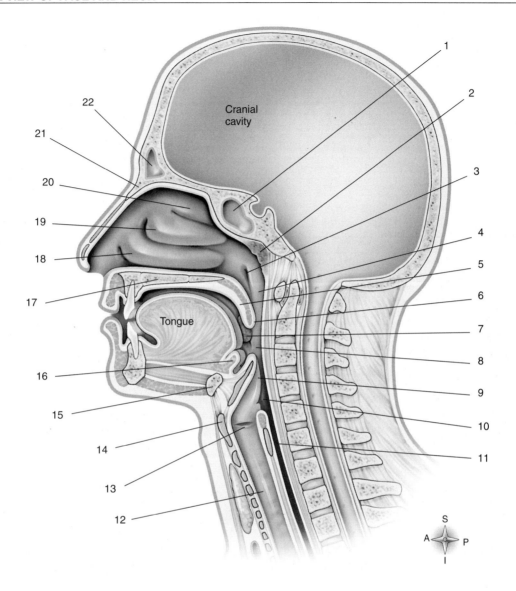

Cranial cavity

Tongue

S
A —✛— P
I

1. _____   12. _____
2. _____   13. _____
3. _____   14. _____
4. _____   15. _____
5. _____   16. _____
6. _____   17. _____
7. _____   18. _____
8. _____   19. _____
9. _____   20. _____
10. _____   21. _____
11. _____   22. _____

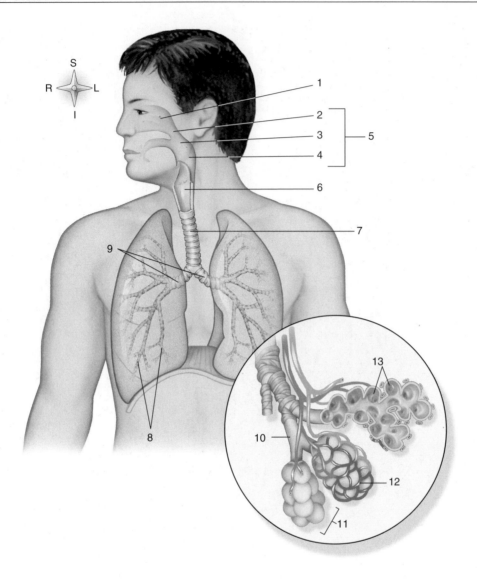

1. _____   8. _____

2. _____   9. _____

3. _____   10. _____

4. _____   11. _____

5. _____   12. _____

6. _____   13. _____

7. _____

PULMONARY VENTILATION VOLUMES

1. _____   4. _____

2. _____   5. _____

3. _____   6. _____

18 Digestive System

Think of the last meal you ate. Imagine the different shapes, sizes, tastes, and textures that you so recently enjoyed. Think of those items circulating in your bloodstream in those same original shapes, sizes, and textures. Impossible? Of course! Because of this impossibility, you can begin to understand and marvel at the close relationship of the digestive system to the circulatory system. It is the digestive system that changes our food, both mechanically and chemically, into a form that can be used by the blood and the body.

This change in food begins the moment you take the very first bite. Digestion starts in the mouth, where food is chewed and mixed with saliva. It then moves down the pharynx and esophagus by peristalsis and enters the stomach. In the stomach it is churned and mixed with gastric juices to become chyme. The chyme goes from the stomach into the duodenum, where it is further broken down chemically by intestinal fluids, bile, and pancreatic juice. Those secretions prepare the food for absorption all along the course of the small intestine. Products that are not absorbed pass on through the entire length of the small intestine (duodenum, jejunum, ileum). From there they enter into the cecum of the large intestine, continue on to the ascending colon, transverse colon, descending colon, and sigmoid colon, and finally into the rectum, and out the anus.

Products that are used in the cells undergo absorption. Absorption allows newly processed nutrients to pass through the walls of the digestive tract and into the bloodstream to be distributed to the cells.

Your review of this system will help you understand the mechanical and chemical processes necessary to convert food into energy sources and compounds necessary for survival.

TOPICS FOR REVIEW

Before progressing to Chapter 19, you should review the structure and function of all the organs of digestion. You should have an understanding of the process of digestion, both chemical and mechanical, and of the processes of absorption and metabolism.

THE DIGESTIVE SYSTEM

ORGANS OF THE DIGESTIVE SYSTEM

Fill in the blanks.

1. The organs of the digestive system form an irregular-shaped tube called the *alimentary canal* or, as it is often called,

   the _____ _____.

2. The churning of food in the stomach is an example of the _____ breakdown of food.

3. _____ breakdown occurs when digestive enzymes act on food as it passes

   through the digestive tract.

4. Waste material resulting from the digestive process is known as _____.

5. Foods undergo three kinds of processing in the body: _____, _____

   _____, and _____.

Identify which are main organs and which are accessory organs of the digestive system. Write the corresponding letter in the answer blank.

A. Main organ   B. Accessory organ

_____ 6. Mouth

_____ 7. Parotids

_____ 8. Liver

_____ 9. Stomach

_____ 10. Cecum

_____ 11. Esophagus

_____ 12. Rectum

_____ 13. Pharynx

_____ 14. Appendix

_____ 15. Teeth

_____ 16. Gallbladder

_____ 17. Pancreas

If you had difficulty with this section, review pages 493-494.

WALL OF DIGESTIVE TRACT

Fill in the blanks.

18. The serosa of the digestive tube is composed of the _____, _____ _____ in the abdominal cavity.

19. The digestive tract extends from the _____ to the _____ _____.

20. The inside or hollow space within the alimentary canal is called the _____.

21. The inside layer of the digestive tract is the _____.

22. The connective tissue layer that lies beneath the lining of the digestive tract is the _____ _____.

MOUTH

TEETH

SALIVARY GLANDS

Circle the correct answer.

23. Which one of the following is *not* a part of the roof of the mouth?
    A. Uvula
    B. Palatine bones
    C. Maxillary bones
    D. Soft palate
    E. All of the above are part of the roof of the mouth

24. The largest of the papillae on the surface of the tongue are the:
    A. filiform
    B. fungiform
    C. circumvallate
    D. taste buds

25. The first baby tooth, on average, appears at:
    A. 2 months
    B. 1 year
    C. 3 months
    D. 1 month
    E. 6 months

26. The portion of the tooth that is covered with enamel is the:
    A. pulp cavity
    B. neck
    C. root
    D. crown
    E. none of the above is correct

27. The wall of the pulp cavity is surrounded by:
    A. enamel
    B. dentin
    C. cementum
    D. connective tissue
    E. blood and lymphatic vessels

28. Which of the following teeth is missing from the deciduous arch?
    A. Central incisor
    B. Canine
    C. Second premolar
    D. First molar
    E. Second molar

191

29. The permanent central incisor erupts between the ages of:
    A. 9 and 13
    B. 5 and 6
    C. 7 and 10
    D. 7 and 8
    E. none of the above

30. The third molar appears between the ages of:
    A. 10 and 14
    B. 5 and 8
    C. 11 and 16
    D. 17 and 24
    E. none of the above

31. A general term for infection of the gums is:
    A. dental caries
    B. leukoplakia
    C. Vincent angina
    D. gingivitis

32. The ducts of the _____ glands open into the floor of the mouth.
    A. sublingual
    B. submandibular
    C. parotid
    D. carotid

33. The volume of saliva secreted per day is about:
    A. one-half pint
    B. one pint
    C. one liter
    D. one gallon

34. Thrush is:
    A. caused by a type of yeast
    B. seen sometimes by adults who are immunosup-pressed
    C. also known as oral candidiasis
    D. all of the above

35. Incisors are used during mastication to:
    A. cut
    B. pierce
    C. tear
    D. grind

36. Another name for the third molar is:
    A. central incisor
    B. wisdom tooth
    C. canine
    D. lateral incisor

37. After food has been chewed, it is formed into a small, rounded mass called a:
    A. moat
    B. chyme
    C. bolus
    D. protease

If you had difficulty with this section, review pages 495-501.

PHARYNX

ESOPHAGUS

STOMACH

Fill in the blanks.

The (38) _____ is a tubelike structure that functions as part of both the respiratory and digestive systems. It connects the mouth with the (39) _____. The pharynx is subdivided into three anatomical components: the (40)_____, the (41)_____, and the (42) _____.

The esophagus serves as a passageway for movement of food from the pharynx to the (43) _____. Food enters the stomach by passing through the muscular (44) _____, _____ at the end of the esophagus. Contraction of the stomach mixes the food thoroughly with the gastric juices and breaks it down into a semisolid mixture called (45) _____. The three divisions of the stomach are the (46) _____, (47) _____, and (48) _____. Food is held in the stomach by the (49) _____ muscle long enough for partial digestion to occur. After food has been in the stomach for approximately 3 hours, the chyme will enter the (50) _____ .

192

Match each term with its corresponding definition.

_____ 51. Stomach folds

_____ 52. Upper right border of stomach

_____ 53. Heartburn

_____ 54. 10-inch passageway

_____ 55. Vomiting

_____ 56. Semisolid mixture of stomach contents

_____ 57. Muscle contractions of the digestive system

_____ 58. Craterlike wound in the digestive system caused by tissue destruction

_____ 59. Stomach pushes through the gap in the diaphragm

_____ 60. Lower left border of stomach

A. Esophagus

B. Chyme

C. Peristalsis

D. Rugae

E. Ulcer

F. Greater curvature

G. Acid indigestion

H. Emesis

I. Hiatal hernia

J. Lesser curvature

If you had difficulty with this section, review pages 501-505.

SMALL INTESTINE

LIVER AND GALLBLADDER

PANCREAS

Circle the correct answer.

61. Which one is *not* part of the small intestine?
    A. Jejunum
    B. Ileum
    C. Cecum
    D. Duodenum

62. Which one of the following structures does *not* increase the surface area of the intestine for absorption?
    A. Plicae
    B. Rugae
    C. Villi
    D. Brush border

63. The union of the cystic duct and hepatic duct forms the:
    A. common bile duct
    B. major duodenal papilla
    C. minor duodenal papilla
    D. pancreatic duct

64. Obstruction of the _____ will lead to jaundice.
    A. hepatic duct
    B. pancreatic duct
    C. cystic duct
    D. none of the above

65. Bile is responsible for the:
    A. final digestion of fats
    B. emulsification of fats
    C. chemical breakdown of fats
    D. chemical breakdown of cholesterol

66. The middle third of the duodenum contains the:
    A. islets
    B. fundus
    C. body
    D. rugae
    E. major duodenal papilla

67. *Cholelithiasis* is the term used to describe:
    A. biliary colic
    B. jaundice
    C. portal hypertension
    D. gallstones

68. The liver is an:
    A. enzyme
    B. endocrine organ
    C. endocrine gland
    D. exocrine gland

69. Fats in chyme stimulate the secretion of the hormone:
    A. lipase
    B. cholecystokinin
    C. protease
    D. amylase

70. The largest gland in the body is the:
    A. pituitary
    B. thyroid
    C. liver
    D. thymus

If you had difficulty with this section, review pages 506-509.

LARGE INTESTINE

APPENDIX

PERITONEUM

True or False

If the statement is true, write "T" in the answer blank. If the statement is false, correct the statement by circling the incorrect term and writing the correct term in the answer blank.

_____ 71. Bacteria in the large intestine are responsible for the synthesis of vitamin E needed for normal blood clotting.

_____ 72. Villi in the large intestine absorb salts and water.

_____ 73. If waste products pass rapidly through the large intestine, constipation results.

_____ 74. The ileocecal valve opens into the sigmoid colon.

_____ 75. The splenic flexure is the bend between the ascending colon and the transverse colon.

_____ 76. The splenic colon is the S-shaped segment that terminates in the rectum.

_____ 77. Appendicitis is the most common of the acute abdominal conditions that require surgery.

_____ 78. Appendicitis is more common in children and young adults because the lumen of the appendix is larger during that period, making it easier for food and fecal material to become trapped.

_____ 79. The visceral layer of the peritoneum lines the abdominal cavity.

_____ 80. The greater omentum is shaped like a fan and serves to anchor the small intestine to the posterior abdominal wall.

_____ 81. Diarrhea is an inflammation of abnormal saclike outpouchings of the intestinal wall.

_____ 82. Crohn disease is a type of autoimmune colitis.

_____ 83. A colostomy is a surgical procedure in which an artificial anus is created on the abdominal wall.

_____ 84. Peritonitis is the abnormal accumulation of fluid in the peritoneal space.

If you had difficulty with this section, review pages 512-516.

DIGESTION

ABSORPTION

Circle the correct answer.

85. Which one of the following substances does *not* contain any enzymes?
    A. Saliva
    B. Bile
    C. Gastric juice
    D. Pancreatic juice
    E. Intestinal juice

86. Which one of the following is a simple sugar?
    A. Maltose
    B. Sucrose
    C. Lactose
    D. Glucose
    E. Starch

194

87. Cane sugar is the same as:
    A. maltose
    B. lactose
    C. sucrose
    D. glucose
    E. none of the above

88. Most of the digestion of carbohydrates takes place in the:
    A. mouth
    B. stomach
    C. small intestine
    D. large intestine

89. Fats are broken down into:
    A. amino acids
    B. simple sugars
    C. fatty acids
    D. disaccharides

If you had difficulty with this section, review pages 518-519.

CHEMICAL DIGESTION

90. **Fill in the blank areas on the chart below.**

Digestive Juices and Enzymes	Substance Digested (or Hydrolyzed)	Resulting Product
Saliva		
1. Amylase	1.	1. Maltose
Gastric Juice		
2. Protease (pepsin) plus hydrochloric acid	2. Proteins	2.
Pancreatic Juice		
3. Protease (trypsin)	3. Proteins (intact or partially digested)	3.
4. Lipase	4.	4. Fatty acids, monoglycerides, and glycerol
5. Amylase	5.	5. Maltose
Intestinal Juice		
6. Peptidases	6.	6. Amino acids
7.	7. Sucrose	7. Glucose and fructose
8. Lactase	8.	8. Glucose and galactose (simple sugars)
9. Maltase	9. Maltose	9.

If you had difficulty with this section, review page 518.

UNSCRAMBLE THE WORDS

91. **SLBOU**

[ ][○][○][ ][ ]

92. **EYCHM**

[○][ ][ ][ ][○]

93. **LLAAPPI**

[ ][○][ ][ ][ ][ ][○]

94. **PMERTEUION**

[○][ ][○][ ][ ][○][ ][ ][ ][ ]

Take the circled letters, unscramble them, and fill in the solution.

What the groom gave his bride after the wedding.

95. [ ][ ][ ][ ] [ ][ ][ ][ ][ ]

APPLYING WHAT YOU KNOW

96. Mr. Amoto is a successful businessman, but he works too hard and is always under great stress. He takes high doses of aspirin, almost daily, to relieve his stress headaches. His doctor cautioned him that if he did not alter his style of living, he would be subject to hyperacidity. What could be a result of hyperacidity?

97. Baby Nicholas has been regurgitating his bottle feeding at every meal. The milk is curdled, but it does not appear to be digested. He has become dehydrated, so his mother, Bobbi, is taking him to the pediatrician. What would you guess is a possible diagnosis, based on what you have learned from your textbook reading?

98. Mr. Lynch has high cholesterol. In an effort to lower his cholesterol, he quickly lost 25 pounds by consuming an ultra-low-fat diet. Since then he has noticed a yellowish cast to his skin and has periodic pain in the right upper quadrant of the abdominopelvic region. What is a possible diagnosis for Mr. Lynch? What is the name of the surgical procedure that may be performed on Mr. Lynch?

99. Word Find

Find and circle 22 terms presented in this chapter. Words may be spelled top to bottom, bottom to top, right to left, left to right, or diagonally.

Absorption	Heartburn	
Appendix	Jaundice	
Cavity	Mastication	
Crown	Mesentery	
Dentin	Metabolism	
Diarrhea	Mucosa	
Digestion	Pancreas	
Duodenum	Papillae	
Emulsify	Peristalsis	
Feces	Stomach	
Fundus	Uvula	

```
X M E T A B O L I S M X X W
R S D P E R I S T A L S I S
E V A M N O I T S E G I D R
E D E E U O Q T W Q O H N Q
Q Z H S R N I N T F E C E S
D H R E C C I T K C J A P E
Q W R N A T N V P Y R M P C
O C A T N R B A P R H O A I
U Y I E O W T A P A O T W D
B O D R L N P B F Q J S V N
N T S Y F I S L U M E E B U
W G J A L U V U N R N W O A
Q S N L X D U O D E N U M J
H C A V I T Y M U C O S A D
Y E A A P H V W S V C Q J C
```

DID YOU KNOW?

- The liver performs over 500 functions and produces over 1,000 enzymes to handle the chemical conversions necessary for survival.
- About 20% of older adults have diabetes, and almost 40% have some impaired glucose tolerance.
- The human stomach lining replaces itself every 3 days.

KNOW YOUR MEDICAL TERMS

Fill in the medical term from the literal translation.

100. Lump _____

101. Blind or hidden/thing _____

102. Break apart/process _____

103. Waste _____

104. Chew/process _____

105. Without/appetite/condition _____

106. Wrinkle _____

107. Worm/shape/hang upon/thing _____

108. Yellow/state _____

109. Decay _____

110. Large intestine/see/activity _____

If you had difficulty with this section, review page 493, and pages 520-524.

DIGESTIVE SYSTEM

Fill in the crossword puzzle.

ACROSS

5. Digested food moves from intestine to blood
8. Semisolid mixture
9. Inflammation of the appendix
11. Rounded mass of food
13. Stomach folds

DOWN

1. Yellowish skin discoloration
2. Process of chewing
3. Fluid stools
4. Movement of food through digestive tract
6. Vomitus
7. Waste product of digestion
10. Intestinal fold
12. Open wound in digestive area acted on by acid juices
14. Prevents food from entering nasal cavities

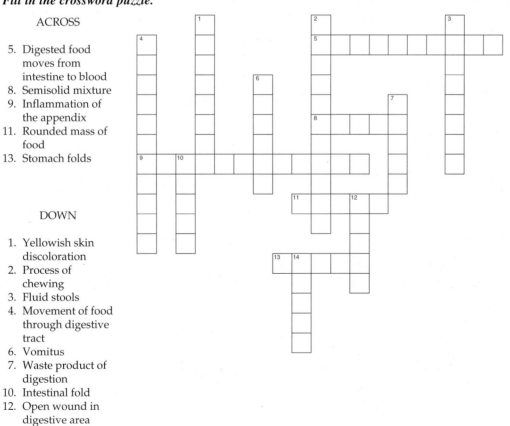

Chapter **18** Digestive System

Multiple Choice

Circle the correct answer.

1. During the process of digestion, *stored* bile is poured into the duodenum by which of the following?
   A. Gallbladder
   B. Liver
   C. Pancreas
   D. Spleen

2. Which portion of the alimentary canal mixes food with gastric juice and breaks it down into a mixture called *chyme*?
   A. Gallbladder
   B. Small intestine
   C. Stomach
   D. Large intestine

3. What is the middle portion of the small intestine called?
   A. Jejunum
   B. Ileum
   C. Duodenum
   D. Cecum

4. The crown of the tooth is covered externally with which of the following?
   A. Cementum
   B. Enamel
   C. Dentin
   D. Pulp

5. What is the layer of tissue that forms the outermost covering of organs found in the digestive tract called?
   A. Mucosa
   B. Serosa
   C. Submucosa
   D. Muscularis

6. Duodenal ulcers appear in which of the following?
   A. Stomach
   B. Small intestine
   C. Large intestine
   D. Esophagus

7. What is an extension of the peritoneum that is shaped like a giant pleated fan?
   A. Omentum
   B. Mesentery
   C. Peritoneal cavity
   D. Ligament

8. Protein digestion begins in the:
   A. esophagus
   B. small intestine
   C. stomach
   D. large intestine

9. The enzyme pepsin is concerned primarily with the digestion of which of the following?
   A. Sugars
   B. Starches
   C. Proteins
   D. Fats

10. The enzyme amylase begins the conversion of which of the following?
    A. Starches to sugars
    B. Sugars to starches
    C. Proteins to amino acids
    D. Fatty acids and glycerol to fats

Completion

Fill in the blanks using the terms listed below. Write the corresponding letter in each blank. Not all letters will be used.

A. Ileum	G. Lower esophageal sphincter	M. Upper esophageal sphincter	S. Premolars
B. Amylase	H. Digestion	N. Sigmoid colon	T. Mucosa
C. Muscularis	I. Incisors	O. Canines	U. Submucosa
D. Metabolism	J. Greater omentum	P. Amino acids	V. Cecum
E. Cholecystokinin	K. Absorption	Q. Duodenum	W. Bile
F. Molars	L. Adventitia	R. Jejunum	X. Serosa

11. The S-shaped portion of the colon is called the _____.

12. The portion of the peritoneum that descends from the stomach and the transverse colon to form a lacy apron of fat over the intestines is called the _____.

13. The "building blocks" of protein molecules and the end products of protein digestion are: _____ _____.

14. The small intestine is made up of three sections called the _____, _____

_____, and _____.

15. Fats that enter into the digestive tract are emulsified when they are acted on by a substance called _____

_____.

16. Foods undergo three kinds of processing in the body: _____, _____

_____ , and _____.

17. Fats in the chyme stimulate the secretion of _____, which stimulates contraction

of the gallbladder to release bile.

18. The four tissue layers that make up the wall of the digestive tract are the _____,

_____, _____, and _____

_____.

19. Food enters the stomach by passing through a muscular structure at the end of the esophagus. This structure is called

the _____.

20. The four major types of teeth found in the human mouth are _____, _____

_____, _____, and _____

_____.

Fill in the Blanks

21. In addition to peristalsis, the GI tract also produces a "back and forth" or "swishing" type of intestinal motility called

_____.

22. Smokers may develop white patches, or _____, which may develop into
malignant tumors.

23. The swallowing of a mass of chewed food is called _____.

24. Gastric and duodenal ulcers usually result from infection with _____.

25. Villi also contain lymphatic capillaries called _____ that absorb fats.

LOCATION OF DIGESTIVE ORGANS

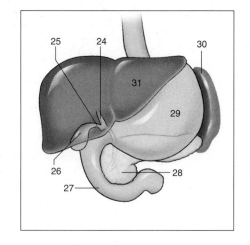

1. _____

2. _____

3. _____

4. _____

5. _____

6. _____

7. _____

8. _____

9. _____

10. _____

11. _____

12. _____

13. _____

14. _____

15. _____

16. _____

17. _____

18. _____

19. _____

20. _____

21. _____

22. _____

23. _____

24. _____

25. _____

26. _____

27. _____

28. _____

29. _____

30. _____

31. _____

Chapter **18   Digestive System**

TOOTH

1. _____
2. _____
3. _____
4. _____
5. _____
6. _____
7. _____

8. _____
9. _____
10. _____
11. _____
12. _____
13. _____

1. _____   4. _____

2. _____   5. _____

3. _____

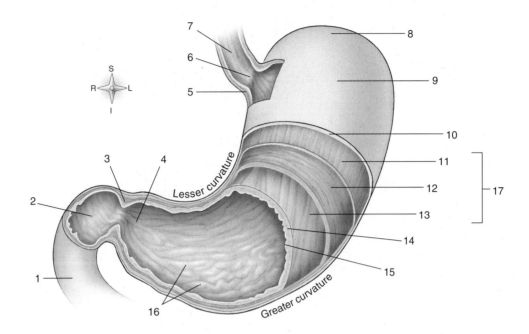

1. _____

2. _____

3. _____

4. _____

5. _____

6. _____

7. _____

8. _____

9. _____

10. _____

11. _____

12. _____

13. _____

14. _____

15. _____

16. _____

17. _____

1. _____

2. _____

3. _____

4. _____

5. _____

6. _____

7. _____

8. _____

9. _____

10. _____

11. _____

12. _____

13. _____

14. _____

THE SMALL INTESTINE

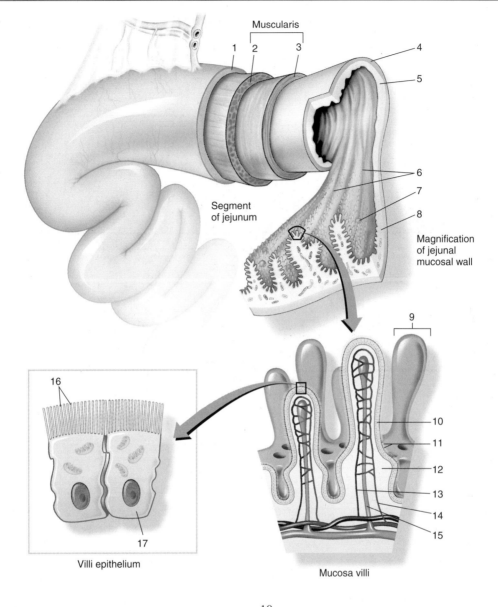

Muscularis

Segment
of jejunum

Magnification
of jejunal
mucosal wall

Villi epithelium

Mucosa villi

1. _____

2. _____

3. _____

4. _____

5. _____

6. _____

7. _____

8. _____

9. _____

10. _____

11. _____

12. _____

13. _____

14. _____

15. _____

16. _____

17. _____

1. _____   10. _____

2. _____   11. _____

3. _____   12. _____

4. _____   13. _____

5. _____   14. _____

6. _____   15. _____

7. _____   16. _____

8. _____   17. _____

9. _____   18. _____

19 Nutrition and Metabolism

Most of us love to eat, but do the foods we enjoy provide us with the basic food types necessary for good nutrition? The body, a finely tuned machine, requires a balance of carbohydrates, fats, proteins, vitamins, and minerals to function properly. These nutrients must be digested, absorbed, and circulated to cells constantly to accommodate the numerous activities that occur throughout the body. The use the body makes of foods once these processes are completed is called *metabolism*.

The liver plays a major role in the metabolism of food. It helps maintain a normal blood glucose level, removes toxins from the blood, processes blood immediately after it leaves the gastrointestinal tract, and initiates the first steps of protein and fat metabolism.

This chapter also discusses basal metabolic rate (BMR). The BMR is the rate at which food is catabolized under basal conditions. This test and the protein-bound iodine (PBI) are indirect measures of thyroid gland functioning. The total metabolic rate (TMR) is the amount of energy, expressed in calories, used by the body each day.

Finally, maintaining a constant body temperature is a function of the hypothalamus and a challenge for the metabolic mechanisms of the body. Review of this chapter is necessary to provide you with an understanding of the "fuel" (nutrition) requirements necessary to maintain this complex homeostatic machine—the body.

TOPICS FOR REVIEW

Before progressing to Chapter 20, you should be able to define and contrast catabolism and anabolism. Your review should include the metabolic roles of carbohydrates, fats, proteins, vitamins, and minerals. Your study should conclude with an understanding of the basal metabolic rate, physiological mechanisms that regulate body temperature, and the common metabolic and eating disorders.

METABOLIC FUNCTIONS OF THE LIVER

Fill in the blanks.

The liver plays an important role in the mechanical digestion of lipids because it secretes (1) _____

_____. It also produces two of the plasma proteins that play an essential role in blood clotting. These

two proteins are (2) _____ and (3) _____.

Additionally, liver cells store several substances, notably vitamins A and D and (4) _____

_____. Finally, the liver is assisted by a unique structural feature of the blood vessels that supply it. This arrangement,

known as the (5) _____ _____ _____

_____, allows toxins to be removed from the bloodstream before nutrients are distributed

throughout the body.

NUTRIENT METABOLISM

Match each term with its corresponding definition. (Answers may be used more than once.)

_____ 6. Used if cells have inadequate amounts of glucose to catabolize

_____ 7. Preferred energy food

_____ 8. Amino acids

_____ 9. Fat soluble

_____ 10. Required for nerve conduction

_____ 11. Glycolysis

_____ 12. Inorganic elements found naturally in the earth

_____ 13. Pyruvic acid

A. Carbohydrate

B. Fat

C. Protein

D. Vitamins

E. Minerals

Circle the term in each word group that does not belong.

14.	Glycolysis	Citric acid cycle	ATP	Bile
15.	Adipose	Amino acids	Triglycerides	Lipid
16.	A	D	M	K
17.	Iron	Proteins	Amino acids	Essential
18.	Hydrocortisone	Insulin	Growth hormone	Epinephrine
19.	Sodium	Calcium	Zinc	Folic acid
20.	Thiamine	Niacin	Ascorbic acid	Riboflavin

If you had difficulty with this section, review pages 534-540.

METABOLIC RATES

Circle the correct answer.

21. The rate at which food is catabolized under basal conditions is the:
    A. TMR
    B. PBI
    C. BMR
    D. ATP

22. The total amount of energy used by the body per day is the:
    A. TMR
    B. PBI
    C. BMR
    D. ATP

23. A/an _____ is the amount of energy needed to raise the temperature of 1 gram of water 1° C.
    A. calorie
    B. kilocalorie
    C. ATP
    D. BMR

24. Which of the following is a factor when determining the BMR?
    A. Sex
    B. Age
    C. Size
    D. All of the above

25. Which of the following is a factor when determining the TMR?
    A. Exercise
    B. Food intake
    C. Environmental temperature
    D. All of the above

If you had difficulty with this section, review page 537, and pages 541-542.

METABOLIC AND EATING DISORDERS

Match each description with its related term. Write the corresponding letter in the answer blank.

_____	26. Insulin deficiency is a symptom of this disorder	A. BMR
_____	27. Behavioral disorder characterized by chronic refusal to eat	B. Diabetes mellitus
_____	28. An advanced form of PCM	C. Anorexia nervosa
_____	29. Results from a deficiency of calories in general and protein in particular	D. Bulimia
_____	30. Hypothyroidism will affect this measurement	E. Obesity
_____	31. Abdominal bloating	F. PCM
_____	32. Symptom of chronic overeating behavior	G. Marasmus
_____	33. Behavioral disorder characterized by insatiable craving for food alternating with periods of self-deprivation	H. Ascites

If you had difficulty with this section, review pages 542-544.

BODY TEMPERATURES

Circle the correct answer.

34. Over _____ of the energy released from food molecules during catabolism is converted to heat rather than being transferred to ATP.
    A. 20%
    B. 40%
    C. 60%
    D. 80%

35. Maintaining thermoregulation is a function of the:
    A. thalamus
    B. hypothalamus
    C. thyroid
    D. parathyroids

36. Transfer of heat energy to the skin and then the external environment is known as:
    A. radiation
    B. conduction
    C. convection
    D. evaporation

37. A flow of heat waves away from the blood is known as:
    A. radiation
    B. conduction
    C. convection
    D. evaporation

38. A transfer of heat energy to air that is continually flowing away from the skin is known as:
    A. radiation
    B. conduction
    C. convection
    D. evaporation

39. Heat that is absorbed by the process of water vaporization is called:
    A. radiation
    B. conduction
    C. convection
    D. evaporation

If you had difficulty with this section, review page 544.

ABNORMAL BODY TEMPERATURE

True or False

If the statement is true, write "T" in the answer blank. If the statement is false, correct the statement by circling the incorrect term and writing the correct term in the answer blank.

_____ 40. Pyrogens cause the thermostatic control centers of the hypothalamus to produce a fever.

_____ 41. Malignant hyperthermia is the inability to maintain a normal body temperature in extremely cold environments.

_____ 42. Frostbite is local damage to tissues caused by extremely low temperatures.

_____ 43. Heat exhaustion is characterized by body temperatures of 41° C or higher.

_____ 44. Dantrium is used to prevent or relieve the effects of frostbite.

If you had difficulty with this section, review pages 545-546.

UNSCRAMBLE THE WORDS

45. **L R I E V**

☐ ⬭ ⬭ ⬭ ☐

46. **T A O B A L I C M S**

☐ ⬭ ⬭ ☐ ⬭ ☐ ☐ ☐ ☐

47. **O M N I A**

⬭ ☐ ⬭ ⬭ ☐

48. **Y P U R C V I**

⬭ ☐ ☐ ☐ ⬭ ☐ ☐

Take the circled letters, unscramble them, and fill in the solution.

How the magician paid his bills.

49. ☐ ☐ ☐ ☐ ☐ ☐ ☐ ☐ ☐ ☐ ☐ ☐ ☐

APPLYING WHAT YOU KNOW

50. Dr. Carey is concerned about Deborah. Her daily food intake provides fewer calories than her TMR. If this trend continues, what will be the result? If it continues over a long time, what eating disorder might Deborah develop?

51. Kathryn has been experiencing fatigue, and a blood test reveals that she is slightly anemic. What mineral will her doctor most likely prescribe? What dietary sources might you suggest that she emphasize in her daily intake?

52. Joe is training daily for an upcoming marathon. Three days before the 25-mile event, he suddenly quits his daily routine of jogging and switches to a diet high in carbohydrates. Why did Joe suddenly switch his routine of training?

53. Word Find

Find and circle 18 terms presented in this chapter. Words may be spelled top to bottom, bottom to top, right to left, left to right, or diagonally.

ATP	Fats	
Adipose	Glycerol	
BMR	Glycolysis	
Bile	Liver	
Carbohydrates	Minerals	
Catabolism	Proteins	
Conduction	Radiation	
Convection	TMR	
Evaporation	Vitamins	

```
C C C B W E F F L J V G G S
A T N L W E U O Z I E L I B
R K K P Z F R I T P O Y K L
B Q M I N E R A L S J C C P
O S S N C X M I D B D O W P
H S I Y O I T X H I N L S N
Y E L N N I K W W D S Y N S
D G O S O W T I U E H S C N
R M B Y T I W C Z N N I A A
A R A Q W A T B E I G S J M
T E T F N I F A E V E W T Y
E V A P O R A T I O N D T E
S I C N E S O P I D A O F E
H L Y K I R E B V P A H C J
I W E E P A D F T E A R G G
```

KNOW YOUR MEDICAL TERMS

Fill in the complete words in the spaces provided for these abbreviations.

54. BMR _____

55. ETS _____

56. TMR _____

57. PCM _____

58. PKU _____

59. MH _____

60. ATP _____

If you had difficulty with this section, review pages 533-535 and pages 547-548.

DID YOU KNOW?

- The amount of energy required for a person to raise a 200-pound man 15 feet in the air is about the amount of energy in one large calorie.
- A recent study indicates that when men crave food, they tend to crave fat and salt. When women crave food, they tend to desire chocolate.
- The human body has enough fat to produce seven bars of soap.

Fill in the crossword puzzle.

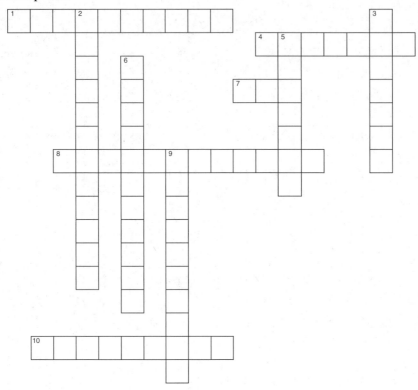

ACROSS

1. Breaks food molecules down, releasing stored energy
4. Amount of energy needed to raise the temperature of 1 gram of water 1° Celsius
7. Rate of metabolism when a person is lying down, but awake (abbreviation)
8. A series of reactions that join glucose molecules together to form glycogen
10. Builds food molecules into complex substances

DOWN

2. Occurs when food molecules enter cells and undergo many chemical changes there
3. Organic molecule needed in small quantities for normal metabolism throughout the body
5. Oxygen-using
6. A unit of measure for heat, also known as a large calorie
9. Takes place in the cytoplasm of a cell and changes glucose to pyruvic acid

CHECK YOUR KNOWLEDGE

Multiple Choice

Circle the correct answer.

1. The citric acid cycle changes acetyl CoA to:
   A. oxygen
   B. carbon dioxide
   C. pyruvic acid
   D. glucose

2. The anabolism of glucose produces which of the following?
   A. Glycogen
   B. Amino acid
   C. Rennin
   D. Starch

3. Which of the following is a major hormone in the body that aids carbohydrate metabolism?
   A. Oxytocin
   B. Epinephrine
   C. Insulin
   D. Growth hormone

4. The total metabolic rate is which of the following?
   A. The amount of fats a person consumes in a 24-hour period
   B. The same as the BMR
   C. The amount of energy expressed in calories used by the body per day
   D. Cannot be calculated

5. When your consumption of calories equals your TMR, your weight will do which of the following?
   A. Increase
   B. Remain the same
   C. Fluctuate
   D. Decrease

6. Which of the following is a normal glucose level?
   A. 40 to 80 mg/100 mL blood
   B. 80 to 120 mg/100 mL blood
   C. 100 to 140 mg/100 mL blood
   D. 180 to 220 mg/100 mL blood

7. When glucose is *not* available, the body will next catabolize which of the following energy sources?
   A. Fats
   B. Proteins
   C. Minerals
   D. Vitamins

8. Maintaining the homeostasis of the body temperature is the responsibility of which of the following?
   A. Hypothalamus
   B. Environmental condition in which we live
   C. Circulatory system
   D. None of the above

9. The liver plays an important role in the mechanical digestion of lipids because it secretes:
   A. glucose molecules
   B. bile
   C. glycogen
   D. citric acid

10. What is the primary molecule the body usually breaks down as an energy source?
   A. Amino acid
   B. Pepsin
   C. Maltose
   D. Glucose

Completion

Complete the following statements using the terms listed below. Write the corresponding letter in the answer blank.

A. Vitamins

B. Insulin

C. Carbohydrates

D. Fats

E. Glycolysis

F. Metabolism

G. ATP

H. Sodium

I. Proteins

J. Citric acid cycle

K. Calcium

L. Glycogen loading

M. Triglycerides

11. Proper nutrition requires the balance of the three basic food types: _____,
    _____ , and _____.

12. The process that changes glucose to pyruvic acid is called _____.

13. Once glucose has been changed to pyruvic acid, another process in which pyruvic acid is changed to carbon dioxide takes place. This reaction is known as the _____.

14. A direct source of energy for doing cellular work is _____.

15. The only hormone that lowers blood glucose level is _____.

16. Fats not needed for catabolism are anabolized to form _____.

17. Some athletes consume large amounts of carbohydrates 2 to 3 days before an athletic event to store glycogen in skeletal muscles. This practice is called _____.

18. Organic molecules needed in small amounts for normal metabolism are _____.

19. Two minerals necessary for nerve conduction and contraction of muscle fibers are _____ _____ and _____.

20. The "use of nutrients" is known as _____.

Fill in the Blanks

21. _____ is when nutrient molecules enter cells and undergo many chemical changes.

22. Catabolism and anabolism together make up the process of _____.

23. _____ _____ _____ _____ are amino acids that must be in the diet.

24. Vitamin E acts as an _____ that prevents highly reactive oxygen molecules called free radicals from damaging DNA and molecules in cell membranes.

25. When exercise and diet are not effective to control blood cholesterol, _____ medications are often used.

20 Urinary System

Living produces wastes. Wherever people live, work, or play, wastes accumulate. To keep these areas healthy, there must be a method of disposing of these wastes such as the services provided by a sanitation department. Wastes also accumulate in your body. The conversion of food and gases into substances and energy necessary for survival results in waste products. A large percentage of these wastes is removed by the urinary system.

Two vital organs, the kidneys, cleanse the blood of the many waste products that are continually produced as a result of the metabolism of nutrients taken into the body cells. They eliminate these wastes in the form of urine.

Urine formation is the result of three processes: filtration, reabsorption, and secretion. These processes occur in successive portions of the microscopic units of the kidneys known as *nephrons*. The amount of urine produced by the nephrons is controlled primarily by the hormones ADH and aldosterone.

After urine is produced, it is drained from the renal pelvis by the ureters to flow into the bladder. The bladder then stores the urine until it is voided through the urethra.

If waste products are allowed to accumulate in the body, they soon become poisonous, a condition called *uremia*. A knowledge of the urinary system is necessary to understand how the body rids itself of waste and avoids toxicity.

TOPICS FOR REVIEW

Before progressing to Chapter 21, you should have an understanding of the structure and function of the organs of the urinary system. Your review should include knowledge of the nephron and its role in urine production. Your study should conclude with a review of the three main processes involved in urine production, the mechanisms that control urine volume, and the major renal and urinary disorders.

KIDNEYS

KIDNEY FUNCTION

Circle the correct answer.

1. The outermost portion of the kidney is known as the:
   A. medulla
   B. papilla
   C. pelvis
   D. pyramid
   E. cortex

2. The saclike structure that surrounds the glomerulus is the:
   A. renal pelvis
   B. calyx
   C. Bowman capsule
   D. cortex
   E. none of the above

3. The renal corpuscle is made up of the:
   A. Bowman capsule and the proximal convoluted tubule
   B. glomerulus and the proximal convoluted tubule
   C. Bowman capsule and the distal convoluted tubule
   D. glomerulus and the distal convoluted tubule
   E. Bowman capsule and the glomerulus

4. Which of the following functions is *not* performed by the kidneys?
   A. Help maintain homeostasis
   B. Remove wastes from the blood
   C. Produce ADH
   D. Remove electrolytes from the blood

Match each descriptive phrase with its related structure. Write the corresponding letter in the answer blank.

_____ 5. Functioning unit of the urinary system

_____ 6. Together with the Bowman capsule forms the renal corpuscle

_____ 7. Division of the renal pelvis

_____ 8. Straight part of renal tubule

_____ 9. Innermost end of a pyramid

_____ 10. Extension of the proximal tubule

_____ 11. Triangular-shaped divisions of the medulla of the kidney

_____ 12. An expansion of the upper end of a ureter

_____ 13. Inner portion of the kidney

_____ 14. Toxic level of waste products in the blood

_____ 15. Cells secrete an enzyme that assists in restoring normal blood pressure and blood volume

_____ 16. Hormone secreted by kidney

_____ 17. Outer portion of kidney

A. Medulla

B. Cortex

C. Pyramids

D. Papilla

E. Pelvis

F. Calyx

G. Nephron

H. Collecting duct

I. Juxtaglomerular apparatus (JG)

J. Uremia

K. Glomerulus

L. Henle loop

M. Erythropoietin

If you had difficulty with this section, review pages 555-560.

FORMATION OF URINE

Match each descriptive phrase with its related structure and write the corresponding letter in the answer blank.

A. Filtration   B. Reabsorption   C. Secretion

18. _____ Begins in the proximal convoluted tubules

19. _____ Occurs to approximately two-thirds of most ions by proximal tubules

20. _____ Plays critical role in maintaining body's fluid, electrolyte, and acid-base balance

21. _____ Occurs in renal corpuscles

22. _____ Nephron loop

23. _____ Occurs at the rate of 125 mL per minute

24. _____ Hydrogen ions, potassium ions, and certain drugs from blood into kidney tubules

25. _____ Transport maximum

If you had difficulty with this section, review pages 560-563.

CONTROL OF URINE VOLUME

True or False

If the statement is true, write "T" in the answer blank. If the statement is false, correct the statement by circling the incorrect term and writing the correct term in the answer blank.

26. _____ The body controls urine volume mainly by controlling the amount of water and dissolved substances reabsorbed by the kidney tubules.

27. _____ ANH is secreted by the posterior pituitary gland.

28. _____ Aldosterone is secreted by the adrenal cortex.

29. _____ ANH has the opposite effect of aldosterone.

30. _____ Aldosterone is the "water-retaining hormone."

31. _____ Oliguria is a scanty amount of urine.

32. _____ Anuria is the absence of urine.

33. _____ Aldosterone increases urine volume.

If you had difficulty with this section, review page 563.

URETERS

URINARY BLADDER

URETHRA

Match each descriptive phrase with its related structure and write the corresponding letter in the answer blank.

A. Ureters   B. Bladder   C. Urethra

_____ 34. Lies between the urinary meatus and bladder

_____ 35. Rugae

_____ 36. Lowest part of the urinary tract

_____ 37. Lining membrane richly supplied with sensory nerve endings

_____ 38. Lies behind the pubic symphysis

_____ 39. Serves a dual function in the male

_____ 40. 1.5 inches long in the female

_____ 41. Drain the renal pelvis

_____ 42. Surrounded by the prostate in the male

_____ 43. Consists of elastic fibers and involuntary muscle fibers

_____ 44. 10 to 12 inches long

_____ 45. Trigone

If you had difficulty with this section, review pages 564-565.

ELIMINATION OF URINE

Fill in the blanks.

The terms (46) _____, (47) _____, and (48) _____ all refer to the passage of urine from the body or the emptying of the bladder. The sphincters guard the bladder. The (49) _____ _____ _____ is the sphincter located at the bladder (50) _____ and is involuntary. The external urethral sphincter encircles the (51) _____ and is under (52) _____ control. As the bladder fills, nervous impulses are transmitted to the spinal cord, and an (53) _____ _____ _____ is initiated. Urine then enters the (54) _____ _____ to be eliminated. Urinary (55) _____ is a condition in which no urine is voided. Urinary (56) _____ is when the kidneys do not produce any urine, but the bladder retains its ability to empty itself. The term (57) _____ _____ is often used to describe the type of urine loss associated with laughing, coughing, or heavy lifting.

If you had difficulty with this section, review pages 565-566.

URINALYSIS

Fill in the blanks.

58. The physical, chemical, and microscopic examination of urine is termed _____.

59. A standard urinalysis is often referred to as a _____ _____ _____ _____.

60. Vitamin supplements may cause the urine to appear _____ in color.

61. Small particles that are often formed by minerals and that may break off in the urine are known as _____ _____.

62. Clinical studies have proven that improper catheterization techniques cause _____ _____ in hospitalized patients.

63. Changes in specific gravity may be due to insufficient _____ intake.

If you had difficulty with this section, review pages 566-568.

RENAL AND URINARY DISORDERS

Match each descriptive phrase with its related disorder. Write the corresponding letter in the answer blank.

_____ 64. Urine backs up into the kidneys, causing swelling of the renal pelvis and calyces

_____ 65. Kidney stones develop

_____ 66. Stage 2 of chronic renal failure

_____ 67. Blood in the urine

_____ 68. Inflammation of the bladder

_____ 69. Inflammation of the renal pelvis and connective tissues of the kidney

_____ 70. An abrupt reduction in kidney function characterized by oliguria and a sharp rise in nitrogenous compounds in the blood

_____ 71. Progressive condition resulting from gradual loss of nephrons

_____ 72. Intense kidney pain caused by obstruction of the ureters by large kidney stones

_____ 73. Most common form of kidney disease caused by a delayed immune response to streptococcal infection

_____ 74. Albumin in the urine

_____ 75. Inflammation of the urethra that commonly results from bacterial infection

A. Pyelonephritis

B. Renal colic

C. Renal calculi

D. Acute glomerulonephritis

E. Proteinuria

F. Hematuria

G. Renal insufficiency

H. Acute renal failure

I. Hydronephrosis

J. Chronic renal failure

K. Cystitis

L. Urethritis

If you had difficulty with this section, review pages 567-573.

UNSCRAMBLE THE WORDS

76. **A Y X L C**

77. **G V N O I D I**

78. **A L P A L I P**

79. **S G U L L O U M R E**

Take the circled letters, unscramble them, and fill in the solution.

What Betty saw while cruising down the Nile.

80.

81. John suffers from low levels of ADH. What primary urinary symptom would he notice?

82. Bud was in a diving accident, and his spinal cord was severed. He was paralyzed from the waist down and, as a result, is incontinent. His physician, Dr. Welch, is concerned about the continuous residual urine buildup. What is the reason for concern?

83. Mrs. Lynch had a prolonged surgical procedure and experienced problems with urinary retention postoperatively. A urinary catheter was inserted into her bladder for the elimination of urine. Several days later Mrs. Lynch developed cystitis. What might be a possible cause of this diagnosis?

84. Mr. Dietz, an accident victim, was admitted to the hospital several hours ago. His chart indicates that he had been hemorrhaging at the scene of the accident. Nurse Petersen has been closely monitoring his urinary output and has noted that it has dropped to 10 mL/hr. (The normal urine output for a healthy adult is approximately 30 to 60 mL/hr.) What might explain this drop in urine output?

85. **Word Find**

Find and circle 18 terms presented in this chapter. Words may be spelled top to bottom, bottom to top, right to left, left to right, or diagonally.

```
H N O I T I R U T C I M N M Y
V E Q N G A L L I P A P S E S
T P M C O L D U J Y S I N D D
L H G O X I O W C G V D I U J
C R F N D B T M T L I M B K L
P O O T X I C A E K A P X L D
Q N U I E G A P R R T C W A O
B J R N T T L L Y T U Y G D M
S D E E R G Y P Y V L L P H Z
I H T N O U X W D S X I U J G
M X E C C Y S T I T I S F S Q
J O R E D D A L B U E S G B S
Y I S E B V L L B H V Q L U L
```

ADH	Filtration	Micturition
Bladder	Glomerulus	Nephron
Calculi	Hemodialysis	Papilla
Calyx	Incontinence	Pelvis
Cortex	Kidney	Pyramids
Cystitis	Medulla	Ureters

KNOW YOUR MEDICAL TERMS

Identify the medical term from the literal translation.

86. _____ Seed pod or cup

87. _____ Strain/process

88. _____ Urinate/process

89. _____ Backward/around/stretched/relating to

90. _____ Bag/see

91. _____ Kidney/substance

92. _____ Kidney/unit

93. _____ Not/urine/condition

A. Micturition

B. Nephron

C. Calyx

D. Anuria

E. Filtration

F. Cystoscope

G. Retroperitoneal

H. Renin

If you had difficulty with this section, review page 555 and pages 574-575.

DID YOU KNOW?

- If the tubules in a kidney were stretched out and untangled, they would measure 70 miles in length.
- One out of every six men will develop prostate cancer in his lifetime, but only one man in every 35 will die from it.
- Half of one kidney could do the work that two kidneys usually do.
- Over 400 gallons of recycled blood is pumped through your kidneys every day.

URINARY SYSTEM

Fill in the crossword puzzle.

ACROSS

3. Bladder infection
7. Absence of urine
8. Passage of a tube into the bladder to withdraw urine
11. Network of blood capillaries tucked into Bowman capsule

DOWN

1. Urination
2. Ultrasound generator used to break up kidney stones
3. Division of the renal pelvis
4. Voiding involuntarily
5. Area on posterior bladder wall free of rugae
6. Glucose in the urine
9. Large amount of urine
10. Scanty urine

CHECK YOUR KNOWLEDGE

Multiple Choice
Circle the correct answer.

1. Which of the following is true of urinary catheterization?
   A. It can be used to treat retention
   B. It requires aseptic technique
   C. It can lead to cystitis
   D. All of the above are true

2. Which of the following processes is used by the artificial kidney to remove waste materials from blood?
   A. Pinocytosis
   B. Hemodialysis
   C. Catheterization
   D. Active transport

3. Failure of the kidneys to remove wastes from the blood will result in which of the following?
   A. Retention
   B. Anuria
   C. Incontinence
   D. Uremia

4. Hydrogen ions are transferred from blood into the urine during which of the following processes?
   A. Secretion
   B. Filtration
   C. Reabsorption
   D. All of the above

5. Which of the following conditions would be expected in an infant less than 2 years of age?
   A. Retention
   B. Cystitis
   C. Incontinence
   D. Anuria

6. Which of the following steps involved in urine formation allows the blood to retain most body nutrients?
   A. Secretion
   B. Filtration
   C. Reabsorption
   D. All of the above

7. Voluntary control of micturition is achieved by the action of which of the following?
   A. Internal urethral sphincter
   B. External urethral sphincter
   C. Trigone
   D. Bladder muscles

8. What is the structure that carries urine from the kidney to the bladder called?
   A. Urethra
   B. Bowman capsule
   C. Ureter
   D. Renal pelvis

9. What are the capillary loops contained within the Bowman capsule called?
   A. Convoluted tubules
   B. Glomeruli
   C. Henle loop limbs
   D. Collecting ducts

10. The triangular divisions of the medulla of the kidney are known as:
    A. pyramids
    B. papillae
    C. calyces
    D. nephrons

11. Which of the following statements about ADH is *not* correct?
    A. It is stored by the pituitary gland
    B. It makes the collecting ducts less permeable to water
    C. It makes the distal convoluted tubules more permeable
    D. It is produced by the hypothalamus

12. Which of the following statements about aldosterone is *not* correct?
    A. It is secreted by the adrenal cortex
    B. It is a water-retaining hormone
    C. It is a salt-retaining hormone
    D. All of the above are correct

13. Which one of the following substances is secreted by diffusion?
    A. Sodium ions
    B. Certain drugs
    C. Ammonia
    D. Hydrogen ions
    E. Potassium ions

14. Glucose reabsorption begins in the:
    A. Henle loop
    B. proximal convoluted tubule
    C. distal convoluted tubule
    D. glomerulus
    E. none of the above

15. _____ % of the glomerular filtrate is reabsorbed.
    A. 20
    B. 40
    C. 75
    D. 85
    E. 99

Matching

Match each term in column A with its corresponding description. (Only one answer is correct for each.)

Column A

_____ 16. Retention

_____ 17. Anuria

_____ 18. Cystitis

_____ 19. Micturition

_____ 20. Oliguria

_____ 21. Polyuria

_____ 22. Incontinence

_____ 23. Hematuria

_____ 24. Suppression

_____ 25. Reabsorption

Column B

A. Involuntary voiding

B. Movement of substance out of renal tubules into blood

C. Absence of urine

D. Urination

E. Bladder does not empty

F. Inflammation of the urinary bladder

G. Traces of blood in the urine

H. Large amount of urine

I. Kidneys not producing urine

J. Scanty amount of urine

1. _____
2. _____
3. _____
4. _____
5. _____
6. _____
7. _____
8. _____

9. _____
10. _____
11. _____
12. _____
13. _____
14. _____
15. _____

KIDNEY

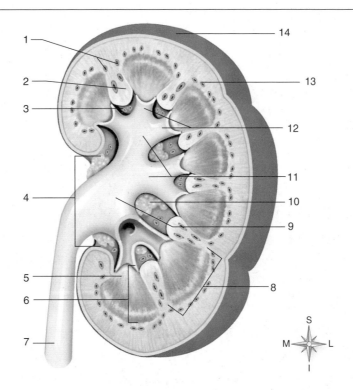

1. _____
2. _____
3. _____
4. _____
5. _____
6. _____
7. _____

8. _____
9. _____
10. _____
11. _____
12. _____
13. _____
14. _____

1. _____   8. _____

2. _____   9. _____

3. _____   10. _____

4. _____   11. _____

5. _____   12. _____

6. _____   13. _____

7. _____   14. _____

21 Fluid and Electrolyte Balance

Referring to the first chapter in your text, you will recall that survival depends on the body's ability to maintain or restore homeostasis. Specifically, *homeostasis* means that the body fluids remain constant within very narrow limits. These fluids are classified as either intracellular fluid (ICF) or extracellular fluid (ECF). As their names imply, intracellular fluid lies within the cells, and extracellular fluid is located outside the cells. A balance between these two fluids is maintained by certain body mechanisms. They are (1) the adjustment of fluid output to fluid intake under normal circumstances; (2) the concentration of electrolytes in the extracellular fluid; (3) the capillary blood pressure; and, finally, (4) the concentration of proteins in the blood.

Comprehension of how these mechanisms maintain and restore fluid balance is necessary for an understanding of the complexities of homeostasis and its relationship to the survival of the individual.

TOPICS FOR REVIEW

Before progressing to Chapter 22, you should review the types of body fluids and their subdivisions. Your study should include the mechanisms that maintain fluid balance and the nature and importance of electrolytes in body fluids. You should be able to give examples of common fluid imbalances, and have an understanding of the role of fluid and electrolyte balance in the maintenance of homeostasis.

BODY FLUID VOLUMES

Circle the correct answer.

1. The largest volume of water in the body by far lies (*inside* or *outside*) cells.

2. Interstitial fluid is (*intracellular* or *extracellular*).

3. Plasma is (*intracellular* or *extracellular*).

4. Obese people have a (*lower* or *higher*) water content per pound of body weight than thin people.

5. Infants have (*more* or *less*) water in comparison to body weight than adults of either sex.

6. There is a rapid (*increase* or *decline*) in the proportion of body water to body weight during the first 10 years of life.

7. The female body contains slightly (*more* or *less*) water per pound of weight.

8. In general, as age increases, the amount of water per pound of body weight (*increases* or *decreases*).

9. Excluding adipose tissue, approximately (*55%* or *85%*) of body weight is water.

10. The term (*fluid balance* or *fluid compartments*) means the volumes of ICF, IF, and plasma and the total volume of water in the body all remain relatively constant.

If you had difficulty with this section, review pages 583-585 and page 587.

MECHANISMS THAT MAINTAIN FLUID BALANCE

Circle the correct answer.

11. Which one of the following is *not* a positively charged ion?
    A. Chloride
    B. Calcium
    C. Sodium
    D. Potassium

12. Which one of the following is *not* a negatively charged ion?
    A. Chloride
    B. Bicarbonate
    C. Phosphate
    D. Sodium

13. The most abundant electrolyte in blood plasma is:
    A. Na
    B. K
    C. HCO₃
    D. Cl
    E. Ca

14. What source contributes the least amount of water in the body?
    A. Water in foods that are eaten
    B. Ingested liquids
    C. Water formed from catabolism
    D. None of the above

15. The greatest amount of water lost from the body comes from the:
    A. lungs
    B. skin by diffusion
    C. skin by sweat
    D. feces
    E. kidneys

16. Which one of the following is *not* a factor that acts as a mechanism for balancing plasma, IF, and ICF volumes?
    A. Regulating fluid output
    B. Regulating fluid input
    C. Exchanging fluids between compartments and from place to place within the body
    D. All of the above are important factors

17. The fluid output source that changes the most is:
    A. water loss in the feces
    B. water loss from the skin
    C. water loss via the lungs
    D. water loss in the urine
    E. none of the above

18. The chief regulators of sodium within the body are the:
    A. lungs
    B. sweat glands
    C. kidneys
    D. large intestine
    E. none of the above

19. Which of the following is *not* correct?
    A. Fluid output must equal fluid intake
    B. ADH increases water output from the body
    C. Water follows sodium
    D. Renal tubule regulation of salt and water is the most important factor in determining urine volume
    E. ANH is a diuretic hormone

20. Diuretics work on all but which one of the following?
    A. Proximal tubule
    B. Nephron loop
    C. Distal tubule
    D. Collecting ducts
    E. Diuretics work on all of the above

21. Of all the sodium-containing secretions, the one with the largest volume is:
    A. saliva
    B. gastric secretions
    C. bile
    D. pancreatic juice
    E. intestinal secretions

22. The higher the capillary blood pressure, the

    _____ the amount of interstitial fluid.
    A. smaller
    B. larger
    C. there is no relationship between capillary blood pressure and volume of interstitial fluid

23. An increase in capillary blood pressure will lead to

    _____ in blood volume.
    A. an increase
    B. a decrease
    C. no change
    D. none of the above

24. Which one of the fluid compartments varies the most in volume?
    A. Intracellular
    B. Interstitial
    C. Extracellular
    D. Plasma

True or False

If the statement is true, write "T" in the answer blank. If the statement is false, correct the statement by circling the incorrect term and writing the correct term in the answer blank.

_____ 25. The three sources of fluid intake are the liquids we drink, the foods we eat, and water formed by the anabolism of foods.

_____ 26. The body maintains fluid balance mainly by changing the volume of urine excreted to match changes in the volume of fluid intake.

_____ 27. Some output of fluid will occur as long as life continues.

_____ 28. ANH decreases urine volume.

_____ 29. Capillary blood pressure is a "water pushing" force.

_____ 30. Excess aldosterone leads to hypovolemia.

_____ 31. When dehydration starts to develop, the ECF volume decreases and the solute concentration of the ECF increases.

_____ 32. Typical daily intake and output totals should be approximately 1,200 mL.

_____ 33. Bile is a sodium-containing internal secretion.

_____ 34. Abnormally large amounts of fluid in the interstitial tissue spaces of the body are known as edema.

If you had difficulty with this section, review pages 586-591.

FLUID IMBALANCES

Fill in the blanks.

(35) _____ is the fluid imbalance seen most often. In this condition, interstitial

fluid volume (36) _____ first, but eventually, if treatment has not been given,

intracellular fluid and plasma volumes (37) _____. (38) _____

_____ can also occur but is much less common. Giving (39) _____

_____ too rapidly or in too large amounts can put too heavy a burden on the

(40) _____. (41) _____ describes a blood

sodium level above 145 mEq/L. (42) _____ is a clinical term used to describe

blood potassium levels above 5.1 mEq/L.

If you had difficulty with this section, review pages 588-592.

UNSCRAMBLE THE WORDS

43. **M D E E A**

44. **D F I L U**

45. **N I O**

46. **S O U I T N V A R E N**

Take the circled letters, unscramble them, and fill in the solution.

What Gary's dad disliked most about his music.

47.

APPLYING WHAT YOU KNOW

48. Mrs. Titus was asked to keep an accurate record of her fluid intake and output. She is concerned because the two did not balance. What is a possible explanation for this?

49. Nurse Briker is caring for a patient who is receiving diuretics. What special nursing implications should be followed for patients being given this therapy?

50. Jack Sprat is 6'5" and weighs 185 lbs. His wife is 5'6" and weighs 185 lbs. Whose body contains more water?

51. Word Find

Find and circle 12 terms presented in this chapter. Words may be spelled top to bottom, bottom to top, right to left, left to right, or diagonally.

```
S T V H O M E O S T A S I S H
I E D E M A S Q A L P U E G L
M M L U F L U I D O Y O I S L
W S B E A E C O L D P N I E R
L I T A C V S H Q O C E H B C
L L X J L T E A W Y B V Q Q O
I O O P E A R U C T C A A R I
N B H R X S N O I I P R T C N
S A O X M G J C L N J T B A H
I N X X D V U D E Y K N Y O C
E A A J Q D I U R E T I C S X
I F C J A M P V E N B E Y F W
V F K T Q X R M D D S I V O T
E T T Z N T R P X I M L J F I
S W Y A P V Q N S K T K W B P
```

Aldosterone	Edema	Imbalance
Anabolism	Electrolyte	Intravenous
Catabolism	Fluid	Ions
Diuretics	Homeostasis	Kidney

KNOW YOUR MEDICAL TERMS

Select the term that matches the definition.

A. Dissociate   D. Cation   G. Anion
B. Nonelectrolyte   E. Electrolyte   H. Ion
C. Hypernatremia   F. Hypercalcemia   I. Overhydration

52. _____ Positively charged particle

53. _____ Action in which a compound breaks apart in solution

54. _____ Compound that does not dissociate into ions in solution

55. _____ Substance that dissociates into ions in solution

56. _____ Negatively charged particle

230

57. _____ Elevation of calcium in the blood

58. _____ Too much fluid input in the body

59. _____ Electrically charged atom

60. _____ Elevation of sodium in the blood

If you had difficulty with this section, review pages 589 and 592.

DID YOU KNOW?

- The best fluid replacement drink is 1/4 teaspoon of table salt added to 1 quart of water.
- If all of the water were drained from the body of an average 160-pound man, the body would weigh 64 pounds.
- An average human drinks about 16,000 gallons of water in a lifetime.

FLUID/ELECTROLYTES

Fill in the crossword puzzle.

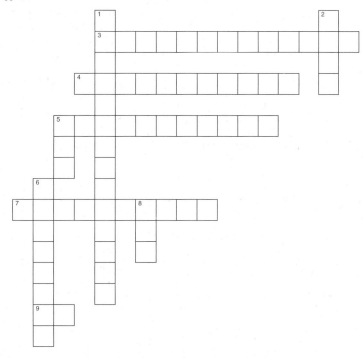

ACROSS

3. Result of rapidly given intravenous fluids
4. Result of large loss of body fluids
5. Compound that dissociates in solution into ions
7. To break up
9. A subdivision of extracellular fluid (abbreviation)

DOWN

1. Organic substance that doesn't dissociate in solution
2. Dissociated particles of an electrolyte that carry an electrical charge
5. Fluid outside cells (abbreviation)
6. "Causing urine"
8. Fluid inside cells (abbreviation)

Multiple Choice

Circle the correct answer.

1. Which of the following statements, if any, is *false*?
   A. The more fat present in the body, the more total water content per unit of weight
   B. The body weight of infants is composed of a higher percentage of water in comparison with the body weight of adults
   C. As age increases, the amount of water per pound of body weight decreases
   D. All of the above statements are true

2. Avenues of fluid output include which of the following?
   A. Skin
   B. Lungs
   C. Kidneys
   D. All of the above

3. Excessive water loss and fluid imbalance can result from which of the following?
   A. Diarrhea
   B. Vomiting
   C. Severe burns
   D. All of the above

4. What factor is primarily responsible for moving water from interstitial fluid into blood?
   A. Aldosterone secretions
   B. Pressure in blood capillaries
   C. Protein concentration of blood plasma
   D. Antidiuretic hormone secretions

5. What is the chief regulator of sodium levels in body fluids?
   A. Kidney
   B. Intestine
   C. Blood
   D. Lung

6. If blood sodium concentration decreases, what is the effect on blood volume?
   A. Increases
   B. Decreases
   C. Remains the same
   D. None of the above

7. Which of the following is true of body water?
   A. It is obtained from the liquids we drink
   B. It is obtained from the foods we eat
   C. It is formed by the catabolism of food
   D. All of the above are true

8. Edema may result from which of the following?
   A. Retention of electrolytes
   B. Decreased blood pressure
   C. Increased concentration of blood plasma proteins
   D. All of the above

9. The most abundant and most important positive plasma ion is which of the following?
   A. Sodium
   B. Chloride
   C. Calcium
   D. Oxygen

10. Which of the following is true when extracellular fluid volume decreases?
    A. Aldosterone secretion increases
    B. Kidney tubule reabsorption of sodium increases
    C. Urine volume decreases
    D. All of the above are true

Completion

Choose from the words below to complete the following statements. Write the corresponding letter in the answer blank.

A. Aldosterone	F. Electrolytes	K. Plasma
B. Edema	G. Positive	L. Urine
C. Proteins	H. Antidiuretic hormone	M. Interstitial fluid
D. Decreases	I. Dehydration	N. Fluid balance
E. Diuretic	J. Extracellular fluid	

11. Any drug that promotes or stimulates the production of urine is called a _____.

12. The presence of abnormally large amounts of fluid in the intercellular tissue spaces of the body is called _____.

13. Water located outside of cells is called _____. It can be divided into two categories. If located in the spaces between the cells, it is called _____; if located in blood vessels, it is called _____.

14. Compounds such as sodium chloride that form ions when placed in solution are called _____.

15. When the adrenal cortex increases its secretion of aldosterone, urine volume _____.

16. Most fluids leave the body in the form of _____.

17. When fluid output is greater than fluid intake, _____ occurs.

18. How much water moves into blood from interstitial fluid depends largely on the concentration of _____ present in blood plasma. These substances act as a water-pulling or water-holding force.

19. Urine volume is regulated primarily by a hormone secreted by the posterior lobe of the pituitary gland called _____ and by a hormone secreted by the adrenal gland called _____.

20. Homeostasis of fluids is also known as _____.

Fill in the Blanks

21. The two main fluid compartments are _____ and _____.

22. A typical daily input and daily output is _____.

23. A type of edema that is often present in congestive heart failure is _____.

24. A compound, such as glucose, that does not dissociate into ions in solution is a _____.

25. As a group _____ are the most commonly used drugs in medicine.

22 Acid-Base Balance

It has been established in previous chapters that equilibrium between intracellular and extracellular fluid volume must exist for homeostasis to be maintained. Equally important to homeostasis is the chemical acid-base balance of the body fluids. The degree of acidity or alkalinity of a body fluid is expressed in pH value. The neutral point, where a fluid would be neither acid nor alkaline, is pH 7. Increasing acidity is expressed as less than 7, and increasing alkalinity as greater than 7. Examples of body fluids that are acidic are gastric juice (1.6) and urine (6.0). Blood, on the other hand, is considered alkaline with a pH of 7.45.

Buffers are substances that prevent a sharp change in the pH of a fluid when an acid or base is added to it. Buffers are just one of several mechanisms that constantly monitor the pH of fluids in the body. If, for any reason, these mechanisms do not function properly, a pH imbalance occurs. The two general types of imbalances are known as *alkalosis* and *acidosis*.

Maintaining the acid-base balance of body fluids is a matter of vital importance. If this balance varies even slightly, necessary chemical and cellular reactions cannot occur. Your review of this chapter is necessary to understand the delicate acid-base balance that is necessary for survival.

TOPICS FOR REVIEW

Before progressing to Chapter 23, you should have an understanding of the pH of body fluids and of the mechanisms that control the pH of these fluids in the body. Your study should conclude with a review of the metabolic and respiratory types of pH imbalances.

pH OF BODY FLUIDS

Identify each of the circumstances or substances as acid or base. Write the corresponding letter in the answer blank.

A. Acid   B. Base

_____   1. Lower concentration of hydrogen ions than hydroxide ions

_____   2. Higher concentration of hydrogen ions than hydroxide ions

_____   3. Gastric juice

_____   4. Saliva

_____   5. Arterial blood

_____   6. Venous blood

_____   7. Baking soda

_____   8. Wine

_____   9. Ammonia

_____   10. Seawater

If you had difficulty with this section, review page 602.

MECHANISMS THAT CONTROL THE pH OF BODY FLUIDS

Circle the correct answer.

11. When carbon dioxide enters the blood, it reacts with the enzyme carbonic anhydrase to form:
    A. sodium bicarbonate
    B. water and carbon dioxide
    C. ammonium chloride
    D. bicarbonate ion
    E. carbonic acid

12. The lungs remove _____ liters of carbonic acid each day.
    A. 10.0
    B. 15.0
    C. 20.0
    D. 25.0
    E. 30.0

13. When a buffer reacts with a strong acid, it changes the strong acid to:
    A. a weak acid
    B. a strong base
    C. a weak base
    D. water
    E. none of the above

14. Which one of the following is *not* a change in the blood that results from the buffering of fixed acids in tissue capillaries?
    A. The amount of carbonic acid increases slightly
    B. The amount of bicarbonate in blood decreases
    C. The hydrogen ion concentration of blood increases slightly
    D. The blood pH decreases slightly
    E. All of the above are changes that result from the buffering of fixed acids in tissue capillaries

15. The most abundant acid in body fluids is:
    A. HCl
    B. lactic acid
    C. carbonic acid
    D. acetic acid
    E. sulfuric acid

16. The normal ratio of sodium bicarbonate to carbonic acid in arterial blood is:
    A. 5:1
    B. 10:1
    C. 15:1
    D. 20:1
    E. none of the above

17. Which of the following would *not* be a consequence of holding your breath?
    A. The amount of carbonic acid in the blood would increase
    B. The blood pH would decrease
    C. The body would develop an alkalosis
    D. No carbon dioxide could leave the body

18. The most effective regulators of blood pH are:
    A. the lungs
    B. the kidneys
    C. buffers
    D. none of the above

19. The pH of the urine may be as low as:
    A. 1.6
    B. 2.5
    C. 3.2
    D. 4.8
    E. 7.4

20. To counter the effect of lactic acid buildup in muscles, some athletes have adopted a technique called:
    A. carbonic acid compensation
    B. bicarbonate loading
    C. buffering
    D. none of the above

21. Which one is *not* a main mechanism for regulating the pH of body fluids?
    A. Urinary mechanisms
    B. Buffer mechanisms
    C. Respiratory mechanisms
    D. Endocrine mechanisms

True or False

If the statement is true, write "T" in the answer blank. If the statement is false, correct the statement by circling the incorrect term and writing the correct term in the answer blank.

_____ 22. More bases than acids are usually added to body fluids.

_____ 23. Buffers consist of two kinds of substances and therefore are often called *duobuffers*.

_____ 24. Black coffee and milk are acidic on the pH scale.

_____ 25. Without buffering, lactic acid buildup results in significant H^+ accumulation over time.

_____ 26. Anything that causes an excessive increase in respiration will, in time, produce acidosis.

_____ 27. Venous blood has a higher pH than arterial blood.

235

_____ 28. More acids than bases are usually excreted by the kidneys because more acids than bases usually enter the blood.

_____ 29. The kidney tubules rid the blood of excess acid and at the same time conserve the bases in it by secreting H^+ ions into the urine while retaining HCO3 in the blood.

_____ 30. Blood levels of carbonic acid can be regulated by the kidneys.

If you had difficulty with this section, review pages 602-606.

pH IMBALANCES

Match each numbered circumstance with its resulting condition. Write the corresponding letter in the answer blank.

_____ 31. Vomiting

_____ 32. Result of untreated diabetes

_____ 33. Chloride-containing solution

_____ 34. Bicarbonate deficit

_____ 35. Occurs during emesis and may result in metabolic alkalosis

_____ 36. Bicarbonate excess

_____ 37. Slow breathing

_____ 38. Carbonic acid excess

_____ 39. Carbonic acid deficit

_____ 40. Used for cardiac arrest

A. Metabolic acidosis

B. Metabolic alkalosis

C. Respiratory acidosis

D. Respiratory alkalosis

E. Emesis

F. Normal saline

G. Uncompensated metabolic acidosis

H. Hypoventilation

I. HCl loss

J. Lactate solution

If you had difficulty with this section, review pages 607-610.

UNSCRAMBLE THE WORDS

41. **ULIFDS**

⬡ □ ⬡ □ □ □

42. **EBTIACNAOBR**

⬡ □ □ □ □ □ □ □ □ □ □

43. **ABSE**

□ □ □ ⬡

44. **XFDEI**

⬡ □ □ □ □

45. **ROGHYNED**

□ □ □ ⬡ □ □ □ □

Take the circled letters, unscramble them, and fill in the solution.

How Sam the "stunt man" used his mattress.

46. □ □ □ □ □ □

APPLYING WHAT YOU KNOW

47. Holly is pregnant and experienced repeated vomiting episodes throughout the day for several days in a row. Her doctor became concerned, admitted her to the hospital, and began intravenous administrations of normal saline. How will this help Holly?

48. Cara has a minor bladder infection. She has heard that this is often the result of the urine being less acidic than necessary and that she should drink cranberry juice to correct the acid problem. She has no cranberry juice, so she decides to substitute orange juice. Why would this substitution not be effective in correcting the acid problem?

49. Mr. Shearer has frequent bouts of hyperacidity of the stomach. Which will assist in neutralizing the acid more promptly: milk or milk of magnesia?

50. Word Find

Find and circle 18 terms presented in this chapter. Words may be spelled top to bottom, bottom to top, right to left, left to right, or diagonally.

```
S I S A T S O E M O H P R G
E C N A L A B D I U L F E F
T S Y E N D I K W T I K A J
Y D M N D E J W L P T D J I
L D N O L H V W O U H D O I
O V E R H Y D R A T I O N S
R E I E E D E M A U R O R Q
T L M T C R U L R F S E O Y
C C U S Z A W E K A T N I X
E O Z O T T A N A U N M F
L F K D P I O I W W Q L G Q
E N I L C O O H O W S B X S
N J X A L N F S U N L J J J
O C U V S A L G T I S C Z X
N I Z L L D Y X Q Q K D C D
```

ADH
Aldosterone
Anions
Cations
Dehydration
Diuretic

Edema
Electrolytes
Fluid balance
Homeostasis
Intake
Kidneys

Nonelectrolytes
Output
Overhydration
Sodium
Thirst
Water

KNOW YOUR MEDICAL TERMS

Fill in the medical term from the literal translation.

51. Sour/condition _____

52. Two/coal/oxygen _____

53. Acetone/chemical _____

54. Cushion/agent _____

55. Coal/relating to (1) _____ without/water/enzyme (2) _____

_____ (2 words)

56. Ashes/condition _____

If you had difficulty with this section, review pages 601 and 611.

DID YOU KNOW?

■ During the nineteenth century, English ships that were at sea for many months at a time carried limes onboard to feed the sailors to protect them from developing scurvy. American ships carried cranberries for this purpose.

ACID-BASE BALANCE

Fill in the crossword puzzle.

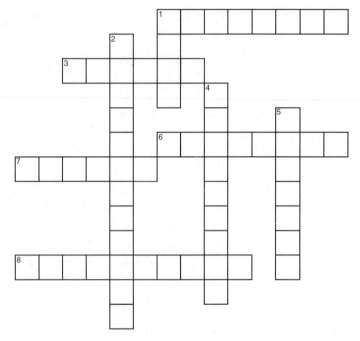

ACROSS

1. Acid-base imbalance
3. Vomitus
6. Substance with a pH higher than 7.0
7. Prevents a sharp change in the pH of fluids
8. Released as a waste product from working muscles (two words)

DOWN

1. Substance with a pH lower than 7.0
2. Results from excessive metabolism of fats in uncontrolled diabetics (two words)
4. Serious complication of vomiting
5. Most effective regulators of blood pH

CHECK YOUR KNOWLEDGE

Multiple Choice

Circle the correct answer.

1. What happens as blood flows through lung capillaries?
   A. Carbonic acid in blood decreases
   B. Hydrogen ions in blood decrease
   C. Blood pH increases from venous to arterial blood
   D. All of the above are true

2. Which of the following organs is considered the most effective regulator of blood carbonic acid levels?
   A. Kidneys
   B. Intestines
   C. Lungs
   D. Stomach

3. Which of the following organs is considered the most effective regulator of blood pH?
   A. Kidneys
   B. Intestines
   C. Lungs
   D. Stomach

4. What is the pH of the blood?
   A. 7.00 to 8.00
   B. 6.25 to 7.45
   C. 7.65 to 7.85
   D. 7.35 to 7.45

5. If the ratio of sodium bicarbonate to carbonate ions is lowered (perhaps 10 to 1) and blood pH is also lowered, what is the condition called?
   A. Uncompensated metabolic acidosis
   B. Uncompensated metabolic alkalosis
   C. Compensated metabolic acidosis
   D. Compensated metabolic alkalosis

6. If a person hyperventilates for an extended time, which of the following will probably develop?
   A. Metabolic acidosis
   B. Metabolic alkalosis
   C. Respiratory acidosis
   D. Respiratory alkalosis

7. What happens when lactic acid dissociates in the blood?
   A. H^+ is added to blood
   B. pH is lowered
   C. Acidosis results
   D. All of the above happen

8. Which of the following is true of metabolic alkalosis?
   A. It occurs in the case of prolonged vomiting
   B. It results when the bicarbonate ion is present in excess
   C. Therapy includes intravenous administration of normal saline
   D. All of the above are true

9. Which of the following is a characteristic of a buffer system in the body?
   A. It prevents drastic changes from occurring in body pH
   B. It picks up both hydrogen and hydroxide ions
   C. It is exemplified by the bicarbonate-carbonic acid system
   D. All of the above are true

10. In the presence of a strong acid (HCl), which of the following is true?
    A. Sodium bicarbonate will react to produce carbonic acid + sodium chloride
    B. Sodium bicarbonate will react to produce more sodium bicarbonate
    C. Carbonic acid will react to produce sodium bicarbonate
    D. Carbonic acid will react to form more carbonic acid

Matching

Match each description in column A with its corresponding term in column B. (Only one answer is correct for each.)

Column A

_____ 11. pH lower than 7.0

_____ 12. pH higher than 7.0

_____ 13. Prevent sharp pH changes

_____ 14. Decrease in respirations

_____ 15. Increase in respirations

_____ 16. Bicarbonate deficit

_____ 17. Bicarbonate excess

_____ 18. "Fixed" acid

_____ 19. Enzyme found in red blood cells

_____ 20. Lower-than-normal ratio of sodium bicarbonate to carbonic acid

Column B

A. Metabolic acidosis

B. Metabolic alkalosis

C. Alkaline solution

D. Lactic acid

E. Respiratory acidosis

F. Respiratory alkalosis

G. Acidic solution

H. Uncompensated metabolic acidosis

I. Buffers

J. Carbonic anhydrase

Fill in the Blanks

21. When blood levels of ketones increase, they "spill over" into the _____ and
can be detected by use of appropriate reagent strips.

22. When reading an analysis of blood gases, the "a" in PaO^2 represents _____.

23. Moving from one unit to the next multiplies the relative H^+ concentration _____
times.

24. _____ is the most abundant acid in the body fluids.

25. From a clinical standpoint, disturbances in acid-base balance can be considered dependent on the relative quantities

(ratio) of _____ and _____ in the
blood.

23 Reproductive Systems

The reproductive system consists of those organs that participate in perpetuating the species. It is a unique body system in that its organs differ between the two sexes, and yet the goal of creating a new being is the same for each gender. Of interest also is the fact that this system is the only one not necessary to the survival of the individual, and yet survival of the species depends on the proper functioning of the reproductive organs.

The male reproductive system is divided into the external genitals, the testes, the duct system, and accessory glands. The testes, or gonads, are considered essential organs because they produce the sex cells, sperm, which join with the female sex cells, ova, to form a new human being. They also secrete the male sex hormone, testosterone, which is responsible for the physical transformation of a boy to a man. Sperm are formed in the testes by the seminiferous tubules. From there they enter a long, narrow duct, the epididymis. They continue onward through the vas deferens into the ejaculatory duct, down the urethra, and out of the body. Throughout this journey, various glands secrete substances that add motility to the sperm and create a chemical environment conducive to reproduction.

The female reproductive system is truly extraordinary and diverse. It produces ova, receives the penis and sperm during intercourse, is the site of conception, houses and nourishes the embryo during prenatal development, and nourishes the infant after birth. Because of its diversity, the physiology of the female is generally considered to be more complex than that of the male. Much of the activity of this system revolves around the menstrual cycle and the monthly preparation that the female undergoes for a possible pregnancy.

The organs of the reproductive systems are divided into essential organs and accessory organs of reproduction. The essential organs of the female are the ovaries. Just as with the male, the essential organs of the female are referred to as the *gonads*. The gonads of both sexes produce the sex cells. In the male, the gonads produce the sperm, and in the female, they produce the ova. The gonads are also responsible for producing the hormones in each gender that are necessary for development of the secondary sex characteristics.

The menstrual cycle of the female typically covers a period of 28 days. Each cycle consists of three phases: the menstrual period, the proliferative phase, and the secretory phase. Changes in the blood levels of the hormones that are responsible for the menstrual cycle also cause physical and emotional changes in the female. Knowledge of these phenomena and this system, in both the male and the female, is necessary to complete your understanding of the reproductive system.

TOPICS FOR REVIEW

Before progressing to Chapter 24, you should familiarize yourself with the structure and function of the organs of the male and female reproductive systems. Your review should include emphasis on the gross and microscopic structure of the testes and on the production of sperm and testosterone. Your study should continue by tracing the pathway of a sperm cell from formation to expulsion from the body.

You should then familiarize yourself with the structure and function of the organs of the female reproductive system. Your review should include emphasis on the development of mature ova from ovarian follicles and should additionally concentrate on the phases and occurrences in a typical 28-day menstrual cycle. Finally, a review of the common disorders occurring in both male and female reproductive systems is necessary to complete the study of this chapter.

SEXUAL REPRODUCTION

MALE REPRODUCTIVE SYSTEM

Match each term on the left with its related term on the right. Write the corresponding letter in the answer blank.

Group A

_____	1. Testes	A. Fertilized ovum
_____	2. Spermatozoa	B. Accessory organ
_____	3. Ovum	C. Male sex cell
_____	4. Penis	D. Gonads
_____	5. Zygote	E. Gamete

241

Group B

_____ 6. Testes   A. Cowper gland

_____ 7. Bulbourethral   B. Scrotum

_____ 8. Asexual   C. Essential organ

_____ 9. External genital   D. Single parent

_____ 10. Prostate   E. Accessory organ

If you had difficulty with this section, review pages 617-618.

TESTES

Circle the correct answer.

11. The testes are surrounded by a tough membrane called the:
    A. ductus deferens
    B. tunica albuginea
    C. septum
    D. seminiferous membrane

12. The _____ lie near the septa that separate the lobules.
    A. ductus deferens
    B. sperm
    C. interstitial cells
    D. nerves

13. Sperm are found in the walls of the _____.
    A. seminiferous tubule
    B. interstitial cells
    C. septum
    D. blood vessels

14. The scrotum provides an environment that is approximately _____ for the testes.
    A. the same as the body temperature
    B. 5 degrees warmer than the body temperature
    C. 3 degrees warmer than the body temperature
    D. 3 degrees cooler than the body temperature

15. The _____ produce(s) testosterone.
    A. seminiferous tubules
    B. prostate gland
    C. bulbourethral gland
    D. pituitary gland
    E. interstitial cells

16. The part of the sperm that contains genetic information that will be inherited is the:
    A. tail
    B. neck
    C. middle piece
    D. head
    E. acrosome

17. Which one of the following is *not* a function of testosterone?
    A. It causes a deepening of the voice
    B. It promotes the development of the male accessory organs
    C. It has a stimulatory effect on protein catabolism
    D. It causes greater muscular development and strength

18. Sperm production is called:
    A. spermatogonia
    B. spermatids
    C. spermatogenesis
    D. spermatocyte

19. The section of the sperm that contains enzymes that enable it to break down the covering of the ovum and permit entry should contact occur is the:
    A. acrosome
    B. midpiece
    C. tail
    D. stem

Fill in the blanks.

The (20) _____ are the gonads of the male. From puberty on, the seminiferous tubules are continuously forming (21) _____. Any of these cells may join with the female sex cell, the (22) _____, to become a new human being. Another function of the testes is to secrete the male hormone (23) _____, which transforms a boy to a man. This hormone is secreted by the (24) _____ _____ of the testes. A good way to remember testosterone's functions is to think of it as "the (25) _____ hormone" and "the (26) _____ _____ hormone."

If you had difficulty with this section, review pages 618-622.

REPRODUCTIVE DUCTS

ACCESSORY OR SUPPORTIVE SEX GLANDS

EXTERNAL GENITALS

Match each description on the left with its corresponding term on the right. Write the letter in the answer blank.

_____ 27. Continuation of ducts that start in the epididymis	A.	Epididymis
_____ 28. Erectile tissue	B.	Vas deferens
_____ 29. Also known as *bulbourethral*	C.	Ejaculatory duct
_____ 30. Narrow tube that lies along the top and behind the testes	D.	Prepuce
_____ 31. Doughnut-shaped gland beneath the bladder	E.	Seminal vesicles
_____ 32. Point where vas deferens joins the duct from the seminal vesicle	F.	Prostate gland
_____ 33. Mixture of sperm and secretions of accessory sex glands	G.	Cowper gland
_____ 34. Contributes 60% of the seminal fluid volume	H.	Corpus spongiosum
_____ 35. Removed during circumcision	I.	Semen
_____ 36. External genitalia	J.	Scrotum

If you had difficulty with this section, review pages 622-624.

DISORDERS OF THE MALE REPRODUCTIVE SYSTEM

Fill in the blanks.

37. Decreased sperm production is called _____.

38. Testes normally descend into the scrotum about _____ _____ _____ before birth.

39. If a baby is born with undescended testes, a condition called _____ results.

40. A common noncancerous condition of the prostate in older men is known as _____ _____ _____ _____.

41. _____ is a condition in which the foreskin fits so tightly over the glans that it cannot retract.

42. Failure to achieve an erection of the penis is called _____.

43. An accumulation of fluid in the scrotum is known as a _____.

44. An _____ _____ results when the intestines push through the weak area of the abdominal wall that separates the abdominopelvic cavity from the scrotum.

45. _____ cancer is the second leading cause of cancer deaths in men.

If you had difficulty with this section, review pages 625-626.

FEMALE REPRODUCTIVE SYSTEM

Match the term on the left with the corresponding term on the right. Write the letter in the answer blank.

_____ 46. Ovaries   A. Genitals

_____ 47. Vagina   B. Accessory sex gland

_____ 48. Bartholin   C. Accessory duct

_____ 49. Vulva   D. Gonads

_____ 50. Ova   E. Sex cell

Identify each of the numbered structures as external or internal. Write the corresponding letter in the answer blank.

A. External structure   B. Internal structure

_____ 51. Mons pubis

_____ 52. Vagina

_____ 53. Labia majora

_____ 54. Uterine tubes

_____ 55. Vestibule

_____ 56. Clitoris

_____ 57. Labia minora

_____ 58. Ovaries

If you had difficulty with this section, review pages 627-633.

OVARIES

Fill in the blanks.

The ovaries are the (59) _____ of the female. They have two main functions. The first is the production of the female sex cell. This process is called (60) _____.

The specialized type of cell division that occurs during sexual cell reproduction is known as (61) _____ _____. The ovum is the body's largest cell and has (62) _____ the number of chromosomes found in other body cells. At the time of (63) _____,

the sex cells from both parents fuse and (64) _____ chromosomes are united. The

second major function of the ovaries is to secrete the sex hormones (65) _____

and (66) _____. Estrogen is the sex hormone that causes the development and maintenance of the female (67) _____ _____

___ _____. Progesterone acts with estrogen to help initiate the (68) _____

_____ _____ in girls entering (69) _____

_____.

If you had difficulty with this section, review pages 627-629.

FEMALE REPRODUCTIVE DUCTS

Match each of the numbered descriptions with its corresponding structure. Write the letter in the answer blank.

A. Uterine tubes   B. Uterus   C. Vagina

_____ 70. Location of most ectopic pregnancies

_____ 71. Lining known as *endometrium*

_____ 72. Birth canal

_____ 73. Site of menstruation

_____ 74. Fringelike projections called *fimbriae*

_____ 75. Consists of a body, fundus, and cervix

_____ 76. Site of fertilization

_____ 77. Also known as *oviduct*

_____ 78. Entranceway for sperm

If you had difficulty with this section, review pages 630-631.

ACCESSORY OR SUPPORTIVE SEX GLANDS

EXTERNAL GENITALS

Match each term on the left with its corresponding description on the right. Write the letter in the answer blank.

Group A

_____ 79. Bartholin glands

_____ 80. Breasts

_____ 81. Alveoli

_____ 82. Lactiferous ducts

_____ 83. Areola

A. Colored area around the nipple

B. Grapelike clusters of milk-secreting cells

C. Drain alveoli

D. Also known as *greater vestibular*

E. Composed primarily of fat tissue

Group B

_____ 84. Mons pubis

_____ 85. Labia majora

_____ 86. Clitoris

_____ 87. Perineum

_____ 88. Episiotomy

A. "Large lips"

B. Area between the vaginal opening and the anus

C. Surgical procedure

D. Composed of erectile tissue

E. Pad of fat over the symphysis pubis

If you had difficulty with this section, review pages 631-633.

245

Copyright © 2018, Elsevier Inc. All rights reserved.

Chapter **23** **Reproductive Systems**

MENSTRUAL CYCLE

True or False

If the statement is true, write "T" in the answer blank. If the statement is false, correct the statement by circling the incorrect term and writing the correct term in the answer blank.

_____ 89. *Climacteric* is the scientific name for the beginning of the menses.

_____ 90. As a general rule, several ovum mature each month during the 30 to 40 years that a woman has menstrual periods.

_____ 91. Ovulation occurs 28 days before the next menstrual period begins.

_____ 92. The first day of ovulation is considered the first day of the cycle.

_____ 93. A woman's fertile period lasts only a few days out of each month.

_____ 94. The control of the menstrual cycle lies in the posterior pituitary gland.

Match the two hormones below to their corresponding descriptions. Write the letter in the answer blank.

A. FSH   B. LH

_____ 95. Ovulating hormone

_____ 96. Secreted during first days of menstrual cycle

_____ 97. Secreted after estrogen level of blood increases

_____ 98. Causes final maturation of follicle and ovum

_____ 99. Suppressed by birth control pills

If you had difficulty with this section, review pages 633-635.

DISORDERS OF THE FEMALE REPRODUCTIVE SYSTEM

Match each numbered description to its corresponding disease or condition. Write the letter in the answer blank.

_____ 100. Often occurs as a result of an STD or a "yeast infection"

_____ 101. Benign tumor of smooth muscle and fibrous connective tissue; also known as a *fibroid tumor*

_____ 102. Yeast infection characterized by leukorrhea

_____ 103. Inflammation of an ovary

_____ 104. Benign lumps in one or both breasts

_____ 105. Venereal diseases

_____ 106. Results from pathogenic organisms transmitted from another person; for example, an STD

_____ 107. Painful menstruation

_____ 108. Asymptomatic in most women and nearly all men

_____ 109. Results from a hormonal imbalance rather than from an infection or disease condition

_____ 110. Screening test for cervical cancer

_____ 111. Causes blisters on the skin of the genitals; the blisters may disappear temporarily but then recur, especially as a result of stress

A. Candidiasis

B. Dysmenorrhea

C. Exogenous infections

D. DUB

E. Myoma

F. Vaginitis

G. Sexually transmitted diseases (STDs)

H. Oophoritis

I. Fibrocystic disease

J. Pap smear

K. Genital herpes

L. Trichomoniasis

If you had difficulty with this section, review pages 632-640.

UNSCRAMBLE THE WORDS

112. **U L A V V**

[ ][ ][◯][◯][ ]

113. **T S T S E E**

[◯][ ][ ][◯][ ][ ]

114. **M N S S E E**

[ ][◯][ ][ ][◯][ ]

115. **A I E I F M B R**

[ ][◯][ ][◯][ ][ ][ ][ ]

116. **C U E R P P E**

[ ][ ][ ][ ][◯][ ][ ]

Take the circled letters, unscramble
them, and fill in the solution.

Where Kathleen displayed the flowers from her husband.

117. [ ][ ][ ][ ][ ][ ][ ][ ][ ][ ][ ]

APPLYING WHAT YOU KNOW

118. Sam is going into the hospital for the surgical removal of his testes. As a result of this surgery, will Sam be impotent?

119. When baby Christopher was born, the pediatrician, Dr. Self, discovered that his left testicle had not descended into the scrotum. If this situation is not corrected soon, might baby Christopher be sterile or impotent?

120. Harlean contracted gonorrhea. By the time she made an appointment to see her doctor, it had spread to her abdominal organs. How is this possible when gonorrhea is a disease of the reproductive system?

121. Dr. Sullivan advises Mrs. Harlan to have a bilateral oophorectomy. Is this a sterilization procedure? Will she experience menopause?

247

122. Vicki had a total hysterectomy. Will she experience menopause?

123. Word Find

Find and circle 18 terms presented in this chapter. Words may be spelled top to bottom, bottom to top, right to left, left to right, or diagonally.

```
M K O V I D U C T S E D H G
S E I R A V O I F U T G L L
I N H Z H M P M K O H I C W
D D V A S D E F E R E N S H
I O A C C I P J V E H Y D S
H M G R R B M N X F G Y I O
C E I O O E Z Y T I C S T E
R T N S T P S D D N O V A D
O R A O U W E B A I J S M Z
T I C M M E Y N E M D L R V
P U A E U D G M I E H I E H
Y M O T C E T A T S O R P B
R P E E R M N E G O R T S E
C O W P E R S I N X K E A P
```

Acrosome	Meiosis	Scrotum
Cowpers	Ovaries	Seminiferous
Cryptorchidism	Oviducts	Sperm
Endometrium	Penis	Spermatids
Epididymis	Pregnancy	Vagina
Estrogen	Prostatectomy	Vas deferens

KNOW YOUR MEDICAL TERMS

Identify the medical term from the literal translation.

124. body/yellow/thing _____

125. within/womb/thing _____

126. offspring/relating to _____

127. lips/large _____

128. months _____

129. egg/cell _____

130. seed _____

131. tunic or coat/white _____

132. within/womb/condition _____

133. painful/month/flow _____

134. not/fruitful/state _____

135. white/flow _____

136. pubic region/cut/action _____

137. vessel/out/cut/action _____

138. tube/inflammation _____

If you had difficulty with this section, review pages 641-644.

DID YOU KNOW?

- The testes produce approximately 50 million sperm per day. Every 2 to 3 months they produce enough cells to populate the entire earth.
- There are an estimated 925,000 daily occurrences of STD transmission and 550,000 daily conceptions worldwide.
- All babies have blue eyes when they are born. Melanin and ultraviolet exposure light are needed to bring out the true color of a baby's eyes.
- Babies are born with 300 bones, but by adulthood we have only 206 in our bodies.
- One in every 2,000 babies is born with a tooth.

REPRODUCTIVE SYSTEMS

Fill in the crossword puzzle.

ACROSS

2. Female erectile tissue
3. Colored area around nipple
5. Male reproductive fluid
6. Sex cells
7. External genitalia
10. Male sex hormone

DOWN

1. Failure to have a menstrual period
2. Surgical removal of foreskin
4. Foreskin
8. Menstrual period
9. Essential organs of reproduction

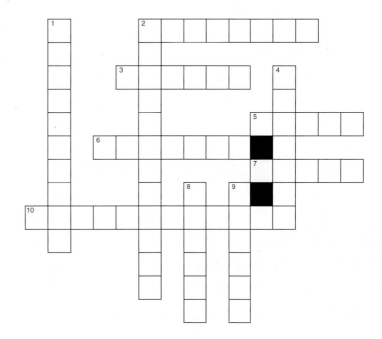

Multiple Choice
Circle the correct answer.

1. What is the membrane that may cover the vaginal opening of the female called?
   A. Hymen
   B. Mons pubis
   C. Labia
   D. Clitoris

2. Which of the following statements is true of the menstrual cycle?
   A. Estrogen levels are lowest at the time of ovulation
   B. Progesterone levels are highest at the time of ovulation
   C. FSH levels are highest during the proliferation phase
   D. None of the above are true

3. A fluid mixture called *semen* could contain which of the following?
   A. Sperm cells
   B. Secretion from the prostate
   C. Secretions from the seminal vesicles
   D. All of the above

4. What is the failure of the testes to descend into the scrotum before birth called?
   A. Cryptococcus
   B. Coccidiomycosis
   C. Cryptorchidism
   D. Cholelithiasis

5. Which of the following is *not* an accessory organ of the female reproductive system?
   A. Breast
   B. Bartholin glands
   C. Ovary
   D. All of the above are accessory organs

6. Which of the following structures can be referred to as *male gonads*?
   A. Testes
   B. Epididymis
   C. Vas deferens
   D. All of the above

7. Sperm cells are suspended outside the body cavity so as to do which of the following?
   A. Protect them from trauma
   B. Keep them at a cooler temperature
   C. Keep them supplied with a greater number of blood vessels
   D. Protect them from infection

8. Surgical removal of the foreskin from the glans penis is called what?
   A. Vasectomy
   B. Sterilization
   C. Circumcision
   D. Ligation

9. What is the colored area around the nipple of the breast called?
   A. Areola
   B. Lactiferous duct
   C. Alveoli
   D. None of the above

10. The female organ that is analogous to the penis in the male is the:
    A. labia minora
    B. labia majora
    C. vulva
    D. clitoris

Completion

Complete the following statements using the terms listed below. Write the corresponding letter in the answer blank.

A. Clitoris   E. Menses   I. FSH (follicle-stimulating hormone)

B. Endometrium   F. Epididymis   J. Ovulation

C. Ectopic   G. Hysterectomy   K. Scrotum

D. Corpus luteum   H. Prostate   L. Testosterone

11. A pregnancy resulting from the implantation of a fertilized ovum in any location other than the uterus is called _____.

12. Interstitial cells of the testes function to produce _____.

13. The doughnut-shaped accessory organ or gland that surrounds the male urethra is called the _____ _____.

14. Surgical removal of the uterus is called _____.

15. The _____ houses sperm cells as they mature and develop their ability to swim.

16. The skin-covered external pouch that contains the testes is called the _____.

17. The lining of the uterus is called _____.

18. The hormone progesterone is secreted by a structure called the _____.

19. Fertilization of an egg by a sperm can only occur around the time of _____.

20. From about the first to the seventh day of the menstrual cycle, the anterior pituitary gland secretes _____ _____.

Fill in the Blanks

21. Sperm exit the epididymis and enter the _____ _____.

22. A complete inability to reproduce is called _____.

23. Cessation of fertility that closely parallels female menopause is referred to as _____.

24. The space between the labia minora is the _____.

25. The _____ phase of the menstrual cycle begins at ovulation and lasts until the next menses begins.

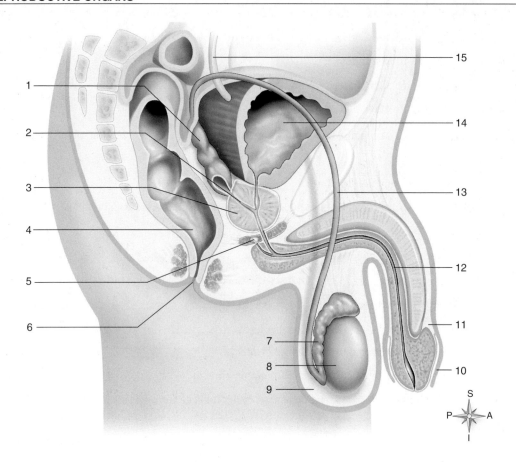

1. _____

2. _____

3. _____

4. _____

5. _____

6. _____

7. _____

8. _____

9. _____

10. _____

11. _____

12. _____

13. _____

14. _____

15. _____

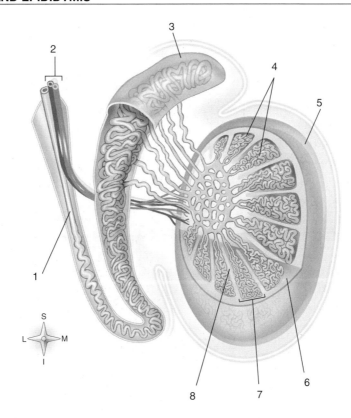

1. _____   5. _____

2. _____   6. _____

3. _____   7. _____

4. _____   8. _____

1. _____

2. _____

3. _____

4. _____

5. _____

6. _____

7. _____

8. _____

9. _____

10. _____

11. _____

12. _____

13. _____

14. _____

15. _____

16. _____

17. _____

18. _____

BREAST

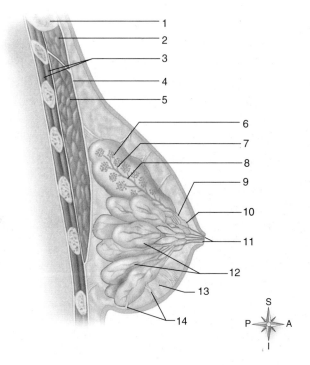

1. _____
2. _____
3. _____
4. _____
5. _____
6. _____
7. _____

8. _____
9. _____
10. _____
11. _____
12. _____
13. _____
14. _____

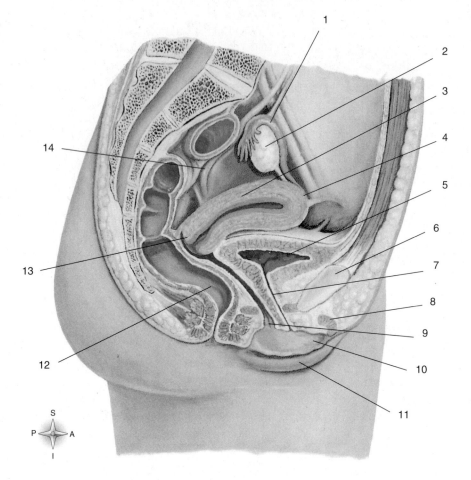

1. _____

2. _____

3. _____

4. _____

5. _____

6. _____

7. _____

8. _____

9. _____

10. _____

11. _____

12. _____

13. _____

14. _____

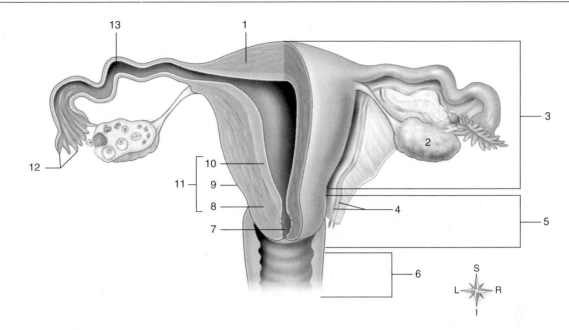

1. _____

2. _____

3. _____

4. _____

5. _____

6. _____

7. _____

8. _____

9. _____

10. _____

11. _____

12. _____

13. _____

Growth and Development

Millions of fragile microscopic sperm swim against numerous obstacles to reach an ovum and create a new life. At birth, the newborn will fill his lungs with air and cry lustily, signaling to the world that he is ready to begin the cycle of life. This cycle will be marked by ongoing changes, periodic physical growth, and continuous development.

This chapter reviews the more significant events that occur in the normal growth and development of an individual from conception to death. Realizing that each person is unique, we nonetheless can discover amid all the complexities of humanity some constants that are understandable and predictable.

Knowledge of human growth and development is essential in understanding the commonalities that influence individuals as they pass through the cycle of life.

TOPICS FOR REVIEW

Before progressing to Chapter 25, you should have an understanding of the concept of development as a biological process. You should familiarize yourself with the major developmental changes from conception through older adulthood. The disorders of pregnancy should be emphasized as you review the chapter. Finally, your study should conclude with a review of the effects of aging on the body systems.

PRENATAL PERIOD

BIRTH OR PARTURITION

Fill in the blanks.

The prenatal stage of development begins at the time of (1) _____ and continues

until (2) _____. The science of the development of an individual before birth is

called (3) _____. Fertilization takes place in the outer third of the (4) _____

_____. The fertilized ovum or (5) _____ begins to divide and in approxi-

mately 3 days forms a solid mass called a (6) _____. By the time it enters the

uterus, it is a hollow ball of cells called a (7) _____. As it continues to develop,

it forms a structure with two cavities. The (8) _____ _____

_____ will become a fluid-filled sac for the embryo. The (9) _____

will develop into an important fetal membrane in the (10) _____.

Match each description on the left with its corresponding term on the right. Write the letter in the answer blank.

_____	11. "Within a glass"	A. Laparoscope
_____	12. Inside germ layer	B. Gestation
_____	13. Before birth	C. Antenatal
_____	14. Length of pregnancy	D. Histogenesis
_____	15. Fiber-optic viewing instrument	E. Apgar score
_____	16. Process of birth	F. Endoderm
_____	17. System used to assess the general condition of a newborn	G. In vitro
_____	18. Study of how the primary germ layers develop into many different kinds of tissues	H. Parturition
_____	19. Term used to describe the developing individual during the first 8 weeks of pregnancy	I. Embryo
_____	20. Monitors progress of developing fetus	J. Ultrasonogram

If you had difficulty with this section, review pages 654-663.

DISORDERS OF PREGNANCY

True or False

If the statement is true, write "T" in the answer blank. If the statement is false, correct the statement by circling the incorrect term and writing the correct term in the answer blank.

_____ 21. Many offspring are lost before implantation occurs, often for unknown reasons.

_____ 22. The most common type of ectopic pregnancy is a tubal pregnancy.

_____ 23. If the placenta grows too closely to the cervical opening, a condition called *abruptio placentae* results.

_____ 24. Separation of the placenta from the uterine wall in a pregnancy of 20 weeks or more is known as *placenta previa*.

_____ 25. Toxemia of pregnancy is also known as *puerperal fever*.

_____ 26. After 20 weeks, delivery of a lifeless infant is termed a *miscarriage*.

_____ 27. Acquired birth defects result from agents called *teratogens* that disrupt normal histogenesis and organogenesis.

If you had difficulty with this section, review pages 662-663.

Circle the correct answer.

28. During the postnatal period:
    A. the head becomes proportionately smaller
    B. thoracic and abdominal contours change from round to elliptical
    C. the legs become proportionately longer
    D. the trunk becomes proportionately shorter
    E. all of the above take place during the postnatal period

29. The period of infancy starts at birth and lasts about:
    A. 4 weeks
    B. 4 months
    C. 10 weeks
    D. 12 months
    E. 18 months

30. The lumbar curvature of the spine appears _____ months after birth.
    A. 1 to 10
    B. 5 to 8
    C. 8 to 12
    D. 11 to 15
    E. 12 to 18

31. During the first 4 months, the birth weight will:
    A. double
    B. triple
    C. quadruple
    D. none of the above

32. At the end of the first year, the weight of the baby will have:
    A. doubled
    B. tripled
    C. quadrupled
    D. none of the above

33. The infant is capable of following a moving object with its eyes at:
    A. 2 days
    B. 2 weeks
    C. 2 months
    D. 4 months
    E. 10 months

34. The infant can lift its head and raise its chest at:
    A. 2 months
    B. 3 months
    C. 4 months
    D. 10 months

35. The infant can crawl at:
    A. 2 months
    B. 3 months
    C. 4 months
    D. 10 months
    E. 12 months

36. The infant can stand alone at:
    A. 2 months
    B. 3 months
    C. 4 months
    D. 10 months
    E. 12 months

37. The permanent teeth, with the exception of the third molar, have all erupted by the age of _____ years.
    A. 6
    B. 8
    C. 12
    D. 14
    E. none of the above

38. Puberty starts at age _____ years in boys.
    A. 10 to 13
    B. 12 to 14
    C. 14 to 16
    D. none of the above

39. Most girls begin breast development at about age:
    A. 8
    B. 9
    C. 10
    D. 11
    E. 12

40. The growth spurt is generally complete by age _____ in males.
    A. 14
    B. 15
    C. 16
    D. 18

41. An average age at which girls begin to menstruate is _____ years.
    A. 10 to 12
    B. 11 to 12
    C. 12 to 13
    D. 13 to 14
    E. 14 to 15

42. The first sign of puberty in boys is:
    A. facial hair
    B. increased muscle mass
    C. pubic hair
    D. deepening of the voice
    E. enlargement of the testicles

Match each description on the left with its corresponding term on the right. Write the letter in the answer blank.

_____ 43. Begins at birth and lasts until death

_____ 44. Study of the diagnosis and treatment of disorders of the newborn

_____ 45. Teenage years

_____ 46. From the end of infancy to puberty

_____ 47. Baby teeth

_____ 48. First 4 weeks of infancy

_____ 49. Age at which secondary sexual characteristics occur

_____ 50. Study of aging

_____ 51. Older adulthood

A. Neonatology

B. Neonatal

C. Adolescence

D. Deciduous

E. Puberty

F. Postnatal

G. Gerontology

H. Childhood

I. Senescence

If you had difficulty with this section, review pages 664-667.

EFFECTS OF AGING

Fill in the blanks.

52. Old bones develop indistinct and shaggy margins with spurs, a process called _____

_____.

53. A degenerative joint disease common in the aged is _____.

54. The number of _____ units in the kidney decreases by almost 50% between the ages of 30 and 75.

55. In old age, respiratory efficiency decreases, and a condition known as _____

_____ results.

56. Fatty deposits accumulate in blood vessels as we age, and the result is _____, which narrows the passageway for the flow of blood.

57. Hardening of the arteries, or _____, occurs during the aging process.

58. Another term for high blood pressure is _____.

59. Hardening of the lens is _____.

60. If the lens becomes cloudy and impairs vision, it is called a _____.

61. _____ causes an increase in the pressure within the eyeball and may result in blindness.

If you had difficulty with this section, review pages 668-670.

UNSCRAMBLE THE WORDS

62. **A N N F C Y I**

[○][ ][○][ ][ ][ ]

63. **N A A L T T S O P**

[ ][ ][ ][○][ ][○][ ][○]

64. **O G S S N E G R A O N E I**

[ ][○][ ][○][ ][ ][○][ ][ ][ ][○]

65. **G T E Y Z O**

[○][ ][ ][○][ ][ ]

66. **H D O O L H C I D**

[ ][○][ ][ ][ ][○][ ][ ]

Take the circled letters, unscramble them, and fill in the solution.

The secret to Farmer Brown's prize pumpkin crop.

67. [ ][ ][ ][ ][ ][ ][ ][ ][ ][ ][ ][ ][ ]

APPLYING WHAT YOU KNOW

68. Billy's mother told the pediatrician during his 1-year visit that Billy had tripled his birth weight, was crawling actively, and could stand alone. Is Billy's development normal, retarded, or advanced?

69. John is 70 years old. He has always enjoyed food and has had a hearty appetite. Lately, however, he has complained that food "just doesn't taste as good anymore." What might be a possible explanation?

70. Mr. Gaylor has noticed hearing problems but only under certain circumstances. He has difficulty with certain tones, especially high or low tones, but has no problem with everyday conversation. What might be a possible explanation?

71. Mrs. Lowell gave birth to twin girls. The obstetrician, Dr. Sullivan, advised Mr. Lowell that even though the girls looked identical, they were really fraternal twins. How was he able to deduce this?

262

72. Word Find

Find and circle 13 terms presented in this chapter. Words may be spelled top to bottom, bottom to top, right to left, left to right, or diagonally.

```
F C M P O D N P P A G M J N Z
K E C N E C S E L O D A G G M
I N R B U X T K D A Y Q T F R
L D L T O M S D W A E Z B F E
Z O B A I S P M A L C E E R P
W D I M P L A N T A T I O N L
H E N M K A I T E P D K S X A
W R G A S A R Z R N T Q P Y C
L M Q S I J O O A U B F G T E
R T N T B N G E S T A T I O N
L A T I N E G N O C I T F Z T
D C B T R L A S G C O O R R A
E N O I T I R U T R A P N S B
N V A S N N E G O T A R E T E
```

Adolescence	Implantation	Placenta
Congenital	Laparoscope	Preeclampsia
Endoderm	Mastitis	Progeria
Fertilization	Parturition	Teratogen
Gestation		

KNOW YOUR MEDICAL TERMS

Indicate whether the medical term is the correct one for the given literal translation by writing "T" (true) or "F" (false).

_____ 73. Adolescence   (grow up/state)

_____ 74. Ectoderm   (outside/skin)

_____ 75. Gestation   (time/deliver)

_____ 76. Neonate   (new/born)

_____ 77. Zygote   (little/egg)

_____ 78. Menopause   (month/cease)

_____ 79. Placenta   (flat/cake)

_____ 80. Glaucoma   (cloud/tumor)

If you had difficulty with this section, review pages 653, and 671-672.

DID YOU KNOW?

- Brain cells do not regenerate. One beer permanently destroys 10,000 brain cells.
- A scientist who weighed people immediately before and after death concluded that the human soul weighs 21 g.
- A fetus acquires fingerprints at the age of 3 months.
- At age seventy, 73% of men are still potent.

GROWTH AND DEVELOPMENT

Fill in the crossword puzzle.

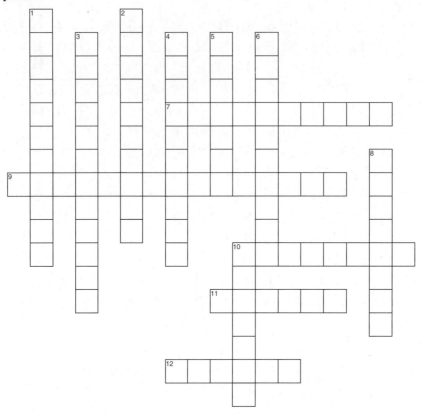

ACROSS

7. Old age
9. Fatty deposit buildup on walls of arteries
10. Cloudy lens
11. Name of zygote after 3 days
12. Fertilized ovum

DOWN

1. Process of birth
2. Science of the development of the individual before birth
3. Study of how germ layers develop into tissues
4. Name of zygote after implantation
5. First 4 weeks of infancy
6. Hardening of the lens
8. Eye disease marked by increased pressure in the eyeball
10. Will develop into a fetal membrane in the placenta

CHECK YOUR KNOWLEDGE

Multiple Choice

Circle the correct answer.

1. When the human embryo is a hollow ball of cells consisting of an outer cell layer and an inner cell mass, what is it called?
   A. Morula
   B. Chorion
   C. Blastocyst
   D. Zygote

2. Degenerative changes in the urinary system that accompany old age include which of the following?
   A. Decreased capacity of the bladder and the inability to empty or void completely
   B. Decrease in the number of nephrons
   C. Less blood flow through the kidneys
   D. All of the above

3. The frontal and maxillary sinuses of the facial region acquire permanent placement or develop fully when the individual is in a stage of development known as which of the following?
   A. Infancy
   B. Childhood
   C. Adolescence
   D. Adulthood

4. The first 4 weeks of human life following birth are referred to as which of the following?
   A. Neonatal
   B. Infancy
   C. Prenatal
   D. Embryonic

5. Which statement regarding labor is *not* true?
   A. It usually lasts from 6 to 24 hours
   B. Expulsion of the placenta is considered part of the labor process
   C. There are 3 stages of labor
   D. A breech birth usually goes through the same stages but requires a slightly longer labor period

6. Which of the following is characteristic of the disorder called *presbyopia*?
   A. It is very characteristic of old age
   B. It causes farsightedness in some individuals
   C. It is characterized by the lens in the eye becoming hard and losing its elasticity
   D. All of the above are true

7. The three most important "low-tech" methods for improving the quality of life as you age are:
   A. a healthy diet, exercise, and stress management
   B. a healthy diet, marriage, and money
   C. a healthy diet, a good job, and living in the suburbs
   D. a healthy diet, weight management, and exercise

8. Which of the following events, if any, is *not* characteristic of adolescence?
   A. Bone closure occurs
   B. Secondary sexual characteristics develop
   C. Very rapid growth occurs
   D. Growth spurts occur in both sexes

9. Which of the following events is *not* characteristic of the prenatal period of development?
   A. Blastocyst is formed
   B. Histogenesis occurs
   C. Bone closure occurs
   D. Amniotic cavity is formed

10. Which of the following structures is derived from ectoderm?
    A. The lining of the lungs
    B. The brain
    C. The kidneys
    D. All of the above

Matching

Match each term in column A with its corresponding definition in column B. (Only one answer is correct for each.)

Column A

_____ 11. Arteriosclerosis

_____ 12. Atherosclerosis

_____ 13. Parturition

_____ 14. Cataract

_____ 15. Adolescence

_____ 16. Amniotic sac

_____ 17. Glaucoma

_____ 18. Senescence

_____ 19. Hypertension

_____ 20. Placenta

Column B

A. High blood pressure

B. Chorion

C. Birth

D. "Bag of waters"

E. Hardening of arteries

F. Degeneration

G. Fat accumulation in arteries

H. Secondary sexual characteristics

I. Clouding of eye lens

J. High eye pressure

Circle the correct answer.

21. At the very beginning of the embryonic stage, all of the cells are (*stem* or *bilayered*).

22. Splitting of embryonic tissue from the same zygote early in development results in (*monozygotic* or *dizygotic*) twins.

23. Puerperal fever is also known as (*childbed fever* or *septicemia*).

24. The period from the time of maximal cervical dilation until the baby exits through the vagina is (*Stage 1* or *Stage 2*) labor.

25. Cessation of the reproductive cycle is (*menarche* or *menopause*).

FERTILIZATION AND IMPLANTATION

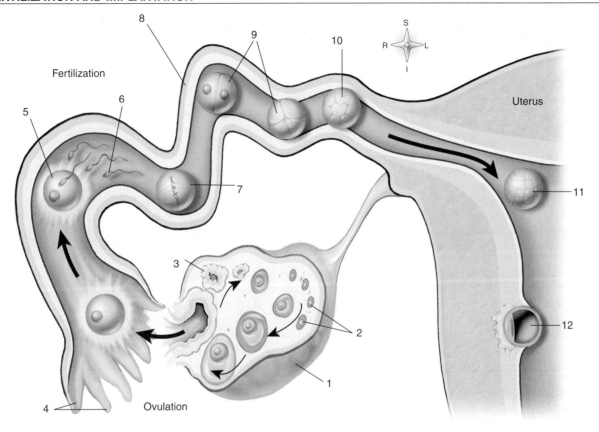

Fertilization

Ovulation

Uterus

1. _____
2. _____
3. _____
4. _____
5. _____
6. _____

7. _____
8. _____
9. _____
10. _____
11. _____
12. _____

Genetics and Genetic Diseases

Look around your classroom and you will notice various combinations of hair color, eye color, body size, skin tone, hair texture, gender, etc. Everyone has unique body features, and this phenomenon alerts us to the marvel of genetics. Independent units, called *genes*, are responsible for the inheritance of biological traits. Genes determine the structure and function of the human body by producing specific regulatory enzymes. Some genes are dominant, and some are recessive. Dominant genes produce traits that appear in the offspring, and recessive genes have traits that do not appear in the offspring when they are masked by a dominant gene.

   Gene therapy is one of the latest advances in science. This revolutionary branch of medicine combines current technology with genetic research to unlock the secrets of the human body. Daily discoveries in the prevention, diagnosis, treatment, and cure of diseases and disorders are being revealed as a result of genetic therapy. Knowledge of genetics is necessary to understand the basic mechanism by which traits are transmitted from parents to offspring.

TOPICS FOR REVIEW

Your review of this chapter should include an understanding of chromosomes, genes, and gene expression. You should continue your study with a knowledge of common genetic diseases. Finally, your review should conclude with an understanding of the prevention and treatment of genetic diseases.

GENETICS AND HUMAN DISEASE

CHROMOSOMES AND GENES

HUMAN GENOME

Match each term on the left with its corresponding description on the right. Write the letter in the answer blank.

_____ 1. Gene	A. DNA molecule
_____ 2. Chromosome	B. Male or female reproductive cell
_____ 3. Gamete	C. Special form of nuclear division
_____ 4. Meiosis	D. Formed by union of sperm and ovum at conception
_____ 5. Zygote	E. Distinct code within a DNA molecule
_____ 6. Genome	F. Adenine
_____ 7. Genomics	G. Entire collection of genetic material in each typical cell
_____ 8. Proteomics	H. Cartoon of a chromosome
_____ 9. Ideogram	I. Analysis of the genome's code
_____ 10. Nucleotide base	J. Analysis of the proteins encoded by the genome

If you had difficulty with this section, review pages 680-681.

GENE EXPRESSION

Fill in the blanks.

After experimentation with pea plants, Mendel discovered that each inherited trait is controlled by two sets of similar (11) _____, one from each parent. He also noted that some genes are (12) _____ and that some are (13) _____.

In the example of albinism, a person with the gene combination of Aa is said to be a genetic (14) _____ _____. If two different dominant genes occur together, a form of dominance called (15) _____ exists. (16) _____ chromosomes do not have matching structures. If an individual has the sex chromosomes XX, that person will have the sexual characteristics of a (17) _____. (18) _____ simply means "change." A (19) _____ _____ is a change in the genetic code.

If you had difficulty with this section, review pages 682-684.

GENETIC DISEASES

Match each description on the left with its corresponding term on the right. Write the letter in the answer blank.

_____ 20. Caused by recessive genes in chromosome pair 7	A.	Single-gene disease
_____ 21. Results in total blindness by age 30	B.	Nondisjunction
_____ 22. Disease conditions that result from the combined effects of inheritance and environmental factors	C.	Monosomy
_____ 23. Results from a failure to produce the enzyme phenylalanine hydroxylase	D.	Leber hereditary optic neuropathy
_____ 24. Presence of only one autosome instead of a pair	E.	Cystic fibrosis
_____ 25. Usually caused by trisomy of chromosome 21	F.	Phenylketonuria
_____ 26. Cystic fibrosis is an example	G.	Down syndrome
_____ 27. Results from nondisjunction of chromosomes and typically has the XXY pattern	H.	Klinefelter syndrome
_____ 28. Term used to describe what happens when a pair of chromosomes fails to separate	I.	Turner syndrome
_____ 29. Sometimes called *XO syndrome*, it is treated with hormone therapy	J.	Genetic predisposition

If you had difficulty with this section, review pages 685-689.

Circle the correct answer.

30. A pedigree is a chart that can be used to determine:
    A. genetic relationships in a family over several generations
    B. the possibility of producing offspring with certain genetic disorders
    C. the possibility of a person developing a genetic disorder late in life
    D. all of the above
    E. none of the above

31. The Punnett square is a grid used to determine:
    A. genetic disorders
    B. the probability of inheriting genetic traits
    C. proper gene replacement therapy
    D. the necessity for amniocentesis

32. Some forms of cancer are thought to be caused, at least in part, by abnormal genes called:
    A. cancercytes
    B. trisomy
    C. oncogenes
    D. autosomes

33. When producing a karyotype, the most common source of cells for the sample is the:
    A. vagina
    B. rectum
    C. lining of the cheek
    D. throat

34. An ultrasound transducer is used during amniocentesis to:
    A. create a sharper image
    B. take measurements during the procedure
    C. prevent damaging rays during the procedure
    D. guide the tip of the needle to prevent placental damage

35. Electrophoresis is a process that:
    A. provides a method for DNA analysis
    B. means electric separation
    C. is the basis for DNA fingerprinting
    D. all of the above

36. The use of genetic therapy began in 1990 with a group of young children who had:
    A. AIDS
    B. adenosine deaminase deficiency
    C. hemophilia
    D. cystic fibrosis

True or False

If the statement is true, write "T" in the answer blank. If the statement is false, correct the statement by circling the incorrect term and writing the correct term in the answer blank.

_____ 37. Chorionic villus sampling is a procedure in which cells that surround a young embryo are collected through the opening of the cervix.

_____ 38. Karyotyping is the process used for DNA fingerprinting.

_____ 39. In amniocentesis, normal genes are introduced with the hope that they will add to the production of the needed protein.

_____ 40. Deficiency of adenosine deaminase results in severe combined immune deficiency.

_____ 41. One hypothesis that may explain some forms of cancer is known as the *tumor suppressor gene* hypothesis.

If you had difficulty with this section, review pages 688 and 690-693.

UNSCRAMBLE THE WORDS

42. **RCRRIEA**

43. **YTSMOIR**

44. **EGNE**

45. **DPEREGIE**

46. **SOEMCROSHOM**

Take the circled letters, unscramble
them, and fill in the solution.

How Bill made his fortune.

47.

APPLYING WHAT YOU KNOW

48. Steve's mother has a dominant gene for dark skin color. Steve's father has a dominant gene for light skin color. What color will Steve's skin most likely be?

49. Mr. and Mrs. Freund both carry recessive genes for cystic fibrosis. Using your knowledge of the Punnett square, estimate the probability of one of their offspring inheriting this condition.

50. Meredith is pregnant and is over 40. She fears her age may predispose her baby to genetic disorders, and she has sought the advice of a genetic counselor. What tests might the counselor suggest to alleviate Meredith's fears?

51. Punnett Square

Mr. Fortner has two dominant genes for brown eyes, and Mrs. Fortner has two recessive genes for blue eyes.

A. The offspring of Mr. and Mrs. Fortner have a _____% chance of having brown eyes and a _____% chance of having blue eyes.

B. Will Mr. and Mrs. Fortner's offspring be carriers of blue eyes?

C. If Mr. and Mrs. Fortner's offspring mates with another offspring who is a carrier of blue eyes, what is the probability of the resulting offspring having blue eyes?

Use the Punnett square identified as Fortner to determine your answer.

Mr. Fortner PP

Mrs. Fortner pp

Mr. and Mrs. Harrington are both carriers for albinism. Using the Punnett square identified as *Harrington*, determine what percentage of Mr. and Mrs. Harrington's offspring will:

A. Have normal pigmentation _____

B. Be carriers _____

C. Have albinism _____

Mrs. Harrington Pp

Mr. Harrington Pp

52. Word Find

Find and circle 14 terms presented in this chapter. Words may be spelled top to bottom, bottom to top, right to left, left to right, or diagonally.

Amniocentesis
Carrier
Chromosomes
Codominance
DNA
Gametes
Gene therapy

Hemophilia
Karyotype
Meiosis
Monosomy
Nondisjunction
Recessive
Zygote

```
N  J  A  T  E  T  O  G  Y  Z  S  F  I  H  Q
M  O  M  D  P  S  I  W  P  L  I  K  Y  E  K
S  M  N  P  E  E  F  Y  A  Z  S  A  X  M  C
F  A  I  D  V  M  M  Z  R  Z  O  R  P  O  L
H  R  O  J  I  O  E  U  E  I  I  Y  D  P  O
I  Q  C  M  S  S  O  L  H  Z  E  O  G  H  X
Y  J  E  O  S  O  J  Z  T  W  M  T  D  I  Q
G  E  N  I  E  M  C  U  E  I  E  Y  X  L  Q
A  O  T  G  C  O  P  K  N  E  J  P  I  I  G
M  P  E  M  E  R  D  A  E  C  P  E  J  A  I
E  D  S  I  R  H  N  C  G  B  T  Z  P  S  Y
T  G  I  D  U  C  G  C  P  X  H  I  F  G  X
E  W  S  R  E  I  R  R  A  C  V  I  O  H  S
S  W  V  B  K  R  C  R  Y  B  V  U  C  N  S
```

KNOW YOUR MEDICAL TERMS

Select the letters that represent the literal translation of the word. Use as many letters as necessary.

A. white
B. single
C. self
D. relating to
E. sexual union
F. gene
G. birth membrane

H. process
I. nucleus
J. retreat
K. idea
L. body
M. characterized by
N. change

O. state
P. kind
Q. entire collection
R. prick
S. produce
T. drawing

_____ 53. Autosome

_____ 54. Gamete

_____ 55. Genome

_____ 56. Recessive

_____ 57. Albinism

_____ 58. Amniocentesis

_____ 59. Ideogram

_____ 60. Monosomy

_____ 61. Mutagen

_____ 62. Karyotype

If you had difficulty with this section, review pages 679 and 694-695.

- Scientists now believe the human body has 50,000 to 100,000 genes packed into just 46 chromosomes.
- If you could unwrap the entire DNA sequence you have in your cells, you could reach the moon 6,000 times.
- If the human genome were a book, it would be equivalent to 800 dictionaries.
- Human DNA is 96% identical to chimpanzee DNA.

GENETICS

Fill in the crossword puzzle.

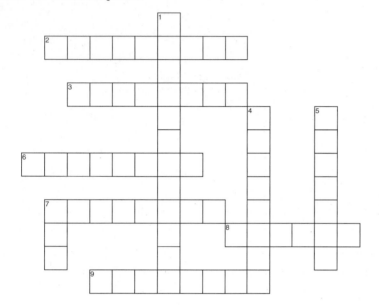

ACROSS

2. Name for the 22 pairs of matched chromosomes
3. Lack of melanin in the skin and eyes
6. Refers to genes that appear in the offspring
7. Chart that illustrates genetic relationships in a family over several generations
8. All genetic material in each cell
9. Scientific study of inheritance

DOWN

1. Trisomy 21 (two words)
4. Agents that cause genetic mutations
5. Triplet of autosomes rather than a pair
7. Excess of phenylketone in the urine (abbreviation)

CHECK YOUR KNOWLEDGE

Multiple Choice

Circle the correct answer.

1. Independent assortment of chromosomes ensures:
   A. each offspring from a single set of parents is genetically unique
   B. at meiosis, each gamete receives the same number of chromosomes
   C. that the sex chromosomes always match
   D. an equal number of males and females are born

2. Which of the following statements is *not* true of a pedigree?
   A. It is useful to genetic counselors in predicting the possibility of producing offspring with genetic disorders
   B. It may allow a person to determine his or her likelihood of developing a genetic disorder later in life
   C. It indicates the occurrence of those family members affected by a trait, as well as carriers of the trait
   D. All of the above are true of a pedigree

3. The genes that cause albinism are:
   A. codominant
   B. dominant
   C. recessive
   D. AA

4. During meiosis, matching pairs of chromosomes line up and exchange genes from their location with genes from the same location on the other side, a process called:
   A. gene linkage
   B. crossing over
   C. cross-linkage
   D. genetic variation

274

5. When a sperm cell unites with an ovum, a _____ is formed.
   A. zygote
   B. chromosome
   C. gamete
   D. none of the above

6. DNA molecules can also be called:
   A. a chromatin strand
   B. a chromosome
   C. A and B
   D. none of the above

7. Nonsexual traits:
   A. show up more often in females than in males
   B. may be carried on sex chromosomes
   C. are the result of genetic mutation
   D. all of the above

8. If a person has only X chromosomes, that person is:
   A. missing essential proteins
   B. abnormal
   C. female
   D. male

9. A karyotype:
   A. can detect trisomy
   B. is useful for diagnosing a tubal pregnancy
   C. is frequently used as a tool in gene augmentation therapy
   D. can detect the presence of oncogenes

10. Which of the following pairs is mismatched?
    A. SCID—gene therapy
    B. Turner syndrome—trisomy
    C. PKU—recessive
    D. Cystic fibrosis—single-gene disease

Completion

Complete the following statements using the terms listed below. Write the corresponding letter in the answer blank.

A. Cystic fibrosis   G. Punnett square

B. Males   H. Oncogenes

C. Phenylketonuria   I. Karyotype

D. Carrier   J. Tay-Sachs disease

E. Genome   K. Amniocentesis

F. Females   L. Hemophilia

11. Abnormal genes called _____ are believed to be related to cancer.

12. Fetal tissue may be collected by a procedure called _____.

13. An abnormal accumulation of phenylalanine results in _____.

14. The entire collection of genetic material in each cell is called the _____.

15. _____ is caused by recessive genes in chromosome pair seven.

16. A _____ is a grid used to help determine the probability of inheriting genetic traits.

17. A _____ is a person who has a recessive gene that is not expressed.

18. Absence of an essential lipid-producing enzyme may result in the recessive condition _____

   _____.

19. _____ is a recessive X-linked disorder.

20. Klinefelter syndrome occurs in _____.

Fill in the Blanks

21. The science of genetics developed from _____ quest to explain how normal biological characteristics are inherited.

22. _____ is the science that describes how environmental and behavioral factors may result in offspring with genetic traits that cannot be explained by genes alone.

23. Trisomy results from a mistake in meiosis called _____ that occurs when a pair of chromosomes fails to separate.

24. Trisomy 21 produces a group of symptoms called _____ _____

    _____.

25. In _____ _____, normal genes are introduced with the hope that they will add to the production of the needed protein.

Answers to Exercises

CHAPTER 1: INTRODUCTION TO THE BODY

Fill in the Blanks

1. Scientific method, p. 4
2. Hypothesis, p. 4
3. Experimentation, p. 4
4. Test group, p. 4
5. Control group, p. 4

Matching

6. D, p. 5
7. E, p. 6
8. A, p. 6
9. C, p. 6
10. B, p. 6

Matching

11. C, p. 7
12. A, p. 7
13. E, p. 7
14. D, p. 7
15. B, p. 7

Crossword

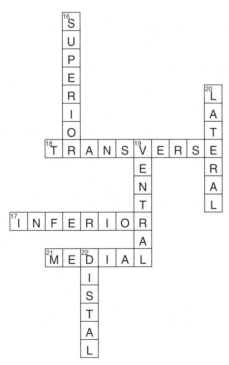

Did you notice that the answers were arranged as they appear on the human body?

Circle the Correct Answer

23. Inferior, p. 7
24. Anterior, p. 7
25. Lateral, p. 7
26. Proximal, p. 7
27. Superficial, p. 7
28. Equal, p. 9
29. Anterior and posterior, p. 9
30. Upper and lower, p. 9
31. Oblique, p. 9

Select the Correct Term

32. A, p. 9
33. B, p. 9
34. A, p. 9
35. A, p. 9
36. A, p. 9
37. B, p. 9
38. A, p. 9

Circle the One That Does Not Belong

39. Extremities (all others are part of the axial portions)
40. Cephalic (all others are part of the arm)
41. Plantar (all others are part of the face)
42. Carpal (all others are part of the leg or foot)
43. Tarsal (all others are part of the skull)

True or False

44. T
45. F (three stages), p. 12
46. T
47. F (they are not usually dissected), p. 12
48. F (during stage 3), p. 12
49. T

Fill in the Blanks

50. Survival, p. 14
51. Internal environment, p. 14
52. Rise, p. 14
53. Developmental processes, p. 16
54. Aging processes, p. 16
55. Negative, positive, p. 15
56. Stabilizing, p. 15
57. Stimulatory, p. 15

Unscramble the Words

58. Axial
59. Physiology
60. Frontal
61. Dorsal
62. Organ

Applying What You Know

63. ① on diagram
64. ② on diagram
65. ③ on diagram

66. **Word Find**

```
N H L T E B W N G N M M Y X A
O O H A V U U C L W E P N G L
I M U N I T S A I D E M W A L
T E R T V C T S I C J S R T K
A O N O P T I A I W A T Y R H
Z S Q S I R L F A T N R G O W
I T W G P R O I R E T S O P F
N A A Z J E E X V E E H L H Z
A S N L M C T P I C P D O Y T
G I C A Y U O X U M N U I V P
R S M R T N U K B S A Y S V M
O R C U R O I R B S Q L Y U G
L H X E M P M E T S Y S H V S
U W L L Q D U Y Y N E E P J B
Q N Z P K D B O D C G I N J A
```

Know Your Medical Terms

67. Hypothesis, p. 17
68. Epigastric, p. 17
69. Antebrachial, p. 3
70. Homeostasis, p. 17
71. Lateral, p. 17
72. Pedal, p. 18
73. Superior, p. 18
74. Diaphragm, p. 17
75. Ventral, p. 18

Check Your Knowledge
Multiple choice

1. A, p. 14
2. D, p. 9
3. B, p. 10
4. D, p. 9
5. A, p. 3
6. C, p. 9
7. C, p. 6
8. A, p. 9
9. C, p. 10
10. B, p. 10
11. D, p. 9
12. B, p. 9
13. C, p. 6
14. A, p. 9
15. D, p. 7
16. C, p. 7
17. D, p. 12
18. D, pp. 9 and 10
19. A, p. 13
20. C, p. 3

Matching

21. F, p. 9
22. B, p. 12
23. J, p. 9
24. G, p. 3
25. H, p. 7
26. C, p. 10
27. D, p. 13
28. I, p. 7
29. A, p. 9
30. E, p. 6

Dorsal and Ventral Body Cavities

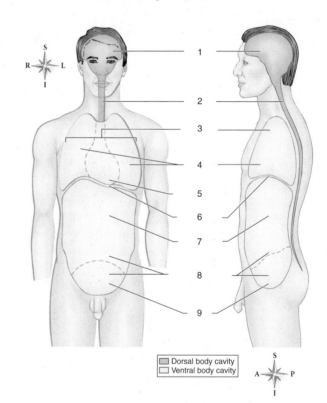

1. Cranial
2. Spinal
3. Thoracic
4. Pleural
5. Mediastinum
6. Diaphragm
7. Abdominal
8. Abdominopelvic
9. Pelvic

278

Directions and Planes of the Body

Sagittal planes

9 Midsagittal

10 Frontal planes

Transverse planes

Oblique planes

1 Superior

3 Posterior 4 Anterior

Proximal

2

5

Distal

Proximal

2
5

Distal

S
P —— A
I

Inferior
6

7 Lateral

Lateral

Frontal plane

Medial Medial
8

S
R —— L
I

1. Superior
2. Proximal
3. Posterior (dorsal)
4. Anterior (ventral)
5. Distal
6. Inferior

7. Lateral
8. Medial
9. Sagittal and Midsagittal
10. Frontal
11. Transverse
12. Oblique

279

Answers to Exercises

Regions of the Abdomen

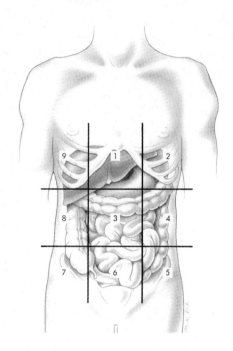

1. Epigastric region
2. Left hypochondriac region
3. Umbilical region
4. Left lumbar region
5. Left iliac (inguinal) region
6. Hypogastric region
7. Right iliac (inguinal) region
8. Right lumbar region
9. Right hypochondriac region

CHAPTER 2: CHEMISTRY OF LIFE

Multiple Choice

1. C, p. 25
2. B, p. 25
3. C, p. 25
4. A, p. 25
5. D, p. 27
6. C, p. 25
7. A, p. 26

True or False

8. T, p. 25
9. F (molecules), p. 25
10. F (uncharged neutrons), p. 25
11. T, p. 25
12. T, p. 26

Multiple Choice

13. C, p. 27
14. B, p. 27
15. A, p. 27
16. B, p. 28
17. A, p. 27
18. C, p. 27

Matching

19. H, p. 29
20. B, p. 29
21. E, p. 29
22. A, p. 29
23. G, p. 29
24. L, p. 29
25. J, p. 29
26. C, p. 30
27. D, p. 30
28. F, p. 30
29. K, p. 30
30. I, p. 31

Matching

31. A, p. 31
32. B, p. 31
33. D, p. 35
34. B, p. 33
35. C, p. 33
36. A, p. 31
37. A, p. 31
38. B, p. 32
39. C, p. 33
40. D, p. 35

Unscramble the Words

41. Protein
42. Base
43. Alkaline
44. Lipid
45. Salt

Crossword

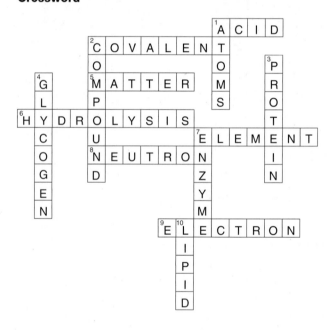

Know Your Medical Terms

46. d. Dissociate, p. 36
47. a. Buffer, p. 36
48. e. Polysaccharide, p. 37
49. c. Cholesterol, p. 36
50. g. Bond, p. 36
51. f. Inorganic compound, p. 37
52. b. Hydrogen, p. 37

Applying What You Know

53. Some fats can become solid at room temperature, such as the fat in butter and lard.
54. Radioactive isotopes will be used to measure Carol's thyroid activity. A diagnosis of hyperthyroidism or hypothyroidism will be based upon how rapidly or slowly the thyroid absorbs the radioactive iodine and emits radiation.
55. The normal pH of blood is 7.35 to 7.45. Blood is slightly alkaline, and therefore India's blood pH results are within the normal range and should be of no concern.

56. Word Find

Check Your Knowledge

Fill in the blanks

1. Formula, p. 27
2. Neutrons, p. 25
3. Higher, p. 25
4. Elements; compounds, p. 26
5. Stable, p. 27
6. Ion, p. 27
7. Inorganic, p. 29
8. Dehydration synthesis, p. 29
9. Chemical equation, p. 30
10. CO_2, p. 30
11. Acids, p. 30
12. Buffers, p. 31
13. Carbohydrate, p. 31
14. Cholesterol, p. 33
15. Structural, p. 34
16. Isotopes, p. 26
17. Enzymes, p. 34
18. Double helix, p. 35
19. Uracil, p. 35
20. Polysaccharides, p. 31

CHAPTER 3: CELLS

Matching
Group A

1. C, p. 44
2. E, p. 44
3. A, p. 44
4. B, p. 44
5. D, p. 48

Group B

6. D, p. 47
7. E, p. 47
8. A, p. 47
9. B, p. 47
10. C, p. 47

Fill in the Blanks

11. Cholesterol, p. 44
12. Tissue typing, p. 45
13. Cilia, p. 49
14. Endoplasmic reticulum, p. 47
15. Ribosomes, p. 47
16. Mitochondria, p. 47
17. Lysosomes, p. 47
18. Golgi apparatus, p. 47
19. Centrioles, p. 48
20. Chromatin granules, p. 50
21. Flagellum, p. 49
22. Microvilli, p. 48

Circle the Correct Answer

23. A, p. 50	29. B, p. 53
24. D, p. 51	30. C, p. 53
25. B, p. 51	31. C, p. 54
26. D, p. 52	32. A, p. 54
27. C, p. 52	33. B, p. 53
28. C, p. 53	34. A, p. 53

Circle the One That Does Not Belong

35. Uracil (RNA contains the base uracil, not DNA)
36. RNA (the others are complementary base pairings of DNA)
37. Anaphase (the others refer to genes and heredity)
38. Thymine (the others refer to RNA)
39. Interphase (the others refer to translation)
40. Prophase (the others refer to anaphase)
41. Prophase (the others refer to interphase)
42. Metaphase (the others refer to telophase)
43. Gene (the others refer to stages of cell division)

Unscramble the Words

44. Interphase	47. Telophase
45. Centriole	48. Organelle
46. Diffusion	49. Translation

Applying What You Know

50.

51. Diffusion
52. Absorption of oxygen into Ms. Bence's blood

53. Word Find

Know Your Medical Terms

54. F, p. 64
55. G, p. 63
56. H, p. 61 and 64
57. C, p. 63
58. A, p. 64
59. E, p. 63
60. B, p. 63
61. D, p. 63

Crossword

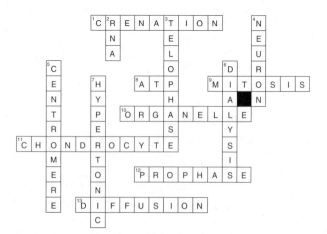

Check Your Knowledge
Multiple choice

1. A, p. 47
2. B, p. 53
3. B, p. 50
4. A, p. 60
5. C, p. 53
6. A, p. 57
7. A, p. 57
8. A, p. 56
9. D, p. 57
10. B, p. 59

Matching

11. F, p. 52
12. G, p. 44
13. J, p. 53
14. C, p. 55
15. A, p. 59
16. B, p. 56
17. I, p. 51
18. H, p. 53
19. D, p. 47
20. E, p. 54

Fill in the blanks

21. Cytoplasm, p. 45
22. Protein, p. 56
23. Interphase, p. 60
24. Apoptosis, p. 47
25. ATP, p. 53

Cell Structure

1. Nucleolus
2. Nuclear envelope
3. Nucleus
4. Nuclear pores
5. Plasma membrane
6. Cytoplasm
7. Centrioles
8. Mitochondrion
9. Lysosome
10. Golgi apparatus
11. Free ribosome
12. Microvilli
13. Cilia
14. Smooth endoplasmic reticulum
15. Ribosome
16. Flagellum
17. Rough endoplasmic reticulum
18. Chromatin

Mitosis

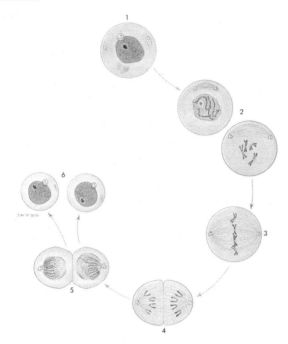

1. Interphase
2. Prophase
3. Metaphase
4. Anaphase
5. Telophase
6. Daughter cells (interphase)

CHAPTER 4: TISSUES

Multiple Choice

1. B, p. 71
2. C, p. 71
3. D, p. 71
4. D, p. 72
5. D, p. 72
6. B, pp 72 and 76
7. B, p. 73
8. B, p. 75
9. C, p. 76

Matching

10. B, p. 75
11. E, p. 73
12. A, p. 73
13. C, p. 75
14. D, p. 76
15. F, p. 76

Labeling

1. Simple columnar epithelium (1. Goblet cell, 2. Columnar epithelial cells)
2. Stratified squamous epithelium (1. Superficial squamous epithelial cell, 2. Basal epithelial cell, 3. Basement membrane)
3. Stratified transitional epithelium (1. Basement membrane, 2. Binucleate cell, 3. Stratified transitional epithelial cells)

Multiple Choice

16. A, p. 78
17. D, p. 79
18. A, p. 80
19. C, p. 80
20. A, p. 79
21. D, p. 76

Labeling

4. Adipose tissue (1. Storage area for fat, 2. Plasma membrane, 3. Nucleus of adipose cell)
5. Dense fibrous connective tissue (1. Nuclei of fiber-producing cells, 2. Bundles of collagenous fibers)
6. Bone tissue (1. Osteon)
7. Blood tissue (1. White blood cell, 2. Matrix (liquid), 3. Red blood cells)

Matching

22. B, p. 82
23. C, p. 82
24. A, p. 82
25. B, p. 81
26. C, p. 82
27. C, p. 82

Labeling

8. Skeletal muscle (1. Striations, 2. Nuclei of muscle fibers, 3. Muscle fiber)
9. Cardiac muscle (1. Nucleus of muscle cell, 2. Intercalated disks)

Matching

28. B, p. 83
29. C, p. 83
30. A, p. 83
31. D, p. 83

Labeling

10. Nervous tissue (1. Nerve cell body, 2. Axon, 3. Dendrites)

32. Fill in the Missing Areas

Tissue	Location	Function
Epithelial		
1.	1.	1a. Absorption by respiratory gases between alveolar air and blood
		1b. Diffusion, filtration, and osmosis
2.	2a. Surface of lining of mouth and esophagus	2.
	2b. Surface of skin	
3.	3. Surface layer of lining of stomach, intestines, and parts of respiratory tract	3.
4. Stratified transitional	4.	4.
5.	5. Surface of lining of trachea	5.
6.	6.	6. Secretion; absorption
Connective		
1.	1. Between other tissues and organs	1.
2. Adipose	2.	2.
3.	3.	3. Flexible but strong connection
4.	4. Skeleton	4.
5.	5. Part of nasal septum, larynx, rings in trachea and bronchi, disks between vertebrae, external ear	5.
6.	6.	6. Transportation
7. Hematopoietic tissue	7.	7.
Muscle		
1.	1. Muscles that attach to bones, eyeball muscles, upper third of esophagus	1.
2. Cardiac	2.	2.
3.	3. Walls of digestive, respiratory, and genitourinary tracts; walls of blood and large lymphatic vessels; ducts of glands; intrinsic eye muscles; arrector muscles of hair	3.
Nervous		
1. Nervous	1. Brain and spinal cord, nerves	1.

Fill in the Blanks

33. Regeneration, p. 84
34. Keloid, p. 84
35. Phagocytic, p. 84
36. Connective, p. 84
37. Nerve, p. 85

Unscramble the Words

38. Dendrite
39. Osteon
40. Squamous
41. Stratified
42. Glia
43. Tissues

Applying What You Know

44. Merrily may have exceeded the 18% to 24% desirable body fat composition. Fitness depends more on the percentage and ratio of specific tissue types than on the overall amount of tissue present.

45. Holly is too lean. Holly should be in the 20% to 22% range to be considered normal. Holly's obsession may put her at risk for other disease conditions because of the stress to her body of being "too lean."

46. Word Find

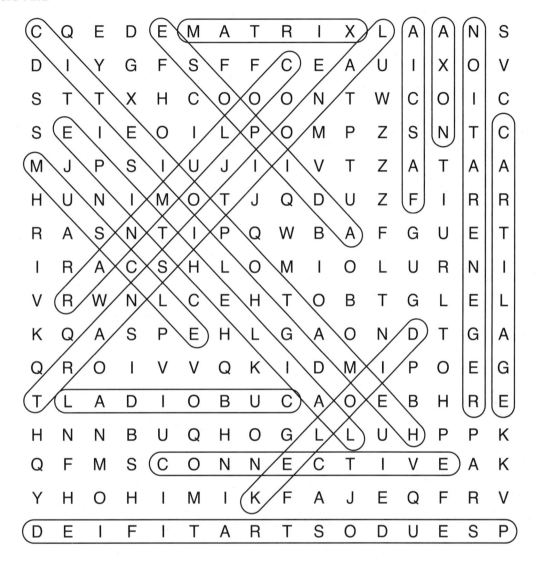

Know Your Medical Terms

47. against; produce, p. 71
48. axon, p. 71
49. chondro; cyte, p. 71
50. colla; gen, p. 71
51. within; secrete, p. 85
52. bone; unit, p. 85
53. gland, p. 85
54. claw; like, p. 86
55. strati; fied, p. 86
56. squam; ous, p. 86

Crossword

```
¹S ²M  O  O  T  H
   A
   T        ³F ⁴A  T
   R     ⁵S    X      ⁶C
   I     T     O      O    ⁷S
⁸E X O  C  R  I  N  E  N    Q
   A              N    U
   T        ⁹S  K  E  L  E  T  A  L
¹⁰G L I  A          C    M
   F              T    O
¹¹K E L  O  I  D      I    U
   E              V    S
¹²C H O  N  D  R  O  C  Y  T  E  S
```

Check Your Knowledge

Labeling

1. Squamous
2. Cuboidal
3. Columnar
4. Simple squamous
5. Simple cuboidal
6. Simple columnar
7. Stratified squamous
8. Pseudostratified columnar

Multiple choice

9. A, p. 81
10. B, p. 76
11. C, p. 73
12. D, p. 81
13. A, p. 84

Fill in the blanks

14. Areola, p. 78
15. Goblet, p. 75
16. Matrix, p. 72
17. Intercalated disks, p. 82
18. Keloid, p. 84
19. Regeneration, p. 84
20. Tissue typing, p. 81
21. Collagen, p. 72
22. Brown, p. 78
23. Cancellous, p. 80
24. Neuroglia or glia, p. 83
25. Fibrocartilage, p. 80

CHAPTER 5: ORGAN SYSTEMS

Matching

Group A

1. A, p. 93
2. E, p. 94
3. D, p. 95
4. B, p. 95
5. C, p. 96

Group B

6. F, p. 96
7. E, p. 97
8. B, p. 99
9. A, p. 98
10. C, p. 98
11. D, p. 100

Circle the One That Does Not Belong

12. Mouth (the others refer to the respiratory system)
13. Rectum (the others refer to the reproductive system)
14. Pancreas (the others refer to the cardiovascular system)
15. Pineal (the others refer to the urinary system)
16. Joints (the others refer to the muscular system)
17. Pituitary (the others refer to the nervous system)
18. Tendons (the others refer to the skeletal system)
19. Appendix (the others refer to the endocrine system)
20. Thymus (the others refer to the integumentary system)
21. Trachea (the others refer to the digestive system)
22. Liver (the others refer to the lymphatic system)

23. Fill in the Missing Areas

System	Organs	Functions
1.	1.	1. Protection, regulation of body temperature, synthesis of chemicals and hormones, serves as a sense organ
2.	2. Bones, joints	2.
3.	3.	3. Movement, maintains body posture, produces heat
4. Nervous	4.	4.
5.	5. Pituitary, thymus, pineal, adrenal, hypothalamus, thyroid, pancreas, parathyroid, ovaries, testes	5.
6.	6.	6. Transportation, immunity, regulation of body temperature
7.	7. Lymph nodes, lymph vessels, thymus, spleen, tonsils	7.
8. Urinary	8.	8.
9.	9. Mouth, pharynx, esophagus, stomach, small and large intestines, rectum, anal canal, teeth, salivary glands, tongue, liver, gallbladder, pancreas, appendix	9.
10. Respiratory	10.	10.
11.	11. Gonads—testes and ovaries	11.

Fill in the Blanks

24. Nonvital organ, p. 101
25. Cochlear implants, p. 103
26. Dialysis machine, p. 103
27. Left ventricular assist systems (LVAS), p. 104
28. Organ transplantation, p. 104
29. Free-flap surgery, p. 105
30. Rejection, p. 104

Unscramble the Words

31. Heart
32. Pineal
33. Nerve
34. Esophagus
35. Nervous

Applying What You Know

36. Endocrinology (endocrine system); gynecology (reproductive system)
37. The skin protects the underlying tissue against invasion by harmful bacteria. With a large percentage of Brian's skin destroyed, he is vulnerable to bacteria, and so he is placed in the cleanest environment possible—isolation. Jenny is required to wear special attire so that the risk of a visitor bringing bacteria to the patient is reduced.
38. Free-flap surgery may be considered as an option. A breast can be formed from skin and muscle taken from other parts of Sheila's body.

39. Word Find

Know Your Medical Terms

40. T, p. 93
41. F, p. 106   Break down/pertaining to/organized whole
42. T, p. 93
43. T, p. 106
44. T, p. 106
45. F, p. 106   On/cover/result of action
46. T, p. 106
47. F, p. 106   Water/relating to/organized whole
48. F, p. 106   Tool or instrument
49. T, p. 107
50. T, p. 107

Crossword

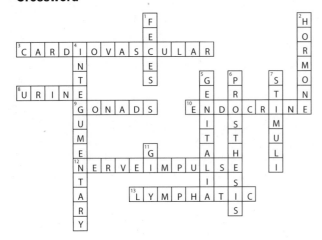

Check Your Knowledge

Multiple choice

1. D, p. 99
2. C, pp. 96 and 100
3. C, p. 98
4. B, p. 95
5. D, p. 94
6. A, p. 99
7. B, p. 95
8. A, p. 93
9. A, p. 98
10. C, p. 93

Matching

11. C, p. 93
12. D, p. 96
13. H, p. 97
14. G, p. 100
15. B, p. 99
16. F, p. 98
17. I, p. 100
18. E, p. 98
19. J, p. 95
20. A, p. 96

Fill in the blanks

21. skeletal, p. 94
22. appendages, p. 93
23. tendon, p. 95
24. peripheral nervous system, p. 95
25. transportation, p. 97

CHAPTER 6: MECHANISMS OF DISEASE

Matching

Group A

1. B, p. 113
2. E, p. 114
3. A, p. 114
4. C, p. 114
5. D, p. 114

Group B

6. C, p. 114
7. A, p. 114
8. D, p. 114
9. B, p. 114
10. E, p. 114

Fill in the Blanks

11. Pathophysiology, p. 115
12. Homeostasis, p. 116
13. Mutated, p. 116
14. Parasite, p. 116
15. Neoplasms, p. 116
16. Self-immunity, p. 116
17. Risk factors, p. 117
18. Centers for Disease Control and Prevention, p. 114
19. Psychogenic, p. 117
20. Secondary, p. 117

Multiple Choice

21. C, p. 118
22. A, p. 120
23. B, p. 119
24. C, p. 120
25. D, p. 121
26. B, p. 123
27. D, p. 123
28. D, p. 124
29. B, p. 125
30. C, p. 125
31. E, p. 125
32. B, p. 127

Circle the Correct Answer

33. Slowly, p. 129
34. Are not, p. 129
35. Papilloma, p. 129
36. Sarcoma, p. 129
37. Anaplasia, p. 130
38. Oncologist, p. 131
39. Biopsy, p. 132
40. Staging, p. 133
41. Appetite, p. 133

Warning Signs of Cancer

42. Sores that do not heal, p. 131
43. Unusual bleeding, p. 131
44. A change in a wart or mole, p. 131
45. A lump or thickening in any tissue, p. 131
46. Persistent hoarseness or cough, p. 131
47. Chronic indigestion, p. 131
48. A change in bowel or bladder function, p. 131
49. Bone pain that wakes the person at night and is located on only one side, p. 131

True or False

50. T
51. F (slowly), p. 135
52. F (white), p. 135
53. T
54. T
55. T
56. T

Unscramble the Words

57. Fungi
58. Oncogene
59. Edema
60. Spore
61. Grading

Applying What You Know

62. No. Trent most likely has a common cold.
63. Pinworm
64. Disinfection
65. A "gene pool" indicates the "risk" of inheriting a disease-causing gene specific to members of a certain ethnic group. The knowledge of a "gene pool" can alert you to early detection of disease.
66. Bill's chosen profession is considered "high risk" because of the paramedic's frequent exposure to body fluids. Hepatitis B is transmitted by body fluids; therefore, vaccination is recommended.

67. Word Find

Know Your Medical Terms

68. Disease, p. 136
69. Swelling, p. 137
70. Change, p. 113
71. Mushroom, p. 136
72. Rotten, p. 136
73. Boil, p. 137
74. Sharp, p. 137

Crossword

Check Your Knowledge
Multiple choice

1. B, p. 114
2. D, p. 114
3. A, p. 127
4. D, p. 114
5. A, p. 122
6. D, p. 115
7. C, p. 115
8. B, p. 133
9. D, p. 118
10. A, p. 123

Matching

11. C, p. 114
12. D, p. 129
13. B, p. 120
14. J, p. 123
15. G, p. 114
16. I, p. 135
17. E, p. 124
18. A, p. 113
19. F, p. 128
20. H, p. 124

Fill in the blanks

21. Psychogenic, p. 117
22. Retrovirus, p. 118
23. Coronavirus, p. 119
24. Nematodes, p. 124
25. Aseptic, p. 125

Major Groups of Pathogenic Bacteria

1. Bacilli (rods)
2. Cocci (spheres)
3. Curved rods
4. Small bacteria

Major Groups of Pathogenic Protozoa

1. Amoebas
2. Flagellates
3. Ciliates
4. Sporozoa

Examples of Pathogenic Animals

1. Nematodes
2. Platyhelminthes
3. Arthropods

Major Groups of Pathogenic Fungi

1. Yeasts
2. Molds

CHAPTER 7: SKIN AND MEMBRANES

Select the Best Answer

1. B, p. 146
2. D, p. 147
3. C, p. 147
4. A, p. 146
5. B, p. 146
6. D, p. 147
7. C, p. 147
8. C, p. 147

Matching
Group A

9. D, p. 148
10. A, p. 148
11. B, p. 148
12. C, p. 149
13. E, p. 148

Group B

14. A, p. 149
15. D, p. 149
16. E, p. 149
17. C, p. 150
18. B, p. 149

Select the Best Answer

19. A, p. 149
20. B, p. 151
21. B, p. 151
22. A, p. 150
23. A, p. 149
24. B, p. 150
25. B, p. 151
26. B, p. 154
27. B, p. 154
28. A, p. 148

Fill in the Blanks

29. Protection, temperature regulation, sense organ activity, excretion, and synthesis of Vitamin D, p. 155
30. Melanin, p. 149
31. Lanugo, p. 151
32. Hair papillae, p. 152
33. Alopecia, p. 152
34. Arrector pili, p. 153
35. Strawberry hemangioma, p. 151
36. Eccrine, p. 154
37. Apocrine, p. 154
38. Sebum, p. 154

Circle the Correct Answer

39. B, p. 156
40. A, p. 156
41. D, p. 158
42. D, p. 159
43. A, p. 161
44. D, p. 161
45. C, p. 161
46. A, p. 164

Circle the Correct Answer

47. Will not, p. 157
48. Will, p. 160
49. Will not, p. 160
50. 11, p. 161
51. Third-, p. 160

Unscramble the Words

52. Epidermis
53. Keratin
54. Hair
55. Lanugo
56. Dehydration
57. Third degree

Applying What You Know

58. 46
59. Pleurisy
60. Sunbathing. Mrs. Collins cannot repair UV damage and thus is very prone to skin cancer.
61. Fingerprints

62. Word Find

Know Your Medical Terms

63. A, p. 145
64. D, p. 166
65. G, p. 145
66. C, p. 145
67. J, p. 165
68. E, p. 166
69. M, p. 166
70. K, p. 166
71. F, p. 166
72. I, p. 167
73. H, p. 167
74. B, p. 166
75. L, p. 166

Crossword

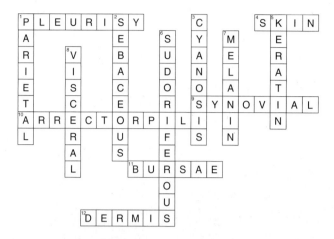

Check Your Knowledge

Multiple choice

1. A, p. 146
2. B, p. 147
3. A, p. 153
4. D, p. 154
5. B, p. 149
6. D, p. 157
7. B, p. 154
8. B, p. 149
9. C, p. 153
10. B, p. 155

Matching

11. C, p. 149
12. D, p. 146
13. B, p. 154
14. G, p. 154
15. I, p. 149
16. H, p. 151
17. J, p. 153
18. E, p. 147
19. A, p. 151
20. F, p. 154

Completion

21. H, p. 154
22. A, p. 161
23. B, p. 154
24. F, p. 160
25. I, p. 152
26. E, p. 148
27. G, p. 146
28. D, p. 147
29. J, p. 154
30. C, p. 147

Longitudinal Section of the Skin

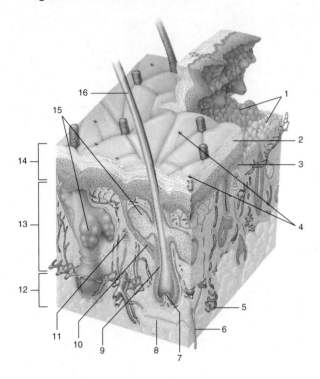

1. Dermal papilla
2. Stratum corneum
3. Stratum germinativum
4. Openings of sweat ducts
5. Sweat gland
6. Cutaneous nerve
7. Papilla of hair
8. Lamellar (Pacini) corpuscle
9. Hair follicle
10. Arrector muscle
11. Tactile (Meissner) corpuscle
12. Subcutaneous tissue
13. Dermis
14. Epidermis
15. Sebaceous (oil) gland
16. Hair shaft

Rule of Nines

CHAPTER 8: SKELETAL SYSTEM

Fill in the Blanks

1. Four, p. 176
2. Medullary cavity, p. 177
3. Articular cartilage, p. 177
4. Endosteum, p. 177
5. Hematopoiesis, p. 176
6. Red bone marrow, p. 176
7. Periosteum, p. 177
8. Long, short, flat, and irregular, p. 176
9. Calcium, p. 176
10. Move, p. 176

Matching
Group A

11. D, p. 177
12. B, p. 177
13. E, p. 177
14. A, p. 177
15. C, p. 177

Group B

16. D, p. 177
17. A, p. 177
18. E, p. 177
19. B, p. 177
20. C, p. 177

True or False

21. T
22. F (epiphyses, not diaphyses), p. 179
23. F (osteoblasts, not osteoclasts), p. 179
24. T
25. T
26. F (juvenile, not adult), p. 179
27. F (diaphysis, not articulation), p. 179
28. T
29. F (ceases, not begins), p. 179
30. T

Multiple Choice

31. A, p. 190
32. D, p. 183
33. A, p. 187
34. D, p. 189
35. C, p. 190
36. C, p. 193
37. D, p. 190
38. D, p. 191 and 194
39. A, p. 193 and 194
40. B, p. 183
41. A, p. 187
42. B, p. 190
43. B, p. 189
44. B, p. 190
45. C, p. 191
46. A, p. 193
47. D, p. 183
48. C, p. 187
49. C, p. 183

Circle the One That Does Not Belong

50. Coxal (all others refer to the spine)
51. Axial (all others refer to the appendicular skeleton)
52. Maxilla (all others refer to the cranial bones)
53. Ribs (all others refer to the shoulder girdle)
54. Vomer (all others refer to the bones of the middle ear)
55. Ulna (all others refer to the coxal bone)
56. Ethmoid (all others refer to the hand and wrist)
57. Nasal (all others refer to cranial bones)
58. Anvil (all others refer to the cervical vertebra)

Choose the Correct Answer

59. A, p. 195	62. A, p. 195
60. B, p. 195	63. B, p. 195
61. B, p. 195	

Matching

64. C, p. 183	71. D, B, p. 183
65. G, p. 190	72. F, p. 183
66. J, L, M, and K, p. 194	73. H, Q, p. 190
67. N, p. 194	74. O, T, p. 194
68. I, p. 190	75. R, p. 183
69. A, p. 183	76. S, E, p. 183
70. P, p. 194	

Circle the Correct Answer

77. Diarthroses, p. 196
78. Synarthrotic, p. 196
79. Diarthrotic, p. 197
80. Ligaments, p. 198
81. Articular cartilage, p. 198
82. Least movable, p. 199
83. Largest, p. 206
84. 2, p. 198
85. Mobility, p. 199
86. Pivot, p. 199

Fill in the Blanks

87. Arthroscopy, p. 208
88. Osteosarcoma, p. 200
89. Osteoporosis, p. 201
90. Osteomalacia, p. 201
91. Paget's disease, p. 202
92. Osteomyelitis, p. 202
93. Simple fractures, p. 203
94. Comminuted fractures, p. 204
95. Osteoarthritis or degenerative joint disease (DJD), p. 204
96. Rheumatoid arthritis, gouty arthritis, and infectious arthritis, p. 205
97. Lyme disease, p. 207

Unscramble the Bones

98. Vertebrae
99. Pubis
100. Scapula
101. Mandible
102. Phalanges
103. Pelvic girdle

Applying What You Know

104. The bones are responsible for the majority of our blood cell formation. Her disease condition might be inhibiting the production of blood cells.
105. Epiphyseal cartilage is present only while a child is still growing. It becomes bone in adulthood. It is particularly vulnerable to fractures in childhood and preadolescence.
106. Osteoporosis
107. Slipped or herniated disk

108. Word Find

Know Your Medical Terms

109. B, p. 209	113. A, p. 211
110. D, p. 210	114. E, p. 211
111. G, p. 210	115. C, p. 210
112. F, p. 209	

Crossword

Check Your Knowledge

Multiple choice

1. A, p. 189	6. D, p. 197
2. C, p. 191	7. C, p. 180
3. A, p. 177	8. C, p. 183
4. C, p. 195	9. D, p. 180
5. C, p. 187	10. A, p. 196

Matching

11. G, p. 198
12. B, p. 177
13. I, p. 196
14. J, p. 183
15. E, p. 194
16. H, p. 177

17. A, p. 177
18. C, p. 183
19. F, p. 194
20. K, p. 176
21. D, p. 177

Fill in the blanks

22. Epiphyseal plate, p. 179
23. Frontal, maxilla, sphenoid, and ethmoid, p. 181
24. Hyoid, p. 183
25. Scoliosis, p. 188

Longitudinal Section of Long Bone

1. Epiphysis
2. Diaphysis
3. Epiphysis
4. Periosteum
5. Yellow marrow
6. Endosteum

7. Medullary cavity
8. Compact bone
9. Red marrow cavities
10. Epiphyseal line
11. Spongy bone
12. Articular cartilage

Anterior View of Skeleton

1. Frontal bone
2. Nasal bone
3. Zygomatic bone
4. Sternum
5. Ribs

6. Vertebral column
7. Ilium
8. Pubis
9. Ischium
10. Greater trochanter

11. Phalanges
12. Metatarsals
13. Tarsals
14. Fibula
15. Tibia
16. Patella
17. Femur
18. Phalanges
19. Metacarpals
20. Carpals

21. Ulna
22. Radius
23. Humerus
24. Xiphoid process
25. Costal cartilage
26. Scapula
27. Manubrium
28. Clavicle
29. Mandible
30. Maxilla

Posterior View of Skeleton

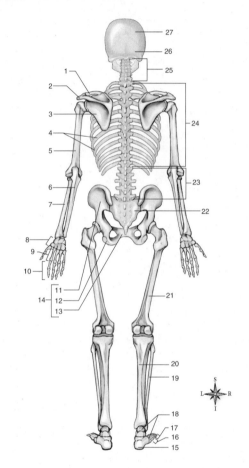

1. Clavicle
2. Acromion process
3. Scapula
4. Ribs
5. Humerus
6. Ulna
7. Radius
8. Carpals
9. Metacarpals
10. Phalanges
11. Ilium
12. Ischium
13. Pubis
14. Coxal (hip) bone

15. Calcaneus (a tarsal bone)
16. Metatarsal bones
17. Phalanges
18. Tarsals
19. Fibula
20. Tibia
21. Femur
22. Sacrum
23. Lumbar vertebrae
24. Thoracic vertebrae
25. Cervical vertebrae
26. Occipital bone
27. Parietal bone

Skull Viewed from the Right Side

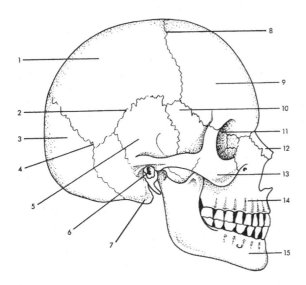

1. Parietal bone
2. Squamous suture
3. Occipital bone
4. Lambdoidal suture
5. Temporal bone
6. External auditory canal
7. Mastoid process
8. Coronal suture
9. Frontal bone
10. Sphenoid bone
11. Ethmoid bone
12. Nasal bone
13. Zygomatic bone
14. Maxilla
15. Mandible

Skull Viewed from the Front

1. Sphenoid bone
2. Ethmoid bone
3. Lacrimal bone
4. Zygomatic bone
5. Vomer
6. Frontal bone
7. Parietal bone
8. Nasal bone
9. Inferior concha
10. Maxilla
11. Mandible

Structure of a Diarthrotic Joint

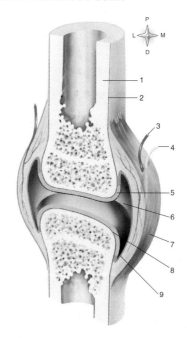

1. Bone
2. Periosteum
3. Blood vessel
4. Nerve
5. Articular cartilage
6. Joint cavity
7. Joint capsule
8. Articular cartilage
9. Synovial membrane

CHAPTER 9: MUSCULAR SYSTEM

Select the Correct Term

1. A, p. 220
2. B, p. 220
3. C, p. 220
4. C, p. 220
5. A, p. 220
6. B, p. 220
7. C and B, p. 220 and Chapter 4
8. A, p. 220
9. C, p. 220
10. C, p. 220

Matching

11. D, p. 220
12. B, p. 220
13. A, p. 220
14. E, p. 220
15. C, p. 220

Matching

16. E, p. 221
17. C, p. 221
18. B, p. 221
19. A, p. 221
20. D, p. 221

Fill in the Blanks

21. Pulling, p. 223
22. Insertion, p. 223
23. Insertion, origin, p. 223
24. Prime mover, p. 223
25. Antagonists, p. 223
26. Synergist, p. 223
27. Tonic contraction, p. 224
28. Muscle tone, p. 224
29. Hypothermia, p. 224
30. ATP, p. 224

True or False

31. F (neuromuscular junction), p. 225
32. T
33. T
34. F (oxygen debt), p. 225
35. T
36. F (lactic acid), p. 224
37. T
38. T
39. F (skeletal muscles), p. 225
40. T

Multiple Choice

41. A, p. 226	46. A, p. 225
42. B, p. 226	47. B, p. 226 and 228
43. B, p. 226	48. C, p. 226
44. C, p. 228	49. B, p. 228
45. D, p. 228	50. D, p. 228

Matching

51. C, p. 229
52. F, p. 229 and A and D, p. 234
53. B, p. 229 and F, p. 234
54. A, p. 229 and 233
55. C, p. 229
56. B and F, p. 229 and 234
57. A, p. 234
58. A and D, p. 229
59. B, p. 229
60. B, p. 229
61. A and E, p. 232
62. B, p. 232
63. D, p. 234

Multiple Choice

64. A, p. 228	67. A, p. 228
65. D, p. 228	68. D, p. 228
66. C, p. 228	69. C, p. 229

Circle the Correct Answer

70. Myalgia, p. 235
71. Myoglobin, p. 235
72. Poliomyelitis, p. 235
73. Muscular dystrophy, p. 236
74. Myasthenia gravis, p. 237

Applying What You Know

75. Bursitis
76. Deltoid area
77. Tendon

78. Word Find

Know Your Medical Terms

79. mouse/little, p. 238
80. muscle/thread/thing, p. 238
81. belly/leg, p. 238
82. breast/relating to/greater, p. 238
83. position, p. 239
84. stiffness/of death, p. 239
85. together/to work/agent, p. 239

Unscramble The Words

86. Flexion	89. Origin
87. Actin	90. Sarcomere
88. Eversion	91. Extension

Crossword

Muscles—Anterior View

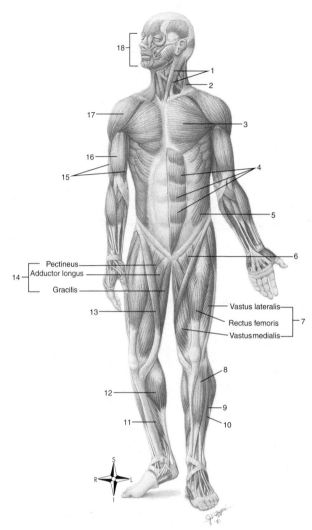

Check Your Knowledge
Multiple choice

1. D, p. 225
2. A, p. 228
3. C, p. 222
4. B, p. 234
5. B, p. 223

6. B, p. 225
7. D, p. 225
8. A, p. 228
9. A, p. 226
10. C, p. 220

True or false

11. T, p. 228
12. T, p. 226
13. F (pronation), p. 228
14. F (hypertrophy), p. 228
15. T, p. 226
16. T, p. 224
17. T, p. 220
18. F (hypothermia), p. 224
19. T, p. 225
20. F (flexion), p. 228

Fill in the blanks

21. Myoglobin, p. 222
22. Eccentric contraction, p. 223
23. Motor neuron, p. 225
24. Inversion, p. 229
25. Triceps brachii, p. 232

1. Sternocleidomastoid
2. Trapezius
3. Pectoralis major
4. Rectus abdominis
5. External abdominal oblique
6. Iliopsoas
7. Quadriceps group
8. Tibialis anterior
9. Fibularis (peroneus) longus

10. Fibularis (peroneus) brevis
11. Soleus
12. Gastrocnemius
13. Sartorius
14. Adductor group
15. Brachialis
16. Biceps brachii
17. Deltoid
18. Facial muscles

Muscles—Posterior View

1. Trapezius
2. External abdominal oblique
3. Gluteus maximus
4. Adductor magnus
5. Soleus
6. Fibularis (peroneus) brevis
7. Fibularis (peroneus) longus
8. Gastrocnemius
9. Hamstring group
10. Latissimus dorsi
11. Triceps brachii
12. Deltoid
13. Sternocleidomastoid

CHAPTER 10: NERVOUS SYSTEM

Matching
Group A

1. B, p. 249
2. C, p. 249
3. D, p. 249
4. A, p. 249

Group B

5. B, p. 250
6. D, p. 250
7. C, p. 250
8. A, p. 250
9. F, p. 253
10. E, p. 253

Select the Best Choice

11. A, p. 250
12. B, p. 250
13. B, p. 251
14. A, p. 250
15. A, p. 250
16. B, p. 252
17. B, p. 252
18. A, p. 250
19. B, p. 252
20. A, p. 250

Fill in the Blanks

21. Two-neuron arc, p. 253
22. Sensory neurons, interneurons, and motor neurons, p. 254
23. Receptors, p. 254
24. Synapse, p. 254
25. Reflex, p. 254
26. Withdrawal reflex, p. 254
27. Ganglion, p. 254
28. Interneurons, p. 254
29. "Knee jerk," p. 254
30. Gray matter, p. 254

Circle the Correct Answer

31. Do not, p. 255
32. Increases, p. 256
33. Excess, p. 256
34. Postsynaptic, p. 256
35. Presynaptic, p. 256
36. Neurotransmitter, p. 257
37. Communicate, p. 257
38. Specifically, p. 257
39. Sleep, p. 258
40. Pain, p. 258

Multiple Choice

41. E, p. 260
42. D, p. 264
43. A, p. 261
44. E, p. 262
45. E, p. 262
46. D, p. 262
47. B, p. 262
48. E, p. 264
49. B, p. 263
50. D, p. 263
51. D, p. 261
52. B, p. 262
53. A, p. 264
54. D, p. 262
55. C, p. 262

Select the Best Choice

56. H, p. 264
57. D, p. 265
58. E, p. 264
59. C, p. 264
60. J, p. 265
61. A, p. 266
62. B, p. 266
63. F, p. 266
64. I, p. 265
65. G, p. 266

True or False

66. F (17 to 18 inches), p. 266
67. F (bottom of the first lumbar vertebra), p. 267
68. F (lumbar punctures), p. 272
69. F (spinal tracts), p. 267
70. T
71. F (one general function), p. 267
72. F (anesthesia), p. 268

Circle the One That Does Not Belong

73. Ventricles (all others refer to meninges)
74. CSF (all others refer to the arachnoid)
75. Pia mater (all others refer to the cerebrospinal fluid)
76. Choroid plexus (all others refer to the dura mater)
77. Brain tumor (all others refer to a lumbar puncture)

Cranial Nerves

78. Fill in the missing areas on the chart below.

Nerve		Conduct Impulses	Function
I	Olfactory		
II			Vision
III		From brain to eye muscles	
IV	Trochlear		
V			Sensations of face, scalp, and teeth, chewing movements
VI		From brain to external eye muscles	
VII			Sense of taste; contraction of muscles of facial expression
VIII	Vestibulocochlear		
IX		From throat and taste buds of tongue to brain; also from brain to throat muscles and salivary glands	
X	Vagus		
XI			Shoulder movements; turning movements of head
XII	Hypoglossal		

Select the Best Choice

79. A, p. 270
80. B, p. 273
81. A, p. 270
82. B, p. 273
83. B, p. 270
84. A, p. 271
85. B, p. 267
86. B, p. 273

Matching

87. D, p. 275
88. E, p. 275
89. F, p. 275
90. B, p. 275
91. A, p. 275
92. C, p. 275

Multiple Choice

93. C, p. 276
94. B, p. 276
95. B, p. 277
96. D, p. 276
97. A, p. 277
98. A, p. 277

Choose the Correct Answer

99. B, p. 277
100. A, p. 277
101. A, p. 277
102. B, p. 277
103. A, p. 277
104. B, p. 277
105. A, p. 277
106. A, p. 277
107. B, p. 277
108. B, p. 277

Fill in the Blanks

109. Acetylcholine, p. 278
110. Adrenergic fibers, p. 278
111. Cholinergic fibers, p. 278
112. Homeostasis, p. 278
113. Heart rate, p. 278
114. Decreased, p. 278
115. Neuroblastoma, p. 279

Unscramble the Words

116. Neurons
117. Synapse
118. Autonomic
119. Smooth muscle
120. Sympathetic

Applying What You Know

121. Right
122. Hydrocephalus
123. Sympathetic
124. Parasympathetic
125. Sympathetic. No, the digestive process is not active during sympathetic control. Bill may experience nausea, vomiting, or discomfort because of this factor. See p. 277.

126. Word Find

Know Your Medical Terms

127. T
128. F, p. 280
129. T
130. T
131. F, p. 280

132. T
133. F, p. 281
134. T
135. T

Crossword

			¹A							⁴T	R	⁵A	C	T		
²R		³R	S									C				
E		E	T					⁶G				E			⁷M	
C		F	R					A				Y			E	
E		L	O			⁸D	E	N	D	R	I	T	E	S	D	
P		E	C					G				L			U	
T		X	Y					L				C			L	
⁹P	O	S	T	G	A	N	G	L	I	O	N	I	C		L	
R		E	E					O				H			A	
S		S	S			¹⁰N	E	U	R	O	G	L	I	A		
								L								
				¹¹M	E	N	I	N	G	E	¹²S					
				Y				N			Y					
				E		¹³N	E	U	R	O	N	S				
				L							A					
				I							P					
			¹⁴A	X	O	N				¹⁵P	N	S				
											E					

Check Your Knowledge

Multiple choice

1. D, p. 250
2. B, p. 269
3. A, p. 268
4. B, p. 261
5. A, p. 277

6. D, p. 278
7. D, p. 250
8. C, p. 256
9. C, p. 267
10. D, p. 275

Matching

11. C, p. 267
12. A, p. 250
13. J, p. 260
14. H, p. 257
15. B, p. 250

16. I, p. 273
17. F, p. 250
18. E, p. 260
19. D, p. 270
20. G, p. 278

Fill in the blanks

21. Multiple sclerosis, p. 252
22. Nerve, p. 253
23. Reflex arc, p. 254

24. Saltatory conduction, p. 256
25. Nitric oxide, p. 258

Neuron

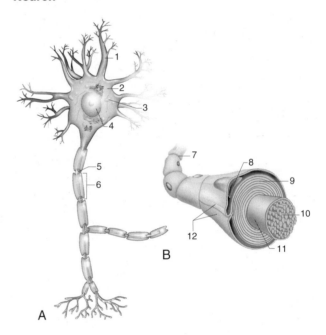

1. Dendrites
2. Cell body
3. Mitochondrion
4. Nucleus
5. Axon
6. Schwann cell
7. Node of Ranvier
8. Nucleus of Schwann cell
9. Myelin sheath
10. Axon
11. Cell membrane of axon
12. Neurilemma (sheath of Schwann cell)

Cranial Nerves

1. Skull
2. Pineal gland
3. Cerebellum
4. Midbrain
5. Spinal cord
6. Medulla
7. Reticular formation
8. Pons
9. Pituitary gland
10. Hypothalamus
11. Cerebral cortex
12. Thalamus
13. Corpus callosum

1. Olfactory nerve (I)
2. Trigeminal nerve (V)
3. Glossopharyngeal nerve (IX)
4. Hypoglossal nerve (XII)
5. Accessory nerve (XI)
6. Vagus nerve (X)
7. Vestibulocochlear nerve (VIII)
8. Facial nerve (VII)
9. Abducens nerve (VI)
10. Oculomotor nerve (III)
11. Optic nerve (II)
12. Trochlear nerve (IV)

The Cerebrum

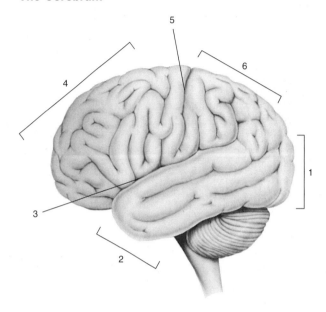

1. Occipital lobe
2. Temporal lobe
3. Lateral fissure
4. Frontal lobe
5. Central sulcus
6. Parietal lobe

Sagittal Section of the Central Nervous System

Neuron Pathways

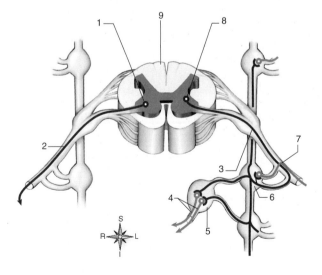

1. Cell body of somatic motor neuron
2. Axon of somatic motor neuron
3. Axon of preganglionic sympathetic neuron

301

4. Postganglionic neuron's axon
5. Collateral ganglion
6. Sympathetic ganglion
7. Postganglionic neuron's axon
8. Cell body of preganglionic neuron
9. Spinal cord

CHAPTER 11: SENSES

Matching

1. D, p. 293
2. B, p. 291
3. A, p. 293
4. E, p. 292
5. C, p. 293

Multiple Choice

6. C, p. 295
7. E, p. 295
8. B, p. 295
9. C, p. 295
10. E, p. 295
11. D, p. 296
12. A, p. 295
13. C, p. 296
14. B, p. 297
15. D, p. 296
16. A, p. 293
17. D, p. 297

Select the Best Answer

18. K, p. 299
19. C, p. 299
20. E, p. 299
21. F, p. 300
22. A, p. 301
23. J, p. 300
24. B, p. 301
25. H, p. 299
26. G, p. 300 and 301
27. I, p. 302
28. D, p. 301

Select the Best Answer

29. B, p. 304
30. C, p. 304
31. B, p. 304
32. A, p. 303
33. C, p. 304
34. A, p. 302
35. C, p. 304
36. B, p. 304
37. A, p. 303
38. C, p. 304

Fill in the Blanks

39. Auricle; external acoustic canal, p. 302
40. Eardrum, p. 303
41. Ossicles, p. 304
42. Oval window, p. 304
43. Otitis media, p. 304
44. Vestibule, p. 304
45. Mechanoreceptors, p. 306
46. Crista ampullaris, p. 306

Select the Best Answer

47. C, p. 307
48. A, p. 307
49. D, p. 307
50. E, p. 307
51. B, p. 307
52. F, p. 307

Circle the Correct Answer

53. Papillae, p. 307
54. Cranial, p. 307
55. Mucus, p. 309
56. Memory, p. 309
57. Chemoreceptors, p. 308

Unscramble the Words

58. Auricle
59. Sclera
60. Papillae
61. Conjunctiva
62. Pupils

Applying What You Know

63. External otitis
64. Cataracts
65. The eustachian tube connects the throat to the middle ear and provides a perfect pathway for the spread of infection.
66. Olfactory

67. Word Find

Know Your Medical Terms

68. Choroid, p. 291
69. Endolymph, p. 310
70. Ganglion, p. 310
71. Chemoreceptor, p. 291
72. Crista ampullaris, p. 310
73. Iris, p. 310
74. Ossicles, p. 310
75. Stapes, p. 311
76. Vestibule, p. 311

Crossword

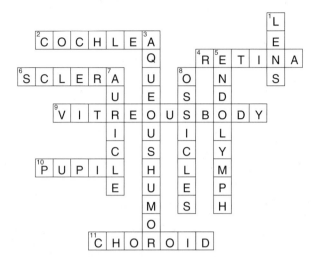

Check Your Knowledge

Multiple choice

1. A, p. 306
2. B, p. 304
3. A, p. 307
4. C, p. 293
5. B, p. 295
6. B, p. 292
7. D, p. 296
8. B, p. 295
9. D, p. 307
10. A, p. 302

True or false

11. T, p. 303
12. F (aqueous humor), p. 301
13. T, p. 299
14. F (malleus, incus, and stapes), p. 304
15. T, p. 299
16. T, p. 295
17. T, p. 296
18. T, p. 295
19. T, p. 308
20. T, p. 306

Fill in the blanks

21. Pain receptors, p. 292
22. Lacrimal gland, p. 295
23. Refracted, p. 297
24. Ceruminous, p. 303
25. Perilymph, p. 304

Eye

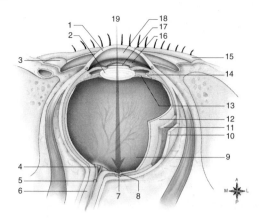

1. Cornea
2. Lens
3. Lacrimal caruncle
4. Optic disc
5. Central artery and vein
6. Optic nerve
7. Fovea
8. Macula
9. Posterior cavity (contains vitreous body)
10. Sclera
11. Choroid
12. Retina
13. Suspensory ligament
14. Ciliary muscle
15. Lower lid
16. Iris
17. Pupil
18. Anterior chamber (contains aqueous humor)
19. Visual (optic) axis

Ear

1. Auricle (pinna)
2. Temporal bone
3. Malleus

4. Incus
5. Stapes
6. Semicircular canals

7. Oval window
8. Vestibular nerve
9. Cochlear nerve
10. Vestibule
11. Cochlea

12. Auditory tube
13. Tympanic membrane
14. External auditory meatus

CHAPTER 12: ENDOCRINE SYSTEM

Matching
Group A
1. D, p. 320
2. C, p. 320
3. E, p. 320

4. A, p. 320
5. B, p. 320

Group B
6. E, p. 324
7. C, p. 325
8. A, p. 325

9. D, p. 320
10. B, p. 320

Fill in the Blanks
11. Second messenger, p. 320
12. Protein, p. 320
13. First messenger, p. 320
14. Target cells, p. 321
15. Cyclic AMP, p. 321
16. Target cells, p. 321
17. Steroid abuse, p. 325

Multiple Choice
18. B, p. 326
19. E, p. 322
20. D, p. 322
21. D, p. 326
22. A, p. 327
23. C, p. 322
24. C, p. 327
25. B, p. 326

26. A, p. 326
27. A, p. 326
28. D, p. 328
29. B, p. 328
30. A, p. 328
31. C, p. 328
32. C, p. 322

Select the Best Answer
33. A, p. 326
34. B, p. 326
35. B, p. 328
36. C, p. 329
37. A, p. 327

38. C, p. 329
39. A, p. 326
40. A, p. 326
41. A, p. 327
42. C, p. 328

Circle the Correct Answer
43. Below, p. 329
44. Calcitonin, p. 329
45. Iodine, p. 329
46. Do not, p. 329
47. Thyroid, p. 329
48. Decreases, p. 330
49. Hypothyroidism, p. 330
50. Cretinism, p. 330
51. PTH, p. 331
52. Increase, p. 331

Fill in the Blanks
53. Adrenal cortex; adrenal medulla, p. 331
54. Corticoids, p. 332
55. Mineralocorticoids, p. 332
56. Glucocorticoids, p. 332
57. Sex hormones, p. 332
58. Gluconeogenesis, p. 332
59. Blood pressure, p. 332
60. Epinephrine; norepinephrine, p. 333
61. Stress, p. 332
62. Virilizing, p. 334

Select the Best Response
63. A, p. 334
64. A, p. 332
65. B, p. 333
66. A, p. 334

67. B, p. 333
68. A, p. 332
69. A, p. 333

Circle the Term That Does Not Belong
70. Beta cells (all others refer to glucagon)
71. Glucagon (all others refer to insulin)
72. Thymosin (all others refer to female sex glands)
73. Chorion (all others refer to male sex glands)
74. Aldosterone (all others refer to the thymus gland)
75. ACTH (all others refer to the placenta)
76. Semen (all others refer to the pineal gland)

Matching
Group A
77. E, p. 334
78. C, p. 335
79. B, p. 336

80. D, p. 336
81. A, p. 336

Group B
82. E, p. 337
83. A, p. 338
84. B, p. 339

85. C, p. 336
86. D, p. 337

Unscramble the Words
87. Corticoids
88. Diuresis
89. Glucocorticoids
90. Steroids
91. Stress

Applying What You Know
92. She was pregnant.
93. The inner zone reticularis of the adrenal cortex
94. Oxytocin

95. Word Find

Know Your Medical Terms

96. Endocrine gland, p. 339
97. Glucagon, p. 339
98. Insulin, p. 340
99. Oxytocin, p. 340
100. Prolactin, p. 340
101. Sella turcica, p. 340
102. Acromegaly, p. 341
103. Dwarfism, p. 341
104. Hypoglycemia, p. 341
105. Pharmacology, p. 341

Crossword

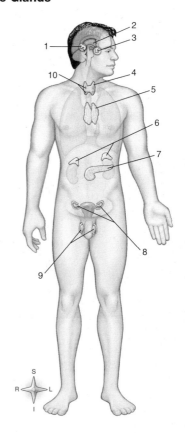

Check Your Knowledge

Multiple choice

1. A, p. 332
2. C, p. 322
3. D, p. 322
4. B, p. 322
5. D, p. 322
6. D, p. 328
7. B, p. 337
8. D, p. 323
9. D, p. 334
10. B, p. 325

Matching

11. J, p. 330
12. G, p. 326
13. H, p. 336
14. I, p. 327
15. B, p. 328
16. F, p. 337
17. A, p. 334
18. D, p. 328
19. E, p. 327
20. C, p. 331

True or false

21. T
22. F (slow), p. 321
23. T
24. F (paracrine), p. 325
25. F (adenohypophysis), p. 326

Endocrine Glands

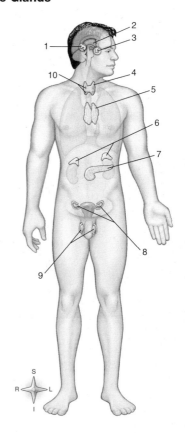

1. Pineal
2. Hypothalamus
3. Pituitary
4. Thyroid
5. Thymus
6. Adrenals
7. Pancreas (islets)
8. Ovaries (female)
9. Testes (male)
10. Parathyroids

Multiple Choice

1. E, p. 350	10. C, p. 352
2. D, p. 350	11. A, p. 352
3. D, p. 350	12. D, p. 352
4. C, p. 351	13. A, p. 352
5. B, p. 350	14. D, p. 353
6. B, p. 352	15. C, p. 353
7. C, p. 351	16. D, p. 353
8. D, p. 351	17. D, p. 354
9. C, p. 352	18. B, p. 353

Fill in the Blank Areas

19.

Blood Type	Antigen Present in Rbc	Antibody Present in Plasma
	A	
		Anti-A
	A, B	
		Anti-A, Anti-B

Fill in the Blanks

20. Antigen, p. 355
21. Antibody, p. 355
22. Agglutinate, p. 355
23. Erythroblastosis fetalis, p. 356
24. Rhesus monkey, p. 356
25. Type O, p. 357
26. Type AB, p. 357

Matching

27. F, p. 359	32. I, p. 360
28. A, p. 358	33. B, p. 356
29. C, p. 360	34. H, p. 360
30. G, p. 359	35. D, p. 358
31. E, p. 360	

Multiple Choice

36. B, p. 361	40. C, p. 362
37. B, p. 361	41. B, p. 362
38. B, p. 362	42. C, p. 353
39. B, p. 362	

Matching

43. C, p. 363	47. H, p. 364
44. E, p. 363	48. G, p. 364
45. A, p. 363	49. D, p. 363
46. B, p. 364	50. F, p. 363

Multiple Choice

51. A, p. 365	54. B, p. 365
52. D, p. 365	55. C, p. 366
53. E, p. 365	

Circle the Correct Response

56. Heart, p. 365	59. HIV/AIDS, p. 368
57. 0.8, p. 366	60. Aspirin, p. 367
58. Hemophilia, p. 367	

Unscramble the Words

61. Phagocyte	64. Fibrin
62. Thrombin	65. Typing
63. Antigen	

Applying What You Know

66. No. If Mrs. Florez were Rh factor negative and her husband were Rh factor positive, it would set up a strong possibility for erythroblastosis fetalis.
67. Both procedures assist the clotting process.
68. Anemia
69. The laboratory test is called the *prothrombin time.* Thromboplastin and calcium are added to a tube of the patient's plasma and a tube containing a normal control solution. The time required for clot formation to occur in both tubes is then determined. A prothrombin time in excess of the control value (7-10 seconds) indicates the level of anticoagulant effect caused by the Coumadin. This information will allow the physician to adjust the dosage required to maintain an appropriate level of anticoagulation.

70. Word Find

Know Your Medical Terms

71. E, p. 368   76. H, p. 349
72. D, p. 369   77. C, p. 369
73. G, p. 368   78. A, p. 368
74. F, p. 369   79. J, p. 370
75. I, p. 368   80. B, p. 369

Crossword

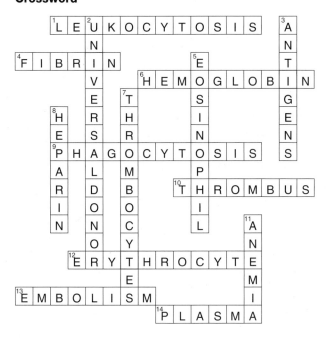

Check Your Knowledge

Multiple choice

1. B, p. 363   6. A, p. 362
2. B, p. 358   7. A, p. 365
3. A, p. 352   8. D, p. 356
4. B, p. 352   9. C, p. 354
5. D, p. 350   10. B, p. 365

Matching

11. D, p. 362   16. C, p. 365
12. F, p. 358   17. B, p. 356
13. H, p. 356   18. E, p. 356
14. A, p. 362   19. I, p. 352
15. G, p. 363   20. J, p. 352

Matching

21. A, p. 356   26. C, p. 366
22. B, p. 361   27. A, p. 354
23. B, p. 362   28. A, p. 355
24. C, p. 365   29. A, p. 353
25. C, p. 366   30. B, p. 362

Human Blood Cells

BODY CELL		FUNCTION
Erythrocyte		Oxygen and carbon dioxide transport
Neutrophil		Immune defense (phagocytosis)
Eosinophil		Defense against parasites
Basophil		Inflammatory response and heparin secretion
B lymphocyte		Antibody production (precursor of plasma cells)
T lymphocyte		Cellular immune response
Monocyte		Immune defenses (phagocytosis)
Thrombocyte		Blood clotting

Blood Typing

Recipient's blood		Reactions with donor's blood			
RBC antigens	Plasma antibodies	Donor type O	Donor type A	Donor type B	Donor type AB
None (Type O)	Anti-A Anti-B				
A (Type A)	Anti-B				
B (Type B)	Anti-A				
AB (Type AB)	(None)				

Normal blood   Agglutinated blood

CHAPTER 14: HEART

Fill in the Blanks

1. Circulatory system, p. 379
2. Apex, p. 380
3. Interatrial septum, p. 381
4. Atria, p. 381
5. Ventricles, p. 381
6. Myocardium, p. 381
7. Endocarditis, p. 381
8. Bicuspid or mitral and tricuspid, p. 383
9. Visceral pericardium or epicardium, p. 381
10. Parietal pericardium, p. 381

Answers to Exercises

11. Pericarditis, p. 381
12. Semilunar valves, p. 383
13. Mitral valve prolapse, p. 383
14. Rheumatic heart disease, p. 383

Select the Best Answer

15. F, p. 384
16. C, p. 385
17. D, p. 385
18. A, p. 384
19. B, p. 384
20. G, p. 385
21. E, p. 386
22. H, p. 386
23. J, p. 384
24. I, p. 386

Multiple Choice

25. B, p. 387
26. C, p. 387
27. A, p. 388
28. C, p. 390
29. A, p. 389
30. D, p. 384
31. C, p. 390
32. A, p. 394
33. B, p. 395
34. C, p. 395
35. A, p. 392
36. D, p. 394

True or False

37. T, p. 387
38. F (able), p. 388
39. F (SA node, AV node, bundle of His, Purkinje fibers), p. 388
40. T, p. 386
41. T, p. 389
42. T, p. 390
43. F (eliminating), p. 392
44. F (ventricle), p. 392
45. F (increases), p. 393
46. T, p. 393
47. T, p. 394

Unscramble the Words

48. Systemic
49. Mitral
50. Heart
51. Thrombus
52. Rhythm

Applying What You Know

53. Coronary bypass surgery
54. Artificial pacemaker
55. The endocardial lining can become rough and abrasive to red blood cells passing over its surface. As a result, a fatal blood clot may be formed.
56. 3   Tricuspid valve
    6   Pulmonary arteries
    9   Bicuspid valve
    1   Vena cava
    4   Right ventricle
    12   Aorta
    7   Pulmonary veins
    5   Pulmonary semilunar valve
    10   Left ventricle
    2   Right atrium
    8   Left atrium
    11   Aortic semilunar valve

57. Word Find

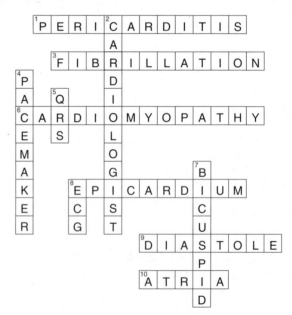

Know Your Medical Terms

58. Atrium, p. 379
59. Chordae tendineae, p. 395
60. Systole, p. 396
61. Angina pectoris, p. 396
62. Cardiomyopathy, p. 396
63. Electrocardiogram, p. 397
64. Endocardium, p. 395
65. Bradycardia, p. 396
66. Embolism, p. 397
67. Fibrillation, p. 397

Crossword

Check Your Knowledge

Multiple choice
1. C, p. 384
2. D, p. 389
3. C, p. 390
4. D, p. 382
5. C, p. 381
6. B, p. 381
7. D, p. 383
8. A, p. 388
9. C, p. 390
10. D, p. 395

Matching
11. F, p. 385
12. G, p. 389
13. H, p. 383
14. I, p. 384
15. J, p. 388
16. B, p. 382
17. C, p. 381
18. A, p. 388
19. D, p. 389
20. E, p. 386
21. Chordae tendineae, p. 383
22. Stenosed valves, p. 383
23. Coronary arteries, p. 385
24. Artificial pacemaker, p. 390
25. Stroke volume, p. 393

The Heart

1. Left common carotid artery
2. Left subclavian artery
3. Arch of aorta
4. Left pulmonary artery
5. Left atrium
6. Left pulmonary veins
7. Great cardiac vein
8. Branches of left coronary artery and cardiac vein
9. Left ventricle
10. Apex
11. Inferior vena cava
12. Right ventricle
13. Auricle of right atrium
14. Right coronary artery and cardiac vein
15. Right pulmonary veins
16. Ascending aorta
17. Right pulmonary artery
18. Superior vena cava
19. Brachiocephalic trunk

Conduction System of the Heart

1. Aorta
2. Pulmonary artery
3. Pulmonary veins
4. Mitral (bicuspid) valve
5. Purkinje fibers
6. Left ventricle
7. Right and left branches of AV bundle block (bundle of His)
8. Inferior vena cava
9. Right ventricle
10. Tricuspid valve
11. Atrioventricular (AV) node
12. Superior (SA) node (pacemaker)
13. Superior vena cava

Normal ECG Deflections

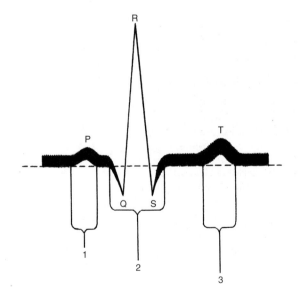

1. Atrial depolarization
2. Ventricular depolarization
3. Ventricular repolarization

309

CHAPTER 15: CIRCULATION OF THE BLOOD

Matching

1. D, p. 405
2. B, p. 406
3. C, p. 405
4. G, p. 404
5. A, p. 404
6. E, p. 404
7. F, p. 404

Matching

8. I, p. 406
9. B, p. 406
10. D, p 406
11. E, p. 406
12. A, p. 406
13. C, p. 406
14. F, p. 408
15. G, p. 408
16. J, p. 408
17. H, p. 407

Multiple Choice

18. D, p. 408
19. C, p. 408
20. B, p. 408
21. B, p. 408
22. D, p. 409
23. B, p. 412
24. B, p. 413
25. A, p. 413
26. D, p. 408

True or False

27. F (highest/arteries; lowest/veins), p. 414
28. F (blood pressure gradient), p. 414
29. F (stop), p. 414
30. F (high blood pressure), p. 414
31. F (decreases), p. 414
32. T
33. T
34. T
35. F (increases blood pressure/weaker heartbeat tends to decrease it), p. 415
36. F (contraction), p. 418
37. F (decreases), p. 416
38. T
39. T
40. F (right), p. 418
41. F (artery), p. 419
42. T
43. T
44. F (brachial), p. 419

Fill in the Blanks

45. Septic shock, p. 421
46. Cardiogenic shock, p. 421
47. Anaphylaxis; anaphylactic shock, p. 421
48. Neurogenic shock, p. 421
49. Low blood volume, p. 421
50. Toxic shock syndrome, p. 421

Unscramble the Words

51. Systemic
52. Venule
53. Artery
54. Pulse
55. Vessel

Applying What You Know

56. Anaphylactic shock
57. Hypovolemic shock
58. Varicose veins; wear support stockings
59. Hemorrhage

60. Word Find

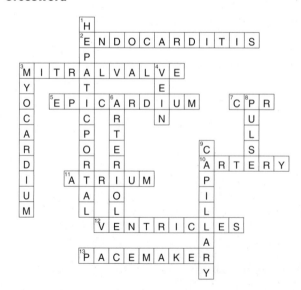

Know Your Medical Terms

61. T
62. T
63. F (widening), p. 422
64. F (gnawing sore), p. 422
65. F (blood flow), p. 422
66. T
67. T
68. T
69. F (swollen veins), p. 423
70. T

Crossword

Check Your Knowledge

Multiple choice

1. C, p. 414
2. A, p. 421
3. C, p. 421
4. C, p. 406
5. C, p. 404
6. B, p. 408
7. A, p. 412
8. A, p. 415
9. D, p. 406
10. B, p. 406

Matching

11. G, p. 404
12. A, p. 406
13. I, p. 411
14. C, p. 413
15. F, p. 406
16. B, p. 408
17. H, p. 408
18. D, p. 406
19. E, p. 404
20. J, p. 421

Fill in the blanks

21. Hemodynamics, p. 414
22. Sinuses, p. 404
23. Arteries, Vein, p. 412
24. Diastolic blood pressure, p. 418
25. Arteries, Veins, p. 414

Hepatic Portal Circulation

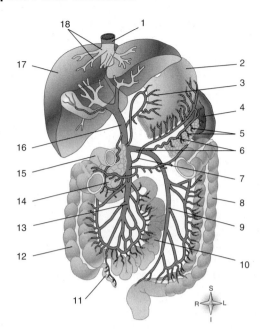

1. Inferior vena cava
2. Stomach
3. Gastric vein
4. Spleen
5. Pancreatic vein
6. Splenic vein
7. Gastroepiploic vein
8. Descending colon
9. Inferior mesenteric vein
10. Small intestine
11. Appendix
12. Ascending colon
13. Superior mesenteric vein
14. Pancreas
15. Duodenum
16. Hepatic portal vein
17. Liver
18. Hepatic veins

Fetal Circulation

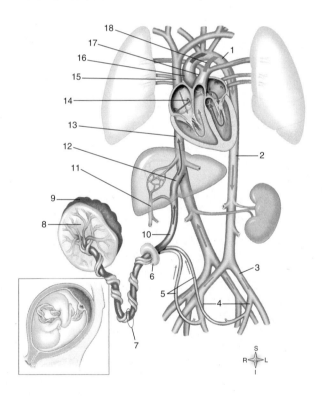

1. Aortic arch
2. Abdominal aorta
3. Common iliac artery
4. Internal iliac arteries
5. Umbilical arteries
6. Fetal umbilicus
7. Umbilical cord
8. Fetal side of placenta
9. Maternal side of placenta
10. Umbilical vein
11. Hepatic portal vein
12. Ductus venosus
13. Inferior vena cava
14. Foramen ovale
15. Superior vena cava
16. Ascending aorta
17. Pulmonary trunk
18. Ductus arteriosus

Principal Arteries of the Body

Principal Veins of the Body

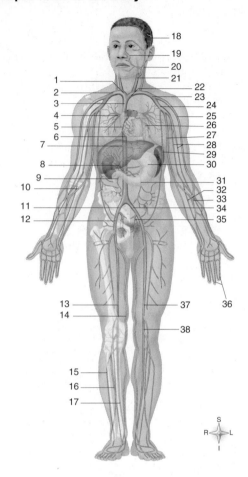

1. Right common carotid	16. Facial
2. Brachiocephalic	17. Internal carotid
3. Right coronary	18. External carotid
4. Axillary	19. Left common carotid
5. Brachial	20. Left subclavian
6. Superior mesenteric	21. Arch of aorta
7. Abdominal aorta	22. Pulmonary
8. Common iliac	23. Left coronary
9. Internal iliac	24. Aorta
10. External iliac	25. Splenic
11. Deep femoral	26. Renal
12. Femoral	27. Celiac
13. Popliteal	28. Inferior mesenteric
14. Anterior tibial	29. Radial
15. Occipital	30. Ulnar

1. Right brachiocephalic	20. External jugular
2. Right subclavian	21. Internal jugular
3. Superior vena cava	22. Left brachiocephalic
4. Right pulmonary	23. Left subclavian
5. Small cardiac	24. Axillary
6. Inferior vena cava	25. Cephalic
7. Hepatic	26. Great cardiac
8. Hepatic portal	27. Basilic
9. Superior mesenteric	28. Brachial veins
10. Median cubital	29. Long thoracic
11. Common iliac	30. Splenic
12. External iliac	31. Inferior mesenteric
13. Femoral	32. Ulnar vein
14. Great saphenous	33. Radial vein
15. Fibular (peroneal)	34. Common iliac
16. Anterior tibial	35. Internal iliac
17. Posterior tibial	36. Digital veins
18. Occipital	37. Femoral
19. Facial	38. Popliteal

CHAPTER 16: LYMPHATIC SYSTEM AND IMMUNITY

Fill in the Blanks

1. Lymph, p. 430
2. Interstitial fluid, p. 431
3. Lymphatic capillaries, p. 431
4. Right lymphatic duct and thoracic duct, p. 431
5. Cisterna chyli, p. 432
6. Lymph nodes, p. 433
7. Afferent, p. 433
8. Efferent, p. 433
9. Lymphedema, p. 432
10. Lymphadenitis, p. 433

Choose the Correct Response

11. B, p. 435
12. C, p. 435
13. C, p. 435
14. A, p. 434
15. C, p. 435
16. A, p. 435
17. A, p. 434

Matching

18. C, p. 436
19. A, p. 436
20. E, p. 437
21. B, p. 436
22. D, p. 438

Matching

23. C, p. 440
24. A, p. 439
25. F, p. 439
26. B, p. 439
27. G, p. 439
28. D, p. 439
29. H, p. 438
30. E, p. 440

Multiple Choice

31. D, p. 441
32. D, p. 442
33. C, p. 442
34. C, p. 442
35. C, p. 442
36. E, p. 442
37. E, p. 442
38. C, p. 442
39. E, p. 443
40. E, p. 443
41. A, p. 443
42. B, p. 443

Circle the Correct Answer

43. Hypersensitivity, p. 445
44. Allergens, p. 445
45. Anaphylactic shock, p. 445
46. Lupus, p. 445
47. Isoimmunity, p. 446
48. HLAs, p. 447

Select the Correct Response

49. B, p. 448
50. A, p. 447
51. A, p. 447
52. B, p. 448
53. A, p. 447

Unscramble the Words

54. Complement
55. Immunity
56. Clones
57. Interferon
58. Memory cells

Applying What You Know

59. Natural active immunity
60. AIDS
61. Baby Wilson has no means of producing T cells, thus making him susceptible to several diseases. Isolation is a means of controlling his exposure to these diseases.

62. Word Find

Know Your Medical Terms

63. vessel/juice, p. 449
64. plant/cutting, p. 449
65. away/carry/relating to, p. 449
66. milk/relating to, p. 449
67. thyme flower, p. 449
68. gland/like, p. 450
69. excessive/able to feel/state, p. 450
70. water/swelling, p. 450
71. cow (cowpox), p. 450
72. tonsil/inflammation, p. 450

Crossword

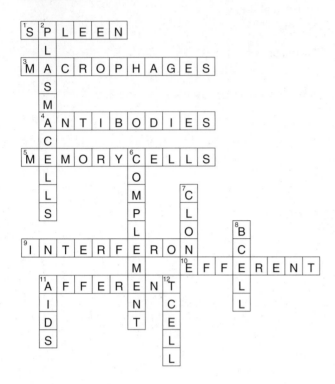

Across / Down grid answers:

1 across: S P L E E N
3 across: M A C R O P H A G E S
4 across: A N T I B O D I E S
5 across: M E M O R Y C E L L S
9 across: I N T E R F E R O N
10 across: E F F E R E N T
11 across: A F F E R E N T

Down answers: SPLEEN, PLASMACELL, COMPLEMENT, CLONE, BCELL, AIDS, TCELL, TONSIL, BCELL

Check Your Knowledge

Multiple choice

1. A, p. 443	6. B, p. 440
2. A, p. 430	7. D, p. 440
3. D, p. 448	8. D, p. 440
4. B, p. 446	9. D, p. 440
5. D, p. 442	10. C, p. 438

Matching

11. E, p. 435	16. B, p. 433
12. D, p. 443	17. A, p. 432
13. I, p. 442	18. J, p. 443
14. H, p. 448	19. C, p. 438
15. G, p. 440	20. F, p. 439

Fill in the blanks

21. Elephantiasis, p. 432
22. Efferent, p. 433
23. Thymosins, p. 435
24. Splenomegaly, p. 435
25. Nonspecific immunity, native immunity, or genetic immunity, p. 436

Principal Organs of the Lymphatic System

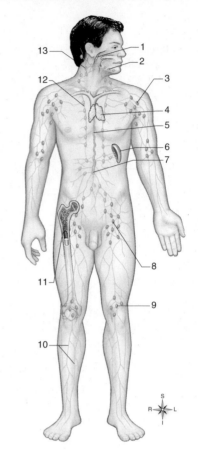

1. Tonsils
2. Submandibular nodes
3. Axillary lymph nodes
4. Thymus
5. Thoracic duct
6. Spleen
7. Cisterna chyli
8. Inguinal lymph nodes
9. Popliteal lymph nodes
10. Lymph vessels
11. Red bone marrow
12. Right lymphatic duct
13. Cervical lymph nodes

CHAPTER 17: RESPIRATORY SYSTEM

Matching

1. J, p. 460	6. F, p. 461
2. G, p. 460	7. C, p. 461
3. A, p. 460	8. H, p. 460
4. I, p. 461	9. D, p. 460
5. B, p. 460	10. E, p. 459

Fill in the Blanks

11. Air distributor, p. 460
12. Gas exchanger, p. 460
13. Filters, p. 459
14. Warms, p. 459
15. Humidifies, p. 459
16. Nose, p. 460
17. Pharynx, p. 460
18. Larynx, p. 460
19. Trachea, p. 460
20. Bronchi, p. 460
21. Lungs, p. 460
22. Alveoli, p. 460
23. Diffusion, p. 460
24. Simple squamous epithelium, p. 461
25. Alveoli, p. 461

Circle the One That Does Not Belong

26. Oropharynx (the others refer to the nose)
27. Conchae (the others refer to paranasal sinuses)
28. Epiglottis (the others refer to the pharynx)
29. Uvula (the others refer to the adenoids)
30. Larynx (the others refer to the eustachian tubes)
31. Tonsils (the others refer to the larynx)
32. Eustachian tube (the others refer to the tonsils)
33. Pharynx (the others refer to the larynx)

Choose the Correct Response

34. A, p. 462
35. B, p. 462
36. A, p. 462
37. A, p. 462
38. A, p. 462
39. B, p. 463
40. B, p. 462
41. C, p. 464
42. A, p. 464
43. B, p. 465
44. A, p. 466

Fill in the Blanks

45. Trachea, p. 466
46. C-rings of cartilage, p. 466
47. Five and Five method, p. 466
48. Primary bronchi, p. 466
49. Alveolar sacs, p. 467
50. Apex, p. 469
51. Pleura, p. 469
52. Pleurisy, p. 470
53. Pneumothorax, p. 470

Fill in the blanks

54. Pneumonia, p. 471
55. Tuberculosis, p. 471
56. Emphysema, p. 472
57. Asthma, p. 472

True or False

58. F (breathing), p. 473
59. F (expiration), p. 474
60. F (down), p. 473
61. F (internal respiration), p. 473
62. T
63. F (1 pint), p. 474
64. T
65. F (vital capacity), p. 475
66. T

Multiple Choice

67. E, p. 473
68. C, p. 481
69. C, p. 481
70. B, p. 473
71. D, p. 475
72. D, p. 475
73. D, p. 475

Matching

74. E, p. 475
75. B, p. 476
76. G, p. 477
77. A, p. 477
78. F, p. 478
79. D, p. 477
80. C, p. 477

Unscramble the Words

81. Pleurisy
82. Bronchitis
83. Epistaxis
84. Adenoids
85. Inspiration

Applying What You Know

86. During the day, Mr. Gorski's cilia are paralyzed because of his heavy smoking. They use the time when Mr. Gorski is asleep to sweep accumulations of mucus and bacteria toward the pharynx. When Mr. Gorski awakens, these collections are waiting to be eliminated.

87. It is difficult for air to travel from the nose into the throat when the tonsils and adenoids are blocking the passageways. The individual may be forced to breathe through the mouth. When the tonsils and adenoids are removed, it will open up the area and allow air to flow freely and not require Penny to breathe through her mouth.

88. During expiration, the alveoli are unable to force out a normal amount of air. Residual volume is increased at the expense of the expiratory reserve volume. Pulmonary infections can cause inflammation and an accumulation of fluid in the air spaces of the lungs. The fluid reduces the amount of space available for air and thus decreases the vital capacity.

89. **Word Find**

Know Your Medical Terms

90. F, p. 459
91. C, p. 482
92. I, p. 483
93. G, p. 483
94. A, p. 482
95. E, p. 483
96. B, p. 484
97. D, p. 483
98. H, p. 484
99. J, p. 484
100. K, p. 484

Crossword

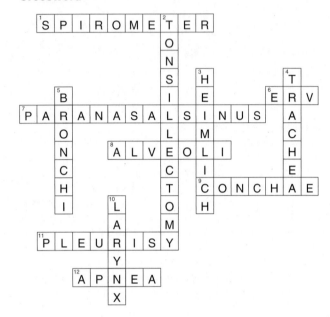

Check Your Knowledge

Multiple choice

1. A, p. 476
2. B, p. 462
3. D, p. 469
4. B, p. 475
5. A, p. 469
6. D, p. 464
7. A, p. 466
8. C, p. 478
9. D, p. 473
10. B, p. 463

Matching

11. E, p. 464
12. I, p. 473
13. A, p. 469
14. G, p. 470
15. D, p. 472
16. B, p. 462
17. C, p. 462
18. H, p. 466
19. F, p. 467
20. J, p. 468

Fill in the blanks

21. Turbinates, p. 462
22. Surfactant, p. 468
23. Pneumonectomy, p. 473
24. Phrenic, p. 473
25. Residual, p. 476

Sagittal View of Face and Neck

1. Sphenoidal sinus
2. Pharyngeal tonsil (adenoids)
3. Opening of auditory (eustachian) tube
4. Nasopharynx
5. Soft palate
6. Uvula
7. Palatine tonsil
8. Oropharynx
9. Epiglottis (part of larynx)
10. Laryngopharynx
11. Esophagus
12. Trachea
13. Vocal cords (part of larynx)
14. Thyroid cartilage (part of larynx)
15. Hyoid bone
16. Lingual tonsil
17. Hard palate
18. Inferior concha
19. Middle nasal concha of ethmoid
20. Superior nasal concha of ethmoid
21. Nasal bone
22. Frontal sinus

Respiratory Organs

1. Nasal cavity
2. Nasopharynx
3. Oropharynx
4. Laryngopharynx
5. Pharynx
6. Larynx
7. Trachea
8. Bronchioles
9. Left and right primary bronchi
10. Alveolar duct
11. Alveolar sac
12. Capillary
13. Alveoli

Pulmonary Ventilation Volumes

1. Total lung capacity
2. Inspiratory reserve volume
3. Tidal volume
4. Expiratory reserve volume
5. Residual volume
6. Vital capacity

CHAPTER 18: DIGESTIVE SYSTEM

Fill in the Blanks

1. Gastrointestinal tract, alimentary canal, digestive tract, or GI tract, p. 494
2. Mechanical, p. 495
3. Chemical, p. 495
4. Feces, p. 495
5. Digestion, absorption, and metabolism, p. 494

Select the Correct Response

6. A, p. 494	12. A, p. 494
7. B, p. 494	13. A, p. 494
8. B, p. 494	14. B, p. 494
9. A, p. 494	15. B, p. 494
10. A, p. 494	16. B, p. 494
11. A, p. 494	17. B, p. 494

Fill in the Blanks

18. Visceral peritoneum, p. 496	20. Lumen, p. 495
19. Mouth; anus, p. 495	21. Mucosa, p. 495
	22. Submucosa, p. 496

Multiple Choice

23. E, p. 496	31. D, p. 501
24. C, p. 497	32. A, p. 499
25. E, p. 497	33. C, p. 498
26. D, p. 498	34. D, p. 501
27. B, p. 498	35. A, p. 497
28. C, p. 498	36. B, p. 498
29. D, p. 498	37. C, p. 497
30. D, p. 497	

Fill in the Blanks

38. Pharynx, p. 501
39. Esophagus, p. 502
40. Nasopharynx, p. 501
41. Oropharynx, p. 501
42. Laryngopharynx, p. 501
43. Stomach, p. 502
44. Lower esophageal sphincter, p. 502
45. Chyme, p. 504
46. Fundus, p. 504
47. Body, p. 504
48. Pylorus, p. 504
49. Pyloric sphincter, p. 505
50. Small intestine, p. 505

Matching

51. D, p. 504	56. B, p. 504
52. J, p. 504	57. C, p. 504
53. G, p. 503	58. E, p. 505
54. A, p. 502	59. I, p. 503
55. H, p. 505	60. F, p. 504

Multiple Choice

61. C, p. 506	66. E, p. 506
62. B, p. 508	67. D, p. 509
63. A, p. 509	68. D, p. 509
64. A, p. 510	69. B, p. 509
65. B, p. 509	70. C, p. 509

317

True or False

71. F (vitamin K), p. 513
72. F (no villi are present in the large intestine), p. 514
73. F (diarrhea), p. 514
74. F (cecum), p. 512
75. F (hepatic), p. 512
76. F (sigmoid), p. 512
77. T
78. T
79. F (parietal), p. 516
80. F (mesentery), p. 516
81. F (diverticulitis), p. 514
82. T
83. T
84. F (ascites), p. 517

Multiple Choice

85. B, p. 518
86. D, p. 518
87. C, p. 518
88. C, p. 518
89. C, p. 519

Chemical Digestion

90. Fill in the blank areas on the chart below.

Digestive Juices and Enzymes	Substance Digested (or Hydrolyzed)	Resulting Product
Saliva		
1.	1. Starch (poly-saccharide)	1.
Gastric Juice		
2.	2.	2. Partially digested proteins
Pancreatic Juice		
3.	3.	3. Peptides and amino acids
4.	4. Fats emulsified by bile	4.
5.	5. Starch	5.
Intestinal Juice		
6.	6. Peptides	6.
7. Sucrase	7.	7.
8.	8. Lactose	8.
9.	9.	9. Glucose

Unscramble the Words

91. Bolus
92. Chyme
93. Papilla
94. Peritoneum
95. Lace apron

Applying What You Know

96. Ulcer
97. Pylorospasm
98. Cholelithiasis; cholecystectomy

99. Word Find

Know Your Medical Terms

100. Bolus, p. 493
101. Cecum, p. 520
102. Digestion, p. 521
103. Feces, p. 521
104. Mastication, p. 521
105. Anorexia, p. 523
106. Rugae, p. 522
107. Vermiform appendix, p. 523
108. Jaundice, p. 524
109. Caries, p. 523
110. Colonoscopy, p. 523

Crossword

Check Your Knowledge

Multiple choice

1. A, p. 509
2. C, p. 504
3. A, p. 506
4. B, p. 498
5. B, p. 495

6. B, p. 505
7. B, p. 516
8. C, p. 518
9. C, p. 518
10. A, p. 499

Completion

11. N, p. 512
12. J, p. 516
13. P, p. 519
14. Q, R, A, p. 506
15. W, p. 509

16. H, K, D, p. 493
17. E, p. 509
18. T, U, C, X, p. 495
19. G, p. 502
20. I, O, S, F, p. 497

Fill in the blanks

21. Segmentation, p. 496
22. Leukoplakia, p. 499
23. Deglutition, p. 502

24. Bacterium, p. 505
25. Lacteals, p. 508

Location of Digestive Organs

1. Parotid gland
2. Submandibular salivary gland
3. Pharynx
4. Esophagus
5. Diaphragm
6. Transverse colon
7. Hepatic flexure of colon
8. Ascending colon
9. Ileum
10. Cecum
11. Vermiform appendix
12. Rectum
13. Anal canal
14. Sigmoid colon
15. Descending colon
16. Splenic flexure of colon
17. Spleen
18. Stomach
19. Liver
20. Trachea
21. Larynx
22. Sublingual salivary gland
23. Tongue
24. Common hepatic duct
25. Cystic duct
26. Gallbladder
27. Duodenum
28. Pancreas
29. Stomach
30. Spleen
31. Liver

Tooth

1. Cusp
2. Enamel
3. Dentin
4. Pulp cavity with nerves and vessels
5. Gingiva (gum)
6. Root canal
7. Periodontal ligament
8. Periodontal membrane
9. Cementum
10. Bone
11. Root
12. Neck
13. Crown

The Salivary Glands

1. Parotid gland
2. Parotid duct
3. Submandibular gland
4. Submandibular duct
5. Sublingual gland

Stomach

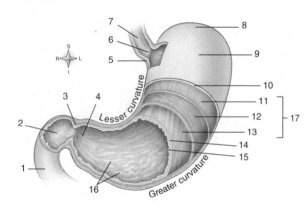

1. Duodenum
2. Duodenal bulb
3. Pyloric sphincter
4. Pylorus
5. Lower esophageal sphincter
6. Gastroesophageal sphincter
7. Esophagus
8. Fundus
9. Body of stomach
10. Serosa
11. Longitudinal muscle layer
12. Circular muscle layer
13. Oblique muscle layer
14. Submucosa
15. Mucosa
16. Rugae
17. Muscularis

Gallbladder and Bile Ducts

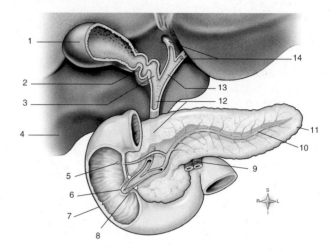

1. Corpus (body) of gallbladder
2. Neck of gallbladder
3. Cystic duct
4. Liver
5. Minor duodenal papilla
6. Major duodenal papilla
7. Duodenum
8. Sphincter muscles
9. Superior mesenteric artery and vein
10. Pancreatic duct
11. Pancreas
12. Common bile duct
13. Common hepatic duct
14. Right and left hepatic ducts

The Small Intestine

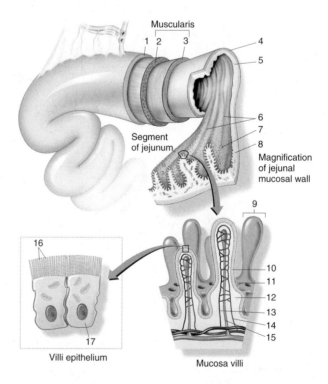

1. Serosa
2. Longitudinal muscle (Answer #2 and answer #3 constitute the "muscularis.")

3. Circular muscle (Answer #2 and answer #3 constitute the "muscularis.")
4. Submucosa
5. Mucosa
6. Plica (fold)
7. Lymph node
8. Mucosa
9. Single villus
10. Epithelium
11. Microvilli
12. Mucosa
13. Vein
14. Artery
15. Lacteal (lymph)
16. Microvilli
17. Epithelial cell

The Large Intestine

1. Aorta
2. Splenic vein
3. Superior mesenteric artery
4. Splenic (left colic) flexure
5. Inferior mesenteric artery and vein
6. Descending colon
7. Sigmoid colon
8. Rectum
9. Mesentery
10. Ileum
11. Vermiform appendix
12. Cecum
13. Ileocecal valve
14. Ascending colon
15. Hepatic (right colic) flexure
16. Transverse colon
17. Inferior vena cava
18. Portal vein

CHAPTER 19: NUTRITION AND METABOLISM

Fill in the Blanks
1. Bile, p. 534
2. Prothrombin, p. 534
3. Fibrinogen, p. 534
4. Iron, p. 534
5. Hepatic portal vein, p. 534

Matching
6. B, p. 537
7. A, p. 535
8. C, p. 538
9. D, p. 539
10. E, p. 540
11. A, p. 535
12. E, p. 540
13. A, p. 535

Circle the Word That Does Not Belong
14. Bile (all others refer to carbohydrate metabolism)
15. Amino acids (all others refer to fat metabolism)
16. M (all others refer to vitamins)
17. Iron (all others refer to protein metabolism)
18. Insulin (all others tend to increase blood glucose)
19. Folic acid (all others are minerals)
20. Ascorbic acid (all others refer to the B-complex vitamins)

Multiple Choice
21. C, p. 541
22. A, p. 541
23. A, p. 537
24. D, p. 542
25. D, p. 542

Choose the Correct Response
26. B, p. 542
27. C, p. 543
28. G, p. 543
29. F, p. 543
30. A, p. 542
31. H, p. 544
32. E, p. 543
33. D, p. 543

Multiple Choice
34. C, p. 544
35. B, p. 544
36. B, p. 544
37. A, p. 544
38. C, p. 544
39. D, p. 544

True or False
40. T
41. F (hypothermia), p. 546
42. T
43. F (heat stroke), p. 546
44. F (malignant hyperthermia), p. 546

Unscramble the Words
45. Liver
46. Catabolism
47. Amino
48. Pyruvic
49. Evaporation

Applying What You Know
50. Weight loss and anorexia nervosa
51. Iron; meat, eggs, vegetables, and legumes
52. He was carbohydrate loading or glycogen loading, which allows the muscles to sustain aerobic exercise for up to 50% longer than usual.

53. Word Find

Know Your Medical Terms

54. Basal metabolic rate, p. 533
55. Electron transport system, p. 547
56. Total metabolic rate, p. 547
57. Protein-calorie malnutrition, p. 548
58. Phenylketonuria, p. 548
59. Malignant hypertension, p. 547
60. Adenosine triphosphate, p. 535

Crossword

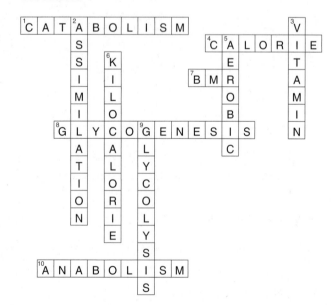

Check Your Knowledge

Multiple choice

1. B, p. 535	6. B, p. 536
2. A, p. 536	7. A, p. 537
3. C, p. 536	8. A, p. 544
4. C, p. 541	9. B, p. 534
5. B, p. 541	10. D, p. 535

Completion

11. C, D, I, p. 534	16. M, p. 538
12. E, p. 535	17. L, p. 536
13. J, p. 535	18. A, p. 538
14. G, p. 535	19. K, H, p. 540
15. B, p. 537	20. F, p. 533

Fill in the blanks

21. Assimilation, p. 533	24. Antioxidant, p. 538
22. Metabolism , p. 533	25. Statin, p. 539
23. Essential amino acids, p. 538	

CHAPTER 20: URINARY SYSTEM

Multiple Choice

1. E, p. 557	3. E, p. 557
2. C, p. 557	4. C, p. 559

Choose the Correct Term

5. G, p. 557	12. E, p. 557
6. K, p. 557	13. A, p. 557
7. F, p. 557	14. J, p. 555
8. H, p. 558	15. I, p. 559
9. D, p. 557	16. M, p. 560
10. L, p. 557	17. B, p. 557
11. C, p. 557	

Choose the Correct Term

18. B, p. 561	22. B, p. 562
19. B, p. 561	23. A, p. 561
20. C, p. 562	24. C, p. 563
21. A, p. 560	25. B, p. 562

True or False

26. T	30. F (ADH), p. 563
27. F (ADH), p. 563	31. T
28. T	32. T
29. T	33. F (reduces), p. 563

Choose the Correct Term

34. C, p. 565	40. C, p. 565
35. B, p. 565	41. A, p. 564
36. C, p. 565	42. C, p. 565
37. A, p. 564	43. B, p. 565
38. B, p. 565	44. A, p. 564
39. C, p. 565	45. B, p. 565

Fill in the Blanks

46. Micturition, p. 565
47. Urination, p. 565
48. Voiding, p. 565

49. Internal urethral sphincter, p. 565
50. Exit, p. 565
51. Urethra, p. 565
52. Voluntary, p. 565
53. Emptying reflex, p. 566
54. Urethra, p. 566
55. Retention, p. 566
56. Suppression, p. 566
57. Stress incontinence, p. 566

Fill in the Blanks

58. Urinalysis, p. 567
59. Routine and microscopic, p. 567
60. Bright yellow, p. 568
61. Casts, p. 568
62. Cystitis or bladder infections, p. 566
63. Fluid, p. 568

Select the Correct Answer

64. I, p. 567
65. C, p. 567
66. G, p. 573
67. F, p. 568
68. K, p. 569
69. A, p. 570
70. H, p. 571
71. J, p. 572
72. B, p. 567
73. D, p. 570
74. E, p. 570
75. L, p. 569

Unscramble the Words

76. Calyx
77. Voiding
78. Papilla
79. Glomerulus
80. Pyramids

Applying What You Know

81. Polyuria
82. Residual urine is often the cause of repeated cystitis.
83. A high percentage of catheterized patients develop cystitis, often because of poor aseptic technique during catheter insertion.
84. Hemorrhage causes a drop in blood pressure, which decreases the urine output and can eventually lead to kidney failure.

85. Word Find

Know Your Medical Terms

86. C, p. 555
87. E, p. 574
88. A, p. 574
89. G, p. 574
90. F, p. 575
91. H, p. 574
92. B, p. 574
93. D, p. 575

Crossword

Check Your Knowledge

Multiple choice

1. D, p. 566
2. B, p. 572
3. D, p. 555
4. A, p. 563
5. C, p. 566
6. C, p. 561
7. B, p. 565
8. C, p. 564
9. B, p. 557
10. A, p. 557
11. B, p. 563
12. D, p. 563
13. C, p. 562
14. B, p. 562
15. E, p. 562

Matching

16. E, p. 566
17. C, p. 563
18. F, p. 569
19. D, p. 565
20. J, p. 563
21. H, p. 563
22. A, p. 566
23. G, p. 568
24. I, p. 566
25. B, p. 560

Urinary System

1. Spleen
2. Renal artery
3. Renal vein
4. Left kidney
5. Inferior vena cava
6. Abdominal aorta
7. Common iliac vein
8. Common iliac artery
9. Urethra
10. Urinary bladder
11. Ureter
12. Right kidney
13. Twelfth rib
14. Liver
15. Adrenal glands

Kidney

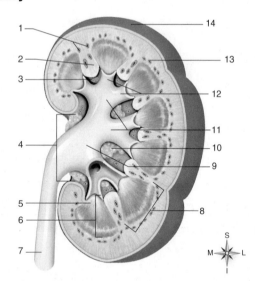

1. Interlobular arteries
2. Renal column
3. Renal sinus
4. Hilum
5. Renal papilla of pyramid
6. Medulla
7. Ureter
8. Medullary pyramid
9. Renal pelvis
10. Fat
11. Major calyces
12. Minor calyces
13. Cortex
14. Capsule (fibrous)

Nephron

1. Proximal convoluted tubule
2. Collecting duct
3. Descending limb of Henle loop
4. Ascending limb of Henle loop
5. Descending limb of Henle loop
6. Artery and vein
7. Distal convoluted tubule
8. Peritubular capillaries
9. Afferent arteriole
10. Juxtaglomerular (JG) apparatus
11. Efferent arteriole
12. Glomerulus
13. Bowman capsule
14. Renal corpuscle

CHAPTER 21: FLUID AND ELECTROLYTE BALANCE

Circle the Correct Answer

1. Inside, p. 584
2. Extracellular, p. 585
3. Extracellular, p. 585
4. Lower, p. 584
5. More, p. 584
6. Decline, p. 584
7. Less, p. 584
8. Decreases, p. 584
9. 55%, p. 584
10. Fluid balance, p. 583 and 587

Multiple Choice

11. A, p. 589
12. D, p. 589
13. A, p. 590
14. C, p. 586
15. E, p. 586
16. D, p. 586
17. D, p. 586
18. C, p. 587
19. B, p. 587
20. D, p. 591
21. E, p. 591
22. B, p. 588
23. B, p. 588
24. B, p. 588

True or False

25. F (catabolism), p. 586
26. T
27. T
28. F (increases), p. 587

29. T
30. F (hypervolemia), p. 587, Figure 21-5
31. T
32. F (2,400 mL), p. 586
33. T
34. T

Fill in the Blanks

35. Dehydration, p. 588
36. Decreases, p. 588
37. Decrease, p. 588
38. Overhydration, p. 589
39. Intravenous fluids, p. 589
40. Heart, p. 589
41. Hypernatremia, p. 592
42. Hyperkalemia, p. 592

Unscramble the Words

43. Edema   46. Intravenous
44. Fluid   47. Volume
45. Ion

Applying What You Know

48. Ms. Titus could not accurately measure water intake created by foods or catabolism; nor could she measure output created by lungs, skin, or the intestines.
49. A careful record of fluid intake and output should be maintained, and the patient should be monitored for signs and symptoms of electrolyte and water imbalance.
50. Jack's body contained more water. Obese people have a lower water content than slender people.

51. Word Find

Know Your Medical Terms

52. D, p. 589   57. F, p. 592
53. A, p. 589   58. I, p. 589
54. B, p. 589   59. H, p. 589
55. E, p. 589   60. C, p. 592
56. G, p. 589

Crossword

Check Your Knowledge
Multiple choice

1. A, p. 584   6. B, p. 590
2. D, p. 586   7. D, p. 586
3. D, p. 588 Review   8. A, p. 590
   chapter 5 Burns   9. A, p. 590
4. C, p. 588   10. D, p. 587
5. A, p. 590

Completion

11. E, p. 591   16. L, p. 586
12. B, p. 590   17. I, p. 588
13. J, M, K, p. 585   18. C, p. 588
14. F, p. 589   19. H and A, p. 587
15. D, p. 587   20. N, p. 583

Fill in the Blanks

21. Extracellular; intracel-   23. Pitting, p. 590
    lular, p. 584   24. Nonelectrolyte, p. 589
22. 2,400 mL, p. 586   25. Diuretics, p. 591

CHAPTER 22: ACID-BASE BALANCE

Choose the Correct Term

1. B, p. 602   6. B, p. 602
2. A, p. 602   7. B, p. 602
3. A, p. 602   8. A, p. 602
4. B, p. 602   9. B, p. 602
5. B, p. 602   10. B, p. 602

Multiple Choice

11. E, p. 602   17. C, p. 606
12. E, p. 603   18. B, p. 606
13. A, p. 603   19. D, p. 606
14. E, p. 605   20. B, p. 606
15. C, p. 605   21. D, p. 602
16. D, p. 605

True or False

22. F (reverse-acids than bases), p. 603
23. F (buffer pairs), p. 604
24. T
25. T
26. F (alkalosis), p. 606
27. F (reverse—arterial blood has a higher pH), p. 602
28. T
29. T
30. F (lungs), p. 603

Matching

31. E, p. 608
32. G, p. 610
33. F, p. 608
34. A, p. 607
35. I, p. 608
36. B, p. 608
37. H, p. 608
38. C, p. 608
39. D, p. 609
40. J, p. 609

Unscramble the Words

41. Fluids
42. Bicarbonate
43. Base
44. Fixed
45. Hydrogen
46. Buffer

Applying What You Know

47. Normal saline contains chloride ions, which replace bicarbonate ions and thus relieve the bicarbonate excess that occurs during severe vomiting.
48. Most citrus fruits, although acid-tasting, are fully oxidized with the help of buffers during metabolism and have little effect on acid-base balance. Cranberry juice is one of the few exceptions.
49. Milk of magnesia. It is a base. Interestingly, milk is slightly acidic.

50. Word Find

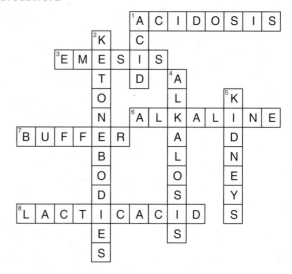

Know Your Medical Terms

51. Acidosis, p. 601
52. Bicarbonate, p. 611
53. Ketone, p. 611
54. Buffer, p. 601
55. Carbonic anhydrase, p. 601
56. Alkalosis, p. 611

Crossword

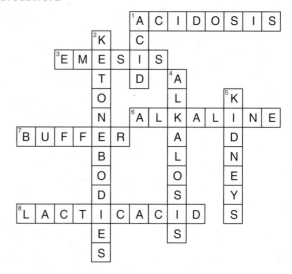

Check Your Knowledge
Multiple choice

1. A, p. 603
2. C, p. 607
3. A, p. 606
4. D, p. 602
5. A, p. 610
6. D, p. 609
7. D, p. 604
8. D, p. 608
9. D, p. 603
10. A, p. 605

Matching

11. G, p. 602
12. C, p. 602
13. I, p. 603
14. E, p. 608
15. F, p. 609
16. A, p. 607
17. B, p. 607
18. D, p. 604
19. J, p. 602
20. H, p. 610

Fill in the blanks

21. Urine, p. 607
22. "Arterial" values, p. 610
23. 10, p. 602
24. Carbonic acid, p. 605
25. Carbonic acid (H_2CO_3) and sodium bicarbonate ($NaHCO_3$), p. 607

CHAPTER 23: REPRODUCTIVE SYSTEMS

Matching
Group A

1. D, p. 618
2. C, p. 618
3. E, p. 618
4. B, p. 618
5. A, p. 618

Group B

6. C, p. 618
7. A, p. 618
8. D, p. 617
9. B, p. 618
10. E, p. 618

Multiple Choice

11. B, p. 619
12. C, p. 619
13. A, p. 619
14. D, p. 619
15. E, p. 619
16. D, p. 621
17. C, p. 622
18. C, p. 619
19. A, p. 621

Fill in the Blanks

20. Testes, p. 619
21. Spermatozoa or sperm, p. 619
22. Ovum, p. 618
23. Testosterone, p. 618
24. Interstitial cells, p. 619
25. Masculinizing, p. 622
26. Anabolic, p. 622

Choose the Correct Term

27. B, p. 622
28. H, p. 624
29. G, p. 623
30. A, p. 622
31. F, p. 623
32. C, p. 623
33. I, p. 623
34. E, p. 623
35. D, p. 624
36. J, p. 623

Fill in the Blanks

37. Oligospermia, p. 625
38. 2 months, p. 625
39. Cryptorchidism, p. 625
40. Benign prostatic hypertrophy, p. 625
41. Phimosis, p. 625
42. Impotence or erectile dysfunction, p. 626
43. Hydrocele, p. 626
44. Inguinal hernia, p. 626
45. Prostate, p. 625

Matching

46. D, p. 627
47. C, p. 627
48. B, p. 631
49. A, p. 627
50. E, p. 627

Choose the Correct Structure

51. A, p. 633
52. B, p. 630
53. A, p. 633
54. B, p. 630
55. A, p. 633
56. A, p. 633
57. A, p. 633
58. B, p. 630

Fill in the Blanks

59. Gonads, p. 627
60. Oogenesis, p. 628
61. Meiosis, p. 628
62. One-half (or 23), p. 628
63. Fertilization, p. 628
64. 46, p. 629
65. Estrogen, p. 629
66. Progesterone, p. 629
67. Secondary sexual characteristics, p. 629
68. Menstrual cycle, p. 629
69. Puberty, p. 629

Choose the Correct Structure

70. A, p. 631
71. B, p. 631
72. C, p. 631
73. B, p. 631
74. A, p. 630
75. B, p. 631
76. A, p. 630
77. A, p. 630
78. C, p. 631

Matching
Group A

79. D, p. 631
80. E, p. 631
81. B, p. 632
82. C, p. 632
83. A, p. 632

Group B

84. E, p. 632
85. A, p. 633
86. D, p. 633
87. B, p. 633
88. C, p. 633

True or False

89. F (menarche), p. 633
90. F (one), p. 634
91. F (14), p. 635
92. F (menstrual period), p. 635
93. T
94. F (anterior), p. 635

Choose the Correct Hormone

95. B, p. 635
96. A, p. 635
97. B, p. 635
98. B, p. 635
99. A, p. 635

Choose the Correct Response

100. F, p. 637
101. E, p. 637
102. A, p. 637
103. H, p. 636
104. I, p. 632
105. G, p. 636
106. C, p. 636
107. B, p. 635
108. L, p. 640
109. D, p. 635
110. J, p. 638
111. K, p. 640

Unscramble the Words

112. Vulva
113. Testes
114. Menses
115. Fimbriae
116. Prepuce
117. Vestibule

Applying What You Know

118. Yes. The testes not only are essential organs of reproduction but also are responsible for producing the "masculinizing" hormone. Without this hormone, Sam will have no desire to reproduce.
119. Sterile. The sperm count may be too low for reproduction, but the remaining testicle will produce enough masculinizing hormone to prevent impotency.

120. The uterine tubes are not attached to the ovaries, and infections can exit at this area and enter the abdominal cavity.

121. Yes. Without the hormones from the ovaries to initiate the menstrual cycle, Mrs. Harlan will no longer have a menstrual cycle and can be considered to be in menopause (cessation of menstrual cycle).

122. No. Vicki still will have her ovaries, which are the source of her hormones. She will not experience menopause because of this procedure.

123. Word Find

```
M K O V I D U C T S E D H G
S E I R A V O I F U T G L L
I N H Z H M P M K O H I C W
D D V A S D E F E R E N S H
I O A C C I P J V E H Y D S
H M G R R B M N X F G Y I O
C E I O O E Z Y T I C S T E
R T N S T P S D D N O V A D
O R A O U W E B A I J S M Z
T I C M M E Y N E M D L R V
P U A E U D G M I E H I E H
Y M O T C E T A T S O R P B
R P E E R M N E G O R T S E
C O W P E R S I N X K E A P
```

Know Your Medical Terms

124. Corpus luteum, p. 641
125. Endometrium, p. 641
126. Gonad, p. 641
127. Labia majora, p. 641
128. Menses, p. 642
129. Oocyte, p. 642
130. Semen or sperm, p. 642
131. Tunica albuginea, p. 642
132. Endometriosis, p. 643
133. Dysmenorrhea, p. 643
134. Infertility, p. 643
135. Leukorrhea, p. 643
136. Episiotomy, p. 643
137. Vasectomy, p. 644
138. Salpingitis, p. 644

Crossword

```
¹A          ²C L I T O R I S
M           I
E     ³A R E O L A      ⁴P
N           U           R
O           C        ⁵S E M E N
R     ⁶G A M E T E S ▓  P
R           I        ⁷V U L V A
H        ⁸M ▓ ⁹G     ▓  C
¹⁰T E S T O S T E R O N E
A           I  N     N
            O  S     A
            N  E     D
            S  S
```

Check Your Knowledge

Multiple choice

1. A, p. 633
2. D, p. 633
3. D, p. 623
4. C, p. 625
5. C, p. 627
6. A, p. 619
7. B, p. 619
8. C, p. 624
9. A, p. 632
10. D, p. 639

Completion

11. C, p. 631
12. L, p. 621
13. H, p. 623
14. G, p. 631
15. F, p. 622
16. K, p. 624
17. B, p. 631
18. D, p. 629
19. J, p. 635
20. I, p. 635

Fill in the blanks

21. Vas Deferens, p. 622
22. Sterility, p. 624
23. Andropause, p. 624
24. Vestibule, p. 633
25. Secretory, p. 633

Male Reproductive Organs

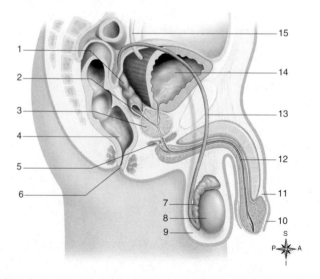

1. Seminal vesicle
2. Ejaculatory duct
3. Prostate gland
4. Rectum
5. Bulbourethral (Cowper) gland
6. Anus
7. Epididymis
8. Testis
9. Scrotum
10. Foreskin (prepuce)
11. Penis
12. Urethra
13. Ductus (vas) deferens
14. Urinary bladder
15. Ureter

1. Mons pubis
2. Pudendal fissure
3. Labium majus
4. Frenulum (of clitoris)
5. Opening of lesser vestibular (Skene) gland
6. Orifice of vagina
7. Hymen
8. Frenulum (of labia)
9. Posterior commissure (of labia)
10. Anus
11. Perineum
12. Greater vestibular (Bartholin) gland
13. Vestibule (clitoral bulb)
14. Vestibule
15. External urinary meatus
16. Labium minus
17. Clitoris (glans)
18. Foreskin (prepuce)

Tubules of Testis and Epididymis

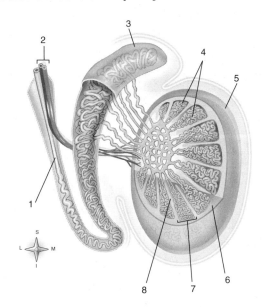

1. Ductus (vas) deferens
2. Nerves and blood vessels in the spermatic cord
3. Epididymis
4. Seminiferous tubules
5. Testis
6. Tunica albuginea
7. Lobule
8. Septum

Vulva

Breast

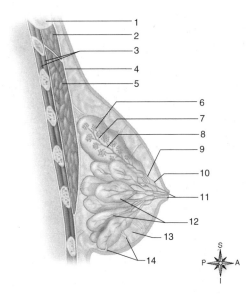

1. Clavicle
2. Pectoralis minor muscle
3. Intercostal muscle
4. Fascia of pectoral muscles
5. Pectoralis major muscle
6. Alveolus
7. Ductule
8. Duct
9. Lactiferous duct
10. Lactiferous sinus
11. Nipple pores
12. Lobes
13. Adipose tissue
14. Suspensory ligaments (of Cooper)

Female Pelvis

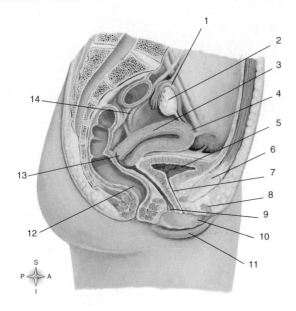

1. Uterine (fallopian) tube
2. Ovary
3. Body of uterus
4. Fundus of uterus
5. Urinary bladder
6. Symphysis pubis
7. Urethra
8. Clitoris
9. Vagina
10. Labium minus
11. Labium majus
12. Rectum
13. Cervix
14. Ureter

Uterus and Adjacent Structures

1. Fundus
2. Ovary
3. Body of uterus
4. Uterine artery and vein
5. Cervix
6. Vagina (cut)
7. Cervical canal
8. Myometrium

9. Perimetrium
10. Endometrium
11. Wall of uterus
12. Fimbriae
13. Uterine (fallopian) tube

CHAPTER 24: GROWTH AND DEVELOPMENT

Fill in the Blanks

1. Conception, p. 654
2. Birth, p. 654
3. Embryology, p. 654
4. Oviduct, fallopian tube, or uterine tube, p. 654
5. Zygote, p. 654
6. Morula, p. 654
7. Blastocyst, p. 654
8. Amniotic cavity, p. 655
9. Chorion, p. 655
10. Placenta, p. 655

Choose the Correct Term

11. G, p. 657
12. F, p. 657
13. C, p. 663
14. B, p. 656
15. A, p. 657
16. H, p. 658
17. E, p. 661
18. D, p. 658
19. I, p. 656
20. J, p. 663

True or False

21. T
22. T
23. F (placenta previa), p. 662
24. F (abruptio placentae), p. 662
25. F (preeclampsia), p. 662
26. F (stillbirth), p. 663
27. T

Multiple Choice

28. E, p. 664
29. E, p. 665
30. E, p. 665
31. A, p. 665
32. B, p. 665
33. C, p. 665
34. B, p. 666
35. D, p. 666
36. E, p. 666
37. D, p. 666
38. A, p. 666
39. C, p. 666
40. C, p. 666
41. C, p. 666
42. E, p. 666

Matching

43. F, p. 664
44. A, p. 665
45. C, p. 666
46. H, p. 666
47. D, p. 666
48. B, p. 665
49. E, p. 666
50. G, p. 667
51. I, p. 667

Fill in the Blanks

52. Lipping, p. 668
53. Osteoarthritis, p. 668
54. Nephron, p. 670
55. Barrel chest, p. 669
56. Atherosclerosis, p. 669
57. Arteriosclerosis, p. 669

330

58. Hypertension, p. 669
59. Presbyopia, p. 669
60. Cataract, p. 669
61. Glaucoma, p. 669

Unscramble the Words

62. Infancy
63. Postnatal
64. Organogenesis
65. Zygote
66. Childhood
67. Fertilization

Applying What You Know

68. Normal
69. Only about 40% of the taste buds present at age 30 remain at age 75.
70. A significant loss of hair cells in the organ of Corti causes a serious decline in ability to hear certain frequencies.
71. Each baby girl had her own placenta.

72. Word Find

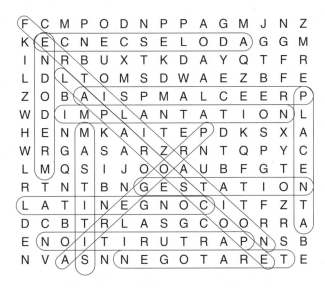

Know Your Medical Terms

73. T, p. 653
74. T, p. 653
75. F (bear/process), p. 671
76. T, p. 671
77. F (union or yolk), p. 671
78. T, p. 672
79. T, p. 671
80. F (gray or silver/tumor), p. 672

Crossword

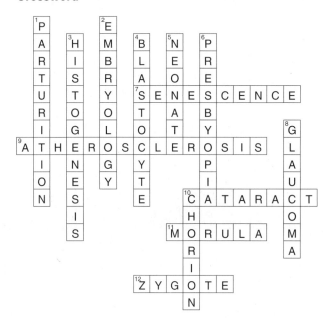

Check Your Knowledge

Multiple choice

1. C, p. 654
2. D, p. 670
3. D, p. 666
4. A, p. 665
5. D, p. 658
6. D, p. 669
7. A, p. 669
8. A, p. 666
9. C, p. 658
10. B, p. 658

Matching

11. E, p. 669
12. G, p. 669
13. C, p. 658
14. I, p. 669
15. H, p. 666
16. D, p. 654
17. J, p. 669
18. F, p. 667
19. A, p. 669
20. B, p. 654

Circle the correct answer

21. Stem, p. 657
22. Monozygotic, p. 661
23. Childbed fever, p. 663
24. Stage 2, p. 661
25. Menopause, p. 670

Fertilization and Implantation

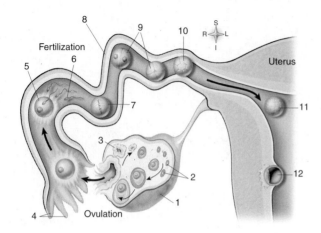

1. Ovary
2. Developing follicles
3. Corpus luteum
4. Fimbriae
5. Discharged ovum
6. Spermatozoa
7. First mitosis
8. Uterine (fallopian) tube
9. Divided zygote
10. Morula
11. Blastocyst
12. Implantation

CHAPTER 25: GENETICS AND GENETIC DISEASES

Matching

1. E, p. 680
2. A, p. 680
3. B, p. 681
4. C, p. 681
5. D, p. 681
6. G, p. 680
7. I, p. 680
8. J, p. 680
9. H, p. 680
10. F, p. 680

Fill in the Blanks

11. Genes, p. 682
12. Dominant, p. 682
13. Recessive, p. 682
14. Carrier, p. 682
15. Codominance, p. 683
16. Sex, p. 683
17. Female, p. 683
18. Mutation, p. 684
19. Genetic mutation, p. 684

Matching

20. E, p. 686
21. D, p. 685
22. J, p. 685
23. F, p. 686
24. C, p. 686
25. G, p. 688
26. A, p. 686
27. H, p. 689
28. B, p. 686
29. I, p. 689

Multiple Choice

30. D, p. 690
31. B, p. 690
32. C, p. 688
33. C, p. 690
34. D, p. 692
35. D, p. 691
36. B, p. 693

True or False

37. T
38. F (electrophoresis), p. 691
39. F (gene augmentation), p. 692
40. T
41. T

Unscramble the Words

42. Carrier
43. Trisomy
44. Gene
45. Pedigree
46. Chromosome
47. Inherited

Applying What You Know

48. In a form of dominance called *codominance*, the effect will be equal, causing "light brown" to occur.
49. One in four or 25%
50. Amniocentesis or chorionic villus sampling. The counselor will then produce a karyotype to determine anomalies.

51. **Punnett Square**

Mr. Fortner PP
Mrs. Fortner pp
A. 100% chance of brown eyes and 0% chance of blue eyes
B. Yes
C. 25%
Mrs. Harrington Pp
Mr. Harrington Pp
A. Normal pigmentation 25%
B. Carriers 50%
C. Albinism 25%

52. **Word Find**

Know Your Medical Terms

53. C, L, p. 679
54. E, p. 679
55. F, Q, p. 679
56. J, D, p. 694
57. A, M, O, p. 695

58. G, R, H, p. 695
59. K, T, p. 695
60. B, L, O, p. 695
61. N, S, p. 695
62. I, P, p. 695

Crossword

Check Your Knowledge

Multiple choice

1. A, p. 682
2. D, p. 690
3. C, p. 682
4. B, p. 682
5. A, p. 681

6. C, p. 680
7. B, p. 683
8. C, p. 683
9. A, p. 690
10. B, p. 689

Completion

11. H, p. 688
12. K, p. 690
13. C, p. 686
14. E, p. 680
15. A, p. 686

16. G, p. 690
17. D, p. 682
18. J, p. 688
19. L, p. 687
20. B, p. 689

Fill in the blanks

21. Mendel's, p. 680 and 685
22. Epigenetics, p. 688
23. Nondisjunction, p. 685

24. Down Syndrome, p. 688
25. Gene augmentation, p. 692